Review of

NEET PG Pattern 2018

Review of
NEET PG Pattern 2018

Model Questions
with
Solved Explanatory Answers

Mukesh Bhatia MBBS, MD (Medicine)
Director
Dr Bhatia Medical Coaching Institute
New Delhi, India

Reetu Dogra MBBS
Academic Director
Dr Bhatia Medical Coaching Institute
New Delhi, India

Contribution by
Rajat Jain
Radiology Faculty
Dr Bhatia Medical Coaching Institute
New Delhi, India

Edited by
DBMI Premiere Faculty

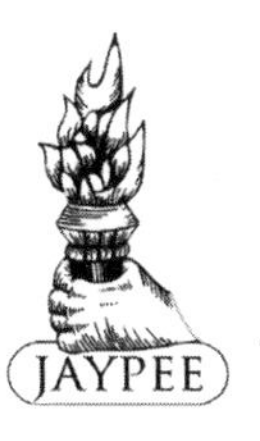

The Health Sciences Publisher
New Delhi | London | Panama

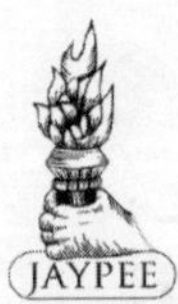

Jaypee Brothers Medical Publishers (P) Ltd

Headquarters

Jaypee Brothers Medical Publishers (P) Ltd
4838/24, Ansari Road, Daryaganj
New Delhi 110 002, India
Phone: +91-11-43574357
Fax: +91-11-43574314
Email: jaypee@jaypeebrothers.com

Overseas Offices

J.P. Medical Ltd
83 Victoria Street, London
SW1H 0HW (UK)
Phone: +44 20 3170 8910
Fax: +44 (0)20 3008 6180
Email: info@jpmedpub.com

Jaypee-Highlights Medical Publishers Inc
City of Knowledge, Bld. 235, 2nd Floor, Clayton
Panama City, Panama
Phone: +1 507-301-0496
Fax: +1 507-301-0499
Email: cservice@jphmedical.com

Jaypee Brothers Medical Publishers (P) Ltd
17/1-B Babar Road, Block-B, Shaymali
Mohammadpur, Dhaka-1207
Bangladesh
Mobile: +08801912003485
Email: jaypeedhaka@gmail.com

Jaypee Brothers Medical Publishers (P) Ltd
Bhotahity, Kathmandu
Nepal
Phone: +977-9741283608
Email: kathmandu@jaypeebrothers.com

Website: www.jaypeebrothers.com
Website: www.jaypeedigital.com

Review of NEET PG Pattern 2018

First Edition: 2018

ISBN: 978-93-5270-510-8

Printed at Rajkamal Electric Press, Plot No. 2, Phase-IV, Kundli, Haryana.

Preface

This book is primarily meant for those students who are preparing for NEET PG Entrance Exams. Our Effort to come up with this current book is due to huge demand by NEET PG aspirants who are in search of quality book with genuine questions, correct options and most authentic answers with relevant references. Every solved question will have a valid answer from a standard textbook or article in order to increase the credibility of the answers. The focussed and detailed explanations should help you solve questions from same topics easily. Our book would serve as a true companion for all hard working PG aspirants with most authentic answers from highly reputed faculties. For making the book authentic we needed crisp explanations and authentic referencing, explaining the picture based questions, each requiring expertise. The only solutions was to seek help. Every chapter in this book was reviewed by the masters in their own subjects.

We have incorporated a systematic approach in solving each and every question which can be appreciated while reading this book. We have tried to put our best effort to give correct explanations in the right contexts covering maximum topics.

The schematic diagrams, tables, illustrations, bulleted key points and references are highlights of this book and will make reading and understanding of the material easier and effective.

All the information have been presented in a pointwise manner making it easy to remember and revise. All these questions have been solved by subject faculty of DBMCI. This is the most important point about the book unlike other books which are written by a single author writing a book on 19 subjects. Hence, similar books by other authors have lot of mistakes and they are not updated also.

Hope we are able to provide you a quality book which can go a long way in helping you prepare for upcoming NEET PG Exam and other PGMEE exams. We hope the students will find this book very useful. Your comments, feedback and suggestions are welcome on our facebook group **'DBMCI 2018 Premiere Group' or in Email id: studentsupport@dbmi.edu.in**

Our job does not end here by providing you the book. We also want to help you throughout your journey. So, we have created a **Facebook Premiere Group,** i.e. **'DBMCI 2018 Premiere Group'** on Facebook which is purely intended to help you all. This group aims to cater to the students directly, in discussing the updates in various subjects related to PG Entrance Exams and solving queries/doubts pertaining to all the subjects of PG Entrance Exams within 2 hours. You can join it by using following link.

https://www.facebook.com/groups/1769262746733609/

Wishing you all the best for a bright future!!!!

Best Wishes
Mukesh Bhatia
Reetu Dogra
Website: *www.dbmci.com*
Email: *studentsupport@dbmi.edu.in*

Acknowledgments

First of all I thank **Lord Krishna** for teaching me the concept of **Gyan Yoga** (importance of always learning) and **Karam Yoga** (to do one's duty with utmost sincerity – Work is Worship!!!).

I am thankful to **Lord Ganpati** whose eternal blessings, divine presence and masterly guidance helps all of us to fulfill our goals.

I am thankful to **my mother and (Late) father** for their constant undemanding love, dedication, sacrifice, inspiring guidance, affectionate encouragement and never-ending enthusiasm; without which this book would not have seen the light of the day. I am thankful to **my wife (Mrs Anu), my son (Dr Nachiketa Bhatia), my daughter (Ms Urvashi)** for their endless support and love.

Mukesh Bhatia

'Without hard work and sacrifices, there is no gain and achievements. So always do hard work, rest is taken care by the God !!!!'

I would like to thank **God, my parents (Dr GL Dogra and Smt Sheela Dogra)** for their immense support for my every decision of life, **my brothers (Mr Rahul and Mr Rohit), my sister (Dr Pooja)**, and **my Friends** for understanding me. Without their belief in me, it would not have been possible.

Lastly, I want to thank **Dr Mukesh Bhatia** who encouraged me to write this book.

Reetu Dogra

We would like to thank all the Faculty of DBMCI for their commitment and hard work throughout the process. I would also like to thank our publishing and Academics team for their relentless efforts in releasing this book out in a short notice, who worked and supported at odd hours to make the book a visual treat.

1. Dr Poonam Goel (Dental Academic Head)
2. Mr Kuldeep Bisht (Sr Academic Manager)
3. Ms Jyoti (Academic Executive)

We are looking forward to hear your feedback and are fully committed in bringing out better editions in the future.

Write to us:
Any observation, suggestions, feedbacks are welcome at:
studentsupport@ dbmi.edu.in

Follow us on Facebook:
https://www.facebook.com/dbmci/?ref=bookmarks

Mukesh Bhatia
Reetu Dogra

Review Board

S.No.	Subject	Faculties	
1	Anatomy	Deepa Singh	
2	Physiology	Ashish Kumar	Soumen Manna
3	Biochemistry	Nilesh Chandra	
4	Pathology	Praveen Kumar	
5	Pharmacology	Saurabh Bhatia	Ankit Kumar
6	Forensic Medicine	Gurudutta	Sumit Tellewar
7	Microbiology	Shivika Juneja	Sonu Panwar
8	Ophthalmology	Pulkit Gupta	
9	ENT	Sanjay	Abhay Anand
10	PSM	Madhu	
11	Medicine	Mukesh Bhatia	
12	Surgery	Jainendra Arora	Rakesh Mittal
13	OBS and Gynecology	Shonali Chandra	
14	Orthopedics	Sushil Vijay	
15	Anesthesia	Ajay Yadav	Amit
16	Psychiatry	Ankit Goel	
17	Radiology	Rajat Jain	
18	Pediatrics	Parul Gupta	Pankaj
19	Skin	Pallavi Ailawadi	Ananta Khurana

Contents

Image-Based Questions

IMAGE-BASED QUESTIONS

1. **What is the action of this Muscle (pointed) at metacarpophalangeal joint?**

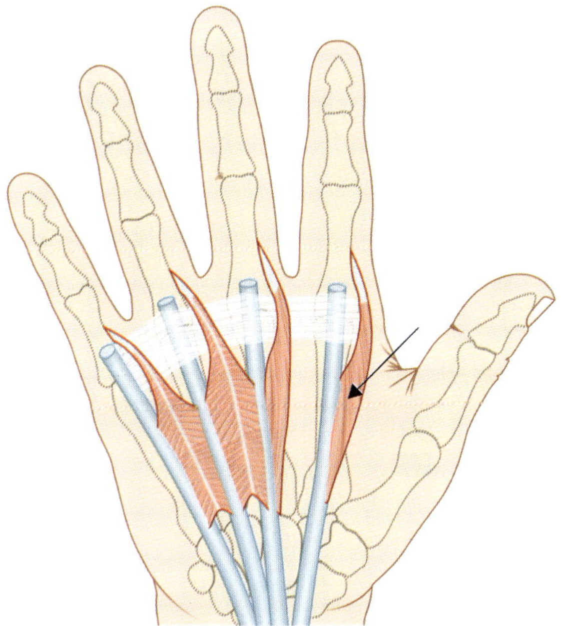

A. Abduction
B. Adduction
C. Flexion
D. Extension

---

1. **Ans. (C) Flexion**

2. What is the feature of the muscle shown in the image below?

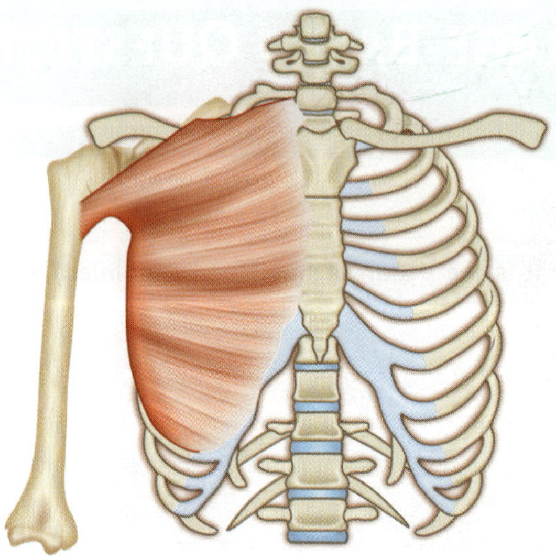

A. Cruciate
B. Multipennate
C. Spiral
D. Unipennate

3. Lesch-Nyhan syndrome is caused due to deficiency of which enzyme?

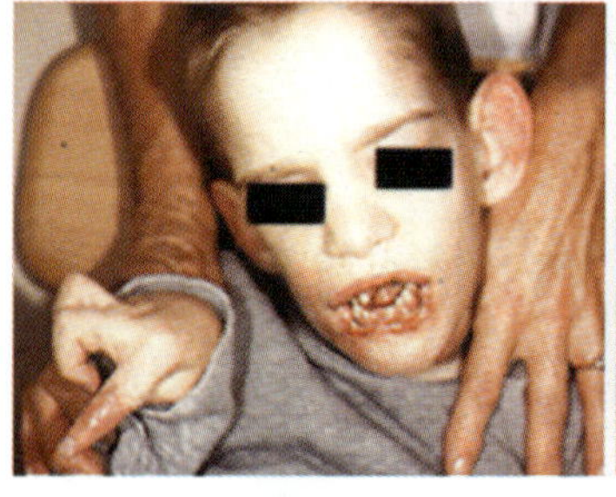

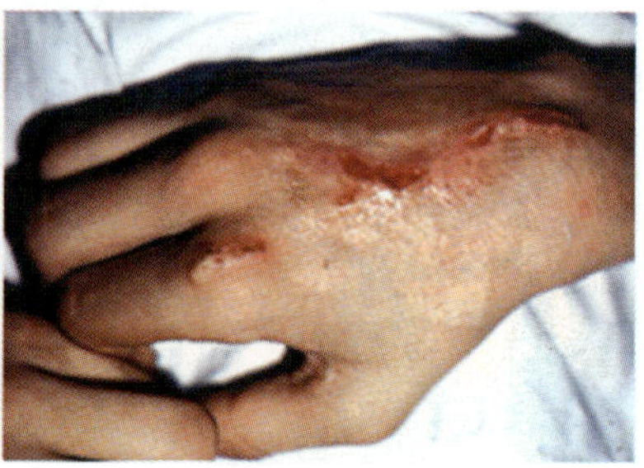

A. HGPRT
B. Tyrosine hydroxylase
C. Xanthine oxidase
D. Uricase

---

2. Ans. (C) Spiral

3. Ans. (A) HGPRT

4. **Section of lung showing what?**

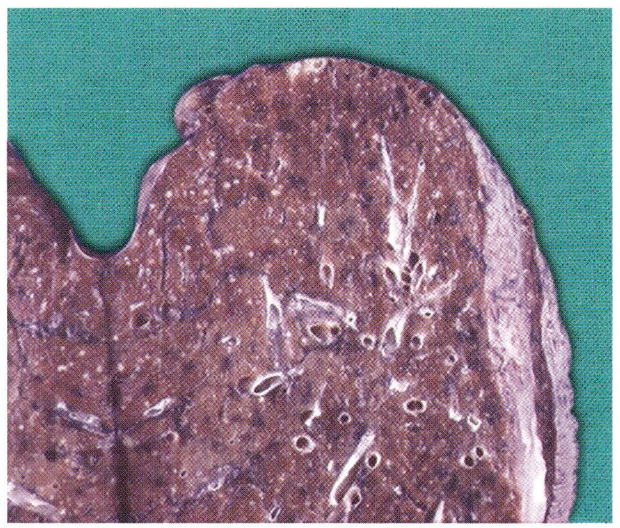

A. Miliary Tb
B. Pneumoconiosis
C. Bronchiectasis
D. Pneumonia

5. **A 38-year-old female with neck swelling shown is gross and histology of the tissue, what is the diagnosis?**

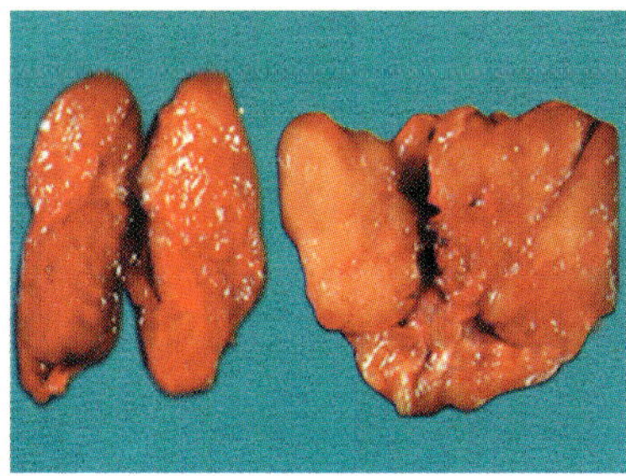

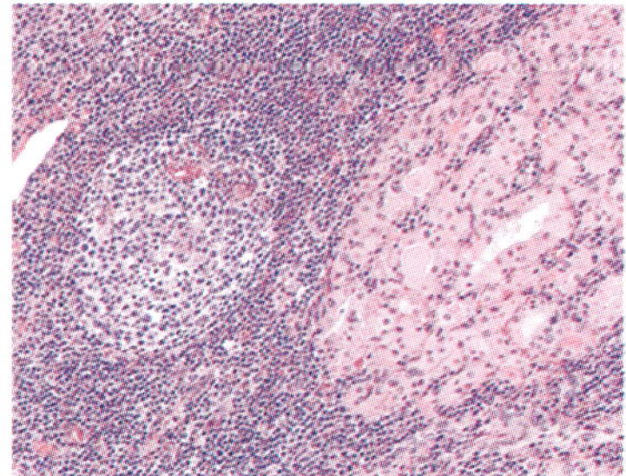

A. NHL
B. MCT
C. Melanoma
D. Hashimoto's thyroiditis

---

4. Ans. (A) Miliary Tb

5. Ans. (D) Hashimoto's thyroiditis

6. A lady died suddenly with pulmonary thromboembolism. A specimen of liver was given. Most likely finding is:

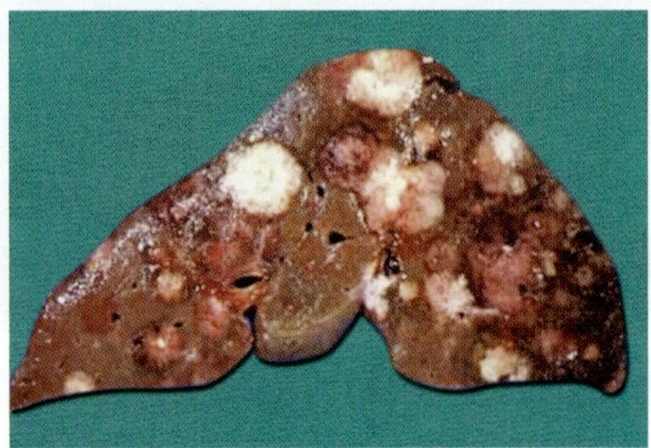

A. Multifocal hepatic adenomas
B. Liver metastasis
C. Invasive angiocarcinoma
D. Metastasis from PE

7. After surgery in Scrotum, tumor specimen obtained is shown below. What is the diagnosis?

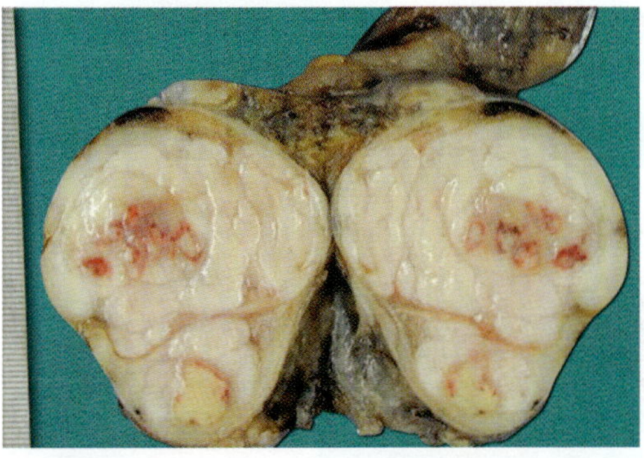

A. Seminoma
B. Teratoma
C. Dysgerminoma
D. Yolk sac tumor

---

6. Ans. (D) Metastasis from PE

7. Ans. (A) Seminoma

8. **In 20-year-old girl reddish brown soft to firm nodule seen on the chest not increasing in size, histopathology image is given, what is the diagnosis?**

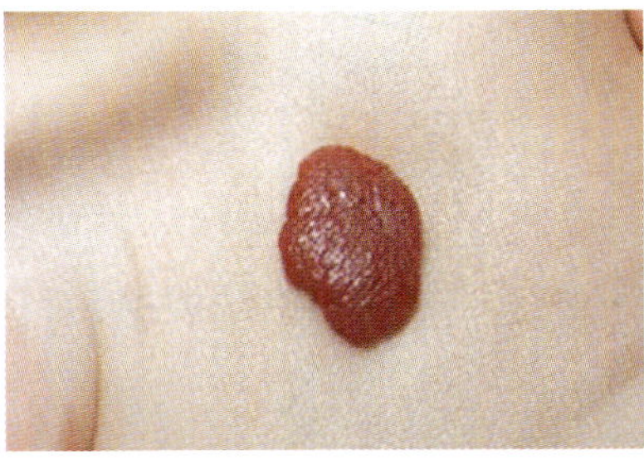

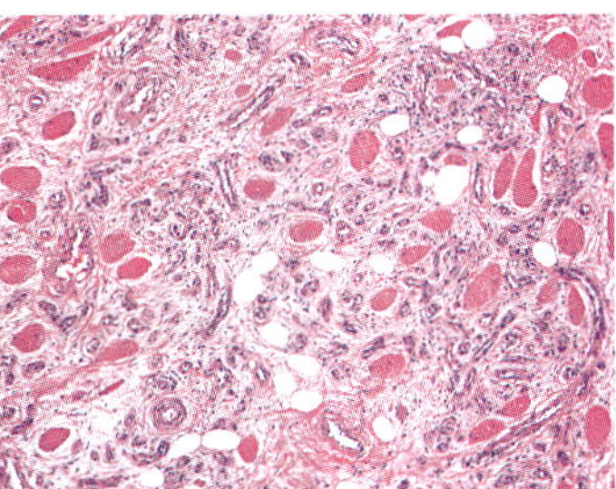

A. Hemangioma
B. Nevus
C. Lipoma
D. Paget's disease

9. **Slide of peripheral blood smear of a patient suffering with fever and chills is shown. Vector for the disease shown in the image is:**

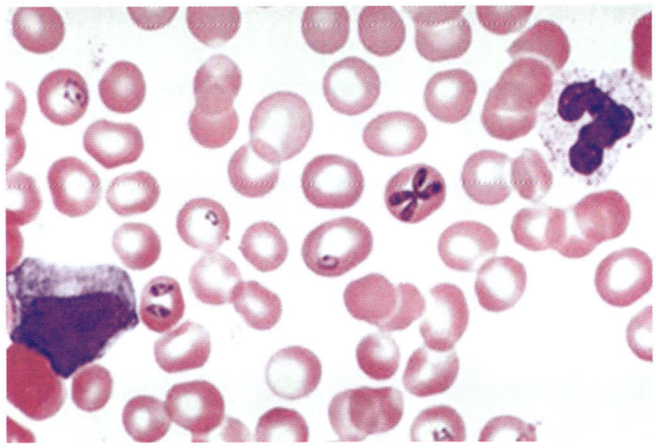

A. Hard tick
B. Anopheles
C. Culex
D. Tsetse fly

---

8. Ans. (A) Hemangioma

9. Ans. (A) Hard tick

10. A patient with history of fall on outstretched hand will most probably have injury to which of the following marked areas in the image?

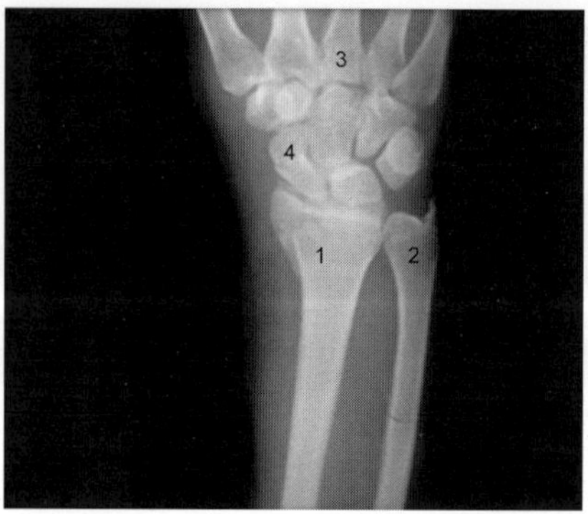

A. 1
B. 2
C. 3
D. 4

11. A 25 years old male having pain and deformity of the tibia as shown in X-ray. He had history of trauma 2 years back. What is the most probable diagnosis?

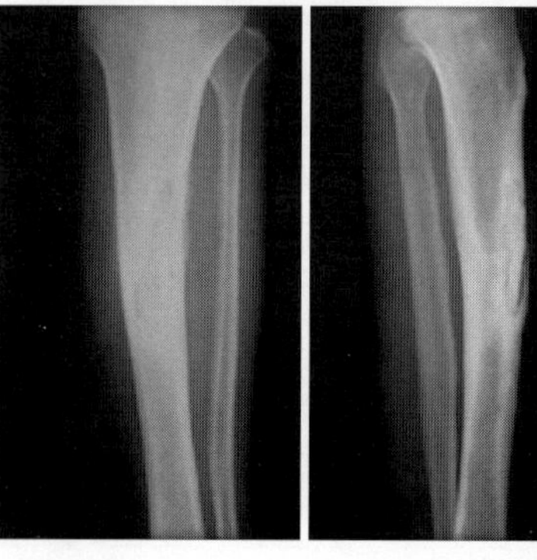

A. Ewing's Sarcoma
B. Chronic osteomyelitis
C. Osteosarcoma
D. Stess fracture tibia

---

10. Ans. (A) 1

11. Ans. (B) Chronic osteomyelitis

12. 70 years old lady 2 days following cataract surgery presents with eye complaints as shown in the image. Next step in its management is?

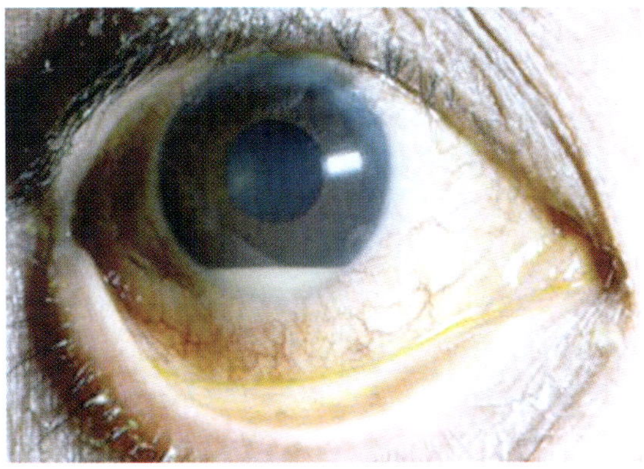

A. Intravitreal antibiotic
B. Intravitreal steroids
C. Eye patch and dressing
D. Intravitreal mannitol

13. Cause of given retina image is:

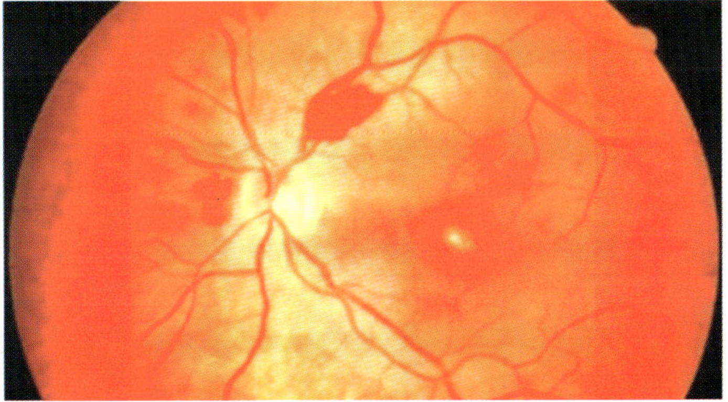

A. Acute leukemia
B. Sickle cell anemia
C. Beta thalassemia
D. Uveal melanoma

---

12. Ans. (A) Intravitreal antibiotic

13. Ans. (A) Acute leukemia

14. A child presents with neurological symptoms and has following feature what test is to be done next?

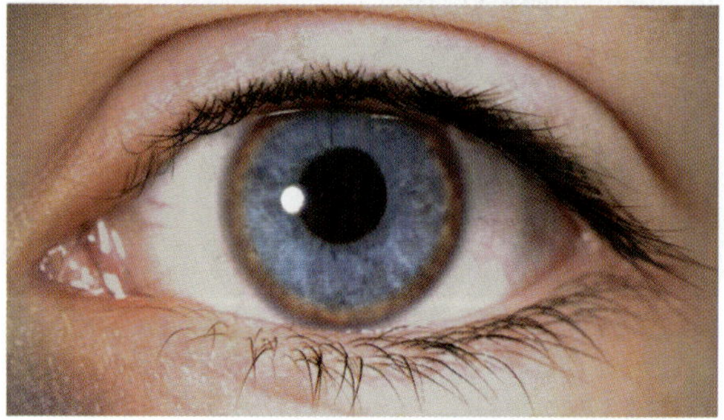

A. Serum ceruloplasmin
B. Karyotyping
C. Serum copper
D. PCR

15. A 55-year-old male having bone pains for the last 2 years with X-ray of skull shown below. Most probable diagnosis is?

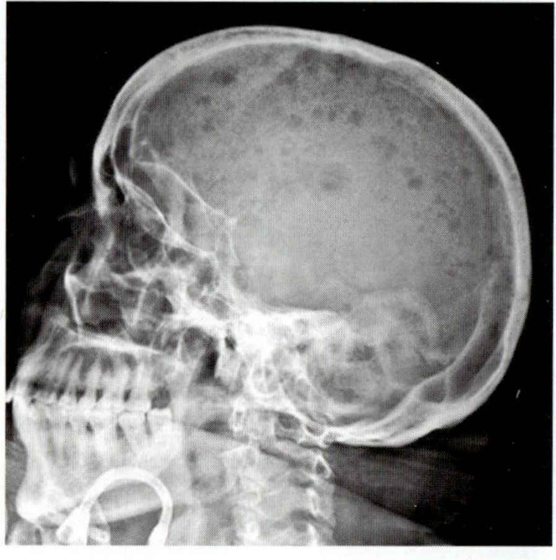

A. Multiple myeloma
B. Paget's disease
C. Hyperparathyroidism
D. Eosinophilic granuloma

---

14. Ans. (A) Serum ceruloplasmin

15. Ans. (A) Multiple myeloma

16. **Plan KUB showing what procedure done?**

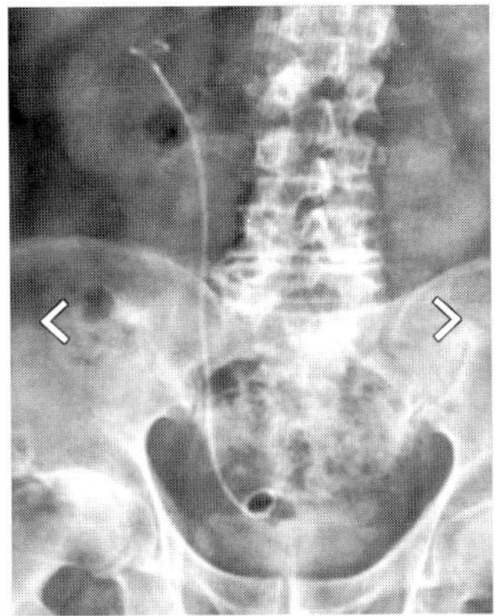

A. ESWL for renal stone
B. ESWL for bladder stones
C. ESWL for renal TB
D. Stent for benign prostatic hyperplasia

17. **A 50-year-old male with symptoms of obstructive uropathy. A retrograde urethrogram was done which shows?**

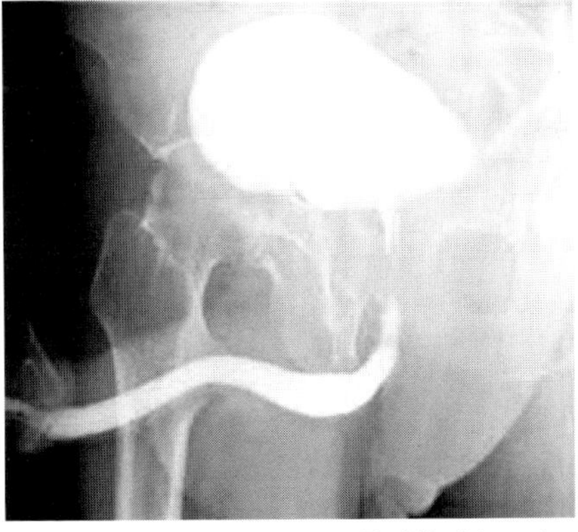

A. Urethral stone
B. Bladder stone
C. Benign prostatic hyperplasia
D. Hydronephrosis

---

16. Ans. (A) ESWL for renal stone

17. Ans. (C) Benign prostatic hyperplasia

18. Identify the retractor?

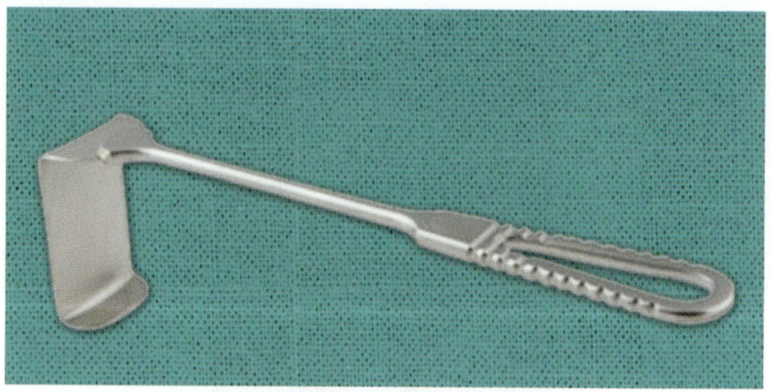

A. Morris retractor
B. Langenbeck retractor
C. Richardson retractor
D. Deaver retractor

19. Which of the following statement is true about suture material in the image?

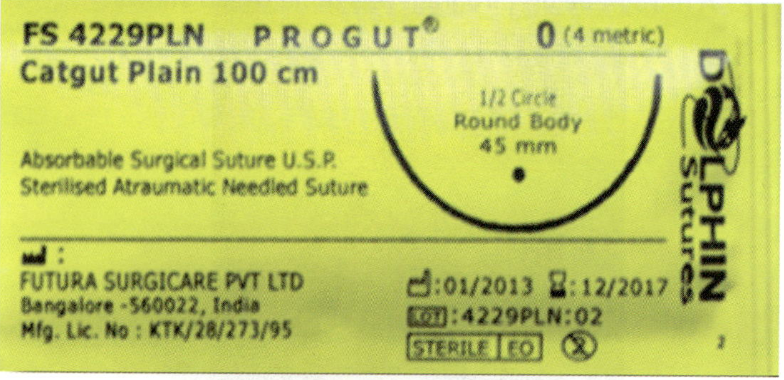

A. Made of rabbit submucosa
B. Made of cat submucosa
C. Not degraded
D. Degraded by enzymatic degradation

---

18. Ans. (A) Morris retractor

19. Ans. (D) Degraded by enzymatic degradation

20. **Female with complaints of infertility, HSG showing what?**

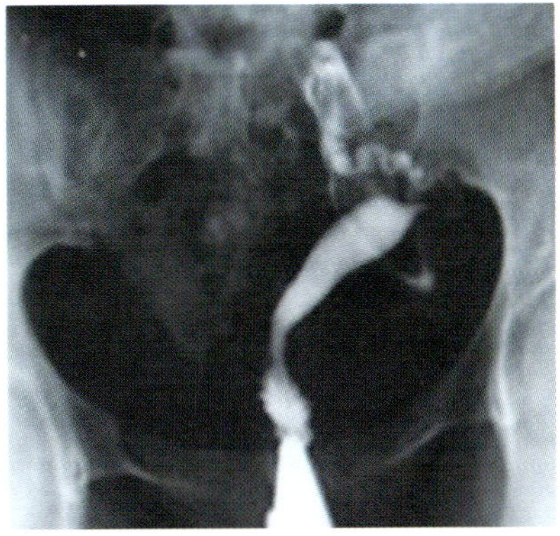

A. Unicornuate uterus
B. Septate uterus
C. Bicornuate uterus
D. Uterus didelphys

21. **Section of uterus showing what?**

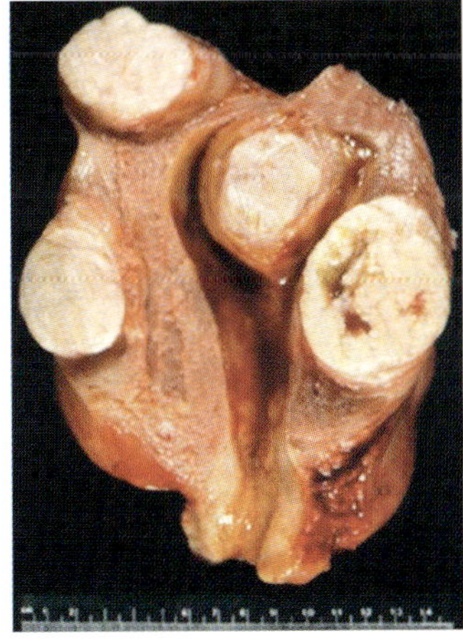

A. Leiomyoma
B. Endometrial polyp
C. Endometriosis
D. Leiomyosarcoma

---

20. Ans. (A) Unicornuate uterus

21. Ans. (A) Leiomyoma

22. A 22-year old male developed pigmentation over upper chest for the last 2 years as shown in image. What is the diagnosis?

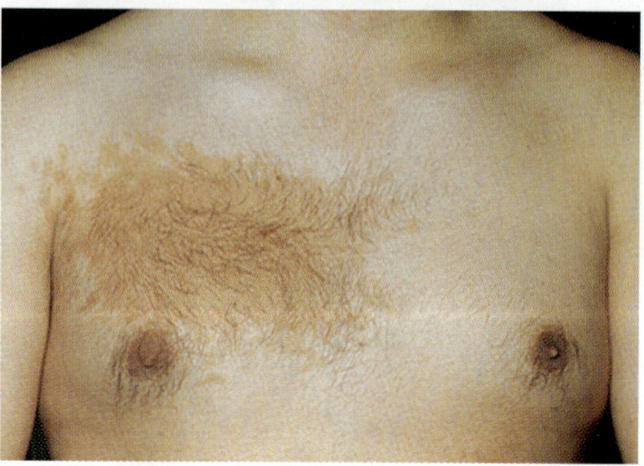

A. Becker nevus
B. Drug reaction
C. Post inflammmatory pigmentation
D. Congenital nevus

23. Identify the nerve thickened here in a leprosy patient?

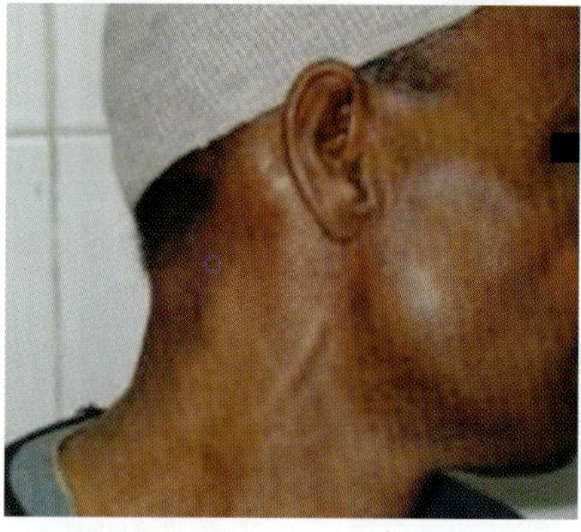

A. Greater auricular nerve
B. Facial nerve
C. Trigemeral nerve
D. Occipital nerve

---

22. Ans. (A) Becker nevus

23. Ans. (A) Greater auricular nerve

24. A child has rash on elbow as shown with family history of asthma. What is the most probable diagnosis?

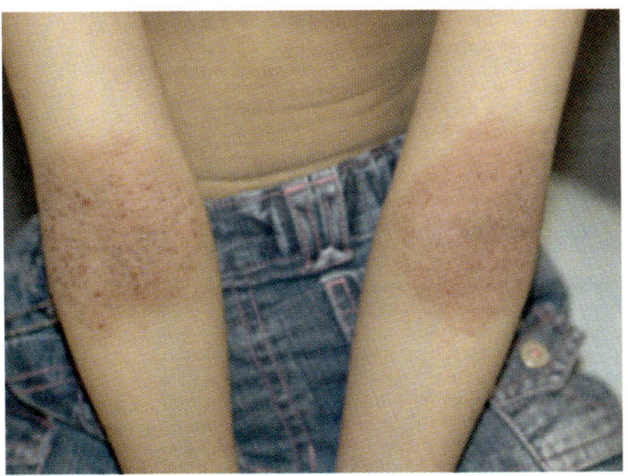

A. Atopic dermatitis
B. Contact dermatitis
C. Allergic dermatitis
D. Seborrheic dermatitis

25. Name the investigation shown in the given image.

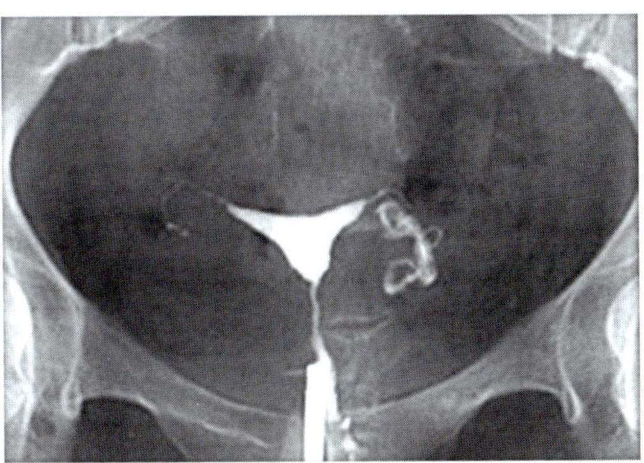

A. MR HSG
B. CT HSG
C. Conventional HSG
D. USG HSG

---

24. Ans. (A) Atopic dermatitis

25. Ans. (C) Conventional HSG

26. Child with bitemporal hemianopia. His IQ is normal. His visual acuity is diminished. The radiological image of this patient is shown below. What is the most likely diagnosis?

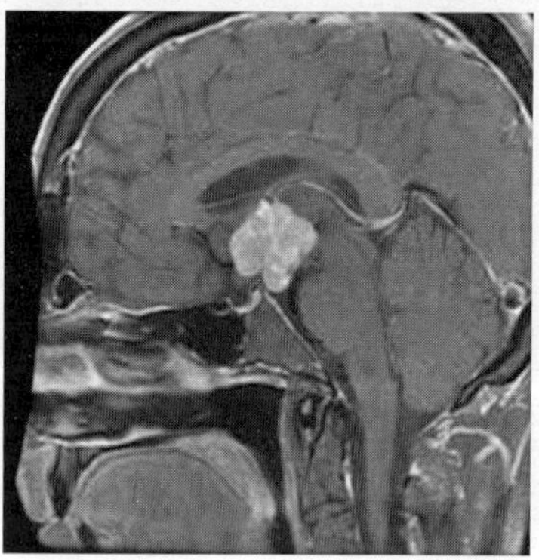

A. Craniopharyngioma
B. Optic glioma
C. Pineal tumor
D. Torus tubaris

27. Identify the condition shown in the CT scan image below:

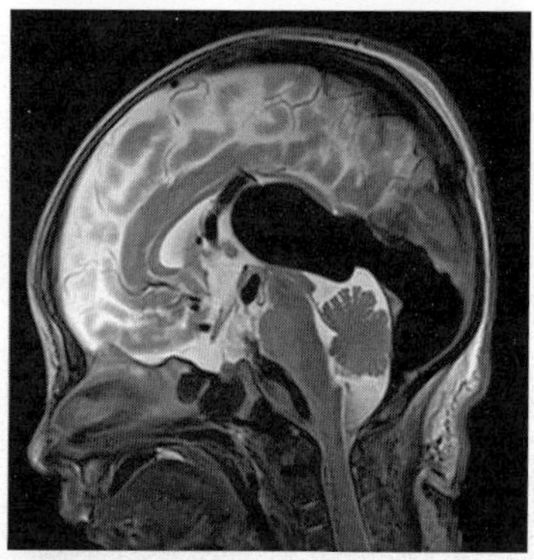

A. Dandy Walker syndrome
B. Vein of Galen malformation
C. Arnold-Chiari malformation
D. Cerebellar vermis malformation

---

26. Ans. (A) Craniopharyngioma

27. Ans. (B) Vein of Galen malformation

28. **Which artery has been shown in the following CT angiographic image?**

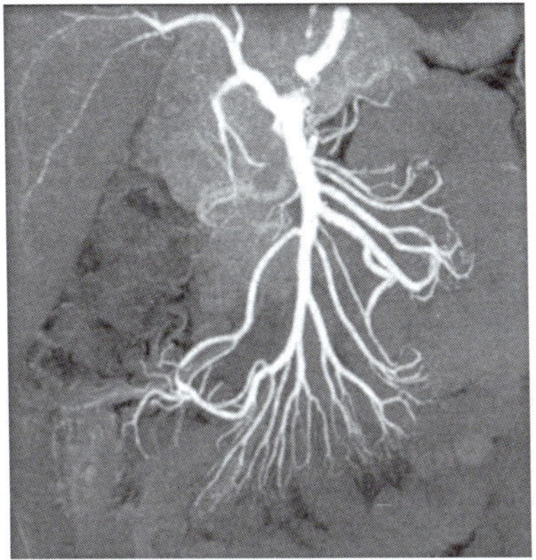

A. Superior mesenteric artery
B. Inferior mesenteric artery
C. Inferior rectal artery
D. Coeliac artery

29. **CT scan of abdomen showing the structure marked is:**

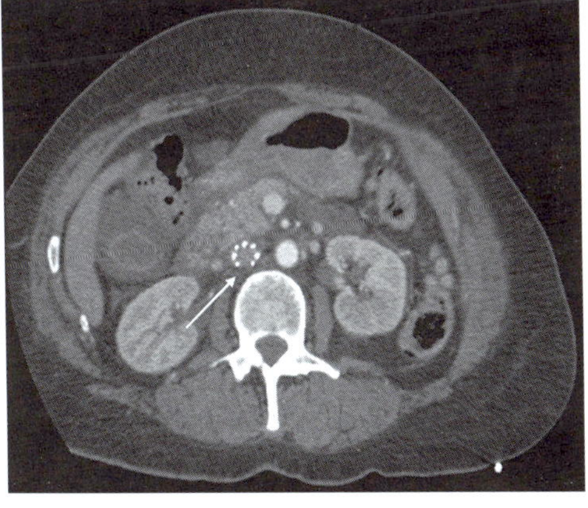

A. SVC
B. IVC
C. Aorta
D. Thoracic duct

---

27. Ans. (A) Superior mesenteric artery

29. Ans. (B) IVC

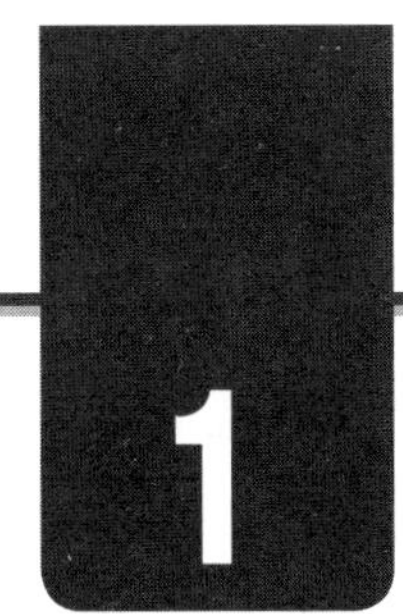

1 Anatomy

1. Nasopharyngeal chordoma arises from:

A. Notochord
B. Endoderm
C. Mesoderm
D. Rathke's pouch

2. Pain referred to ear in tonsillitis is due to:

A. Facial nerve
B. Trigeminal nerve
C. Glossopharyngeal nerve
D. Vagus nerve

3. About Sibson's fascia all are true except:

A. Attached to the inner border of 2nd rib
B. Subclavian vein runs over it
C. Formed by scalenus anterior muscle
D. Covers apex of the lung

4. Structure not passing through aortic opening:

A. Thoracic duct
B. IVC
C. Aorta
D. Azygos vein

5. What is the action of this Muscle (pointed) at metacarpophalangeal joint?

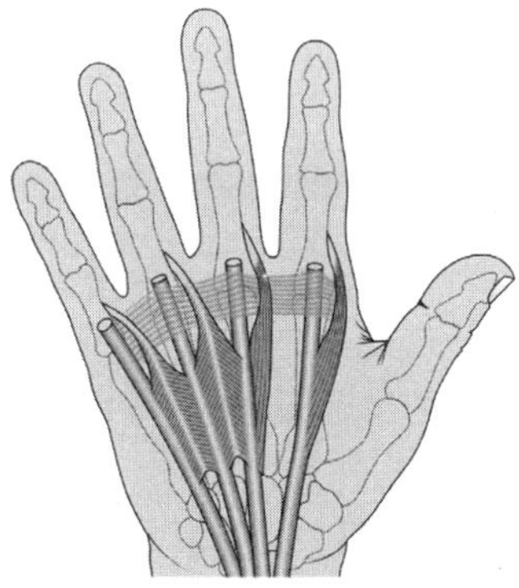

A. Abduction
B. Adduction
C. Flexion
D. Extension

6. Special visceral efferent fiber is not seen in:

A. Trigeminal nerve
B. Facial nerve
C. Nucleus ambigus
D. Vagus nerve

7. Nerves supplying pharyngeal arches are developed from:

A. Mesoderm
B. Neural crest
C. Endoderm
D. Notochord

8. Broca's area is situated in:

A. Inferior frontal gyrus
B. Superior temporal gyrus
C. Inferior temporal gyrus
D. Angular gyrus

9. Ureteric bud develops from?

A. Metanephros
B. Mesonephric duct
C. Mesonephros
D. Genital sinus

10. What is the feature of the muscle shown in the image below:

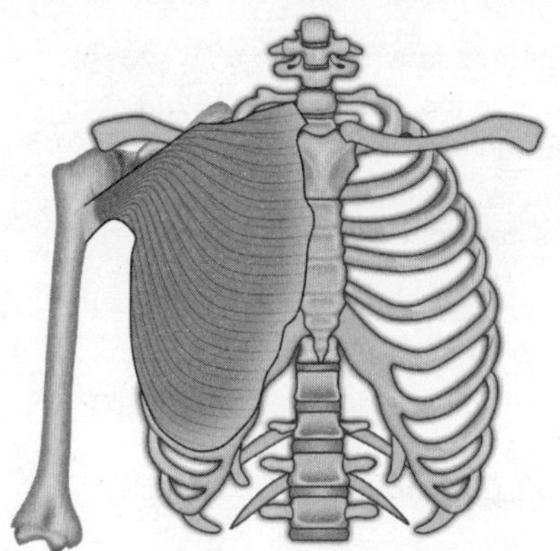

A. Cruciate
B. Multipennate
C. Spiral
D. Unipennate

11. Which of the following statements is not true about iliolumbar ligament?

A. Upper fibers attached to the iliac crest
B. Lower fibers attached to the base of sacrum
C. Help in maintaining the lumbosacral joint stability
D. Upper attachment to transverse process of T12

12. Which of the following structure develops from dorsal mesentery?

A. Greater omentum
B. Lesser omentum
C. Liver
D. Diaphragm

Answers with Explanations

1. **Ans. (A) Notochord**
   - Chordoma is a rare slowgrowing neoplasm thought to arise from cellular remnants of the notochord.
   - There are three histological variants of chordoma: Classical (or "conventional"), chondroid and dedifferentiated.
   - The histological appearance of classical chordoma is of a lobulated tumor composed of groups of cells separated by fibrous septa. The cells have small round nuclei and abundant vacuolated cytoplasm, sometimes described as physaliferous (having bubbles or vacuoles).
   - Chondroid chordomas histologically show features of both chordoma and chondrosarcoma.
   - Chordomas can arise from bone in the skull base and anywhere along the spine. The two most common locations are cranially at the clivus and in the sacrum at the bottom of the spine.
   - A possible association with tuberous sclerosis complex (TSC1 or TSC2) has been suggested.
   - In most cases, complete surgical resection followed by radiation therapy offers the best chance of long-term control.
   - Chordomas are relatively radioresistant, requiring high doses of radiation to be controlled. The proximity of chordomas to vital neurological structures such as the brainstem and nerves, limits the dose of radiation that can safely be delivered. Therefore, highly focused radiation such as proton therapy and carbon ion therapy are more effective than conventional X-ray radiation.
   - The PDGFR inhibitor Imatinib and sirolimus can be used but only modest response.
2. **Ans. (C) Glossopharyngeal nerve**

   Referred (secondary) pain in ear causes are:
   - Via Trigeminal nerve [cranial nerve V]: Oral cavity carcinoma can also cause referred ear pain via this pathway.
   - Via Facial nerve [cranial nerve VII]: This can come from the teeth, temporomandibular joint (due to its close relation to the ear canal), or the parotid gland.

- Via Glossopharyngeal nerve [cranial nerve IX]: This comes from the oropharynx, and can be due to pharyngitis, pharyngeal ulceration, tonsillitis, or to carcinoma of the oropharynx (base of tongue, soft palate, pharyngeal wall, tonsils).
- Via Vagus nerve [cranial nerve X]: This can arise from the laryngopharynx in carcinoma of this area, or from the esophagus in GERD.
- Via the second and third spinal segments, C2 and C3.

3. **Ans. (A) Attached to the inner border of 2nd rib**

The **suprapleural membrane** is also known as **Sibson's fascia.**

Suprapleural membrane is:

- Dome-shaped musculo – fascial expansion
- Muscular part – scalenus minimus muscle
- Fascial part – endothoracic fascia.

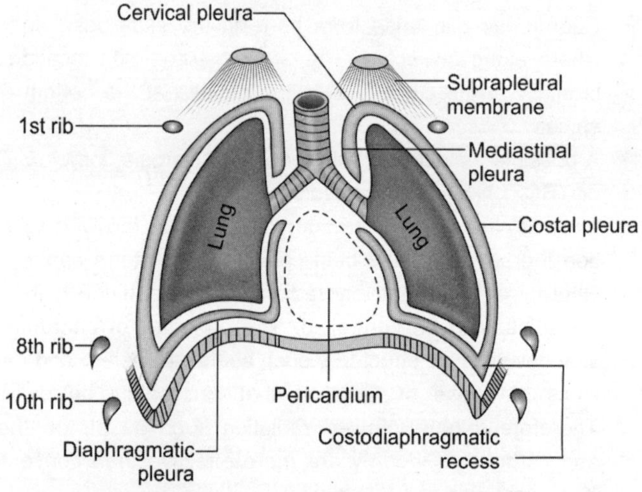

- Attachments:
  - In front—Inner border of the 1st rib
  - Behind—Tip of the transverse process of the 7th cervical vertebra
  - Medially—Continuous with the pretracheal fascia by the side of the trachea.
- Protects the apex of the lung and cervical pleura from the structures of the root of the neck.

4. Ans. (B) IVC

Opening	*Vertebral level*	*Location*	*Structures passing through*
Vena caval hiatus	T8	Central tendon of diaphragm	• Inferior vena cava • Right phrenic nerve
Esophageal hiatus	T10	Muscular part at the right crus of the diaphragm	• Esophagus • Vagus nerve • Left inferior phrenic vessels
Aortic hiatus	T12	Between the diaphragm and vertebral column	• Aorta • Azygos vein • Thoracic duct

5. Ans. C. Flexion

- The lumbricals perform movements of the second to fifth finger. Their contraction leads to flexion at the metacarpophalangeal joints (MCP) and extension at both proximal (PIP) and distal interphalangeal joints (DIP).
- The reason for the opposite actions is that the tendons cross the MCP on the palmar side, but distally insert at the dorsal side of the finger.
- These combined movements support a strong hand grip (e.g. holding a pen).
- The muscle pointed is the first lumbrical which will flex the second MCP joint and extend the PIP and DIP joints of the index finger.

6. Ans. (C) Nucleus ambigus

- Special visceral efferent (SVE) fibers are the efferent nerve fibers that provide motor innervation to the muscles of the pharyngeal arches in humans.
- The only nerves containing SVE fibers are: Trigeminal nerve (V), facial nerve (VII), glossopharyngeal nerve (IX), vagus nerve (X) and accessory nerve (XI).
- Nucleus ambiguus contains the cell bodies of nerves that innervate the muscles of the soft palate, pharynx, and larynx which are strongly associated with speech and swallowing.
- The axons of these cell bodies will form the tract and run in the ninth, tenth and eleventh cranial nerves.

7. Ans. (B) Neural crest

Nerves supplying pharyngeal arches are developed from the cranial neural crest. The cranial neural crest arises in the cranial part of the embryo and populates the face and the pharyngeal arches giving rise to bones, cartilage, nerves and connective tissue. The endocranium and facial bones of the skull are ultimately derived from crest cells.

Other places of Migration of cranial neural crest are:

- Into the pharyngeal arches and play an inductive role in thymus development.
- Into the pharyngeal arches and form the parafollicular cell or ultimobranchial bodies of the thyroid gland.
- Into the pharyngeal arches and play an inductive role in the parathyroid gland development.
- Facial ectomesenchyme of the pharyngeal arches forming skeletal muscle, bone, and cartilage in the face.
- Odontoblasts (dentin-producing cells) of the teeth.
- Around the optic vesicle and the developing eye and contributes to many eye elements such as choroid, sclera, iris, and ciliary body. It also contributes to the attaching skeletal muscles of the eye.
- Into the otic placode and participates in the inner ear development.
- Sensory ganglia of the fifth, seventh, ninth and tenth cranial nerves.
- Schwann cells

8. Ans. (A) Inferior frontal gyrus

The inferior frontal gyrus includes the following areas:

- Brodmann area 44
- Brodmann area 45
- Brodmann area 47

Brodmann area 44 corresponds to Broca's area (sometimes Broca's area is taken to encompass Brodmann's areas 44 and 45) — for the dominant hemisphere of the brain.

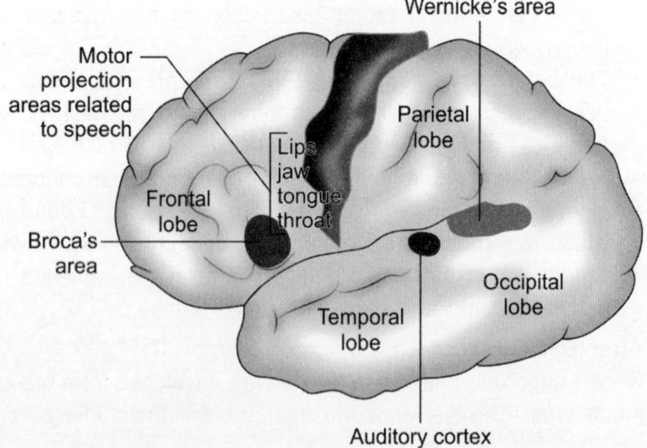

9. Ans. (B) Mesonephric duct

The ureteric bud also known as the metanephrogenic diverticulum is a protrusion from the mesonephric duct. It later develops into a conduit for urine drainage from the kidneys which in contrast originate from the metanephric blastema.

10. Ans. (C) Spiral

- The muscle in the image is pectoralis major, which has spiral/twisted fascicular arrangement.
- Spiral or twisted fibers are also found in trapezius, latissimus dorsi and supinator.
- Pectoralis major may also be called as a convergent muscle (the fascicles extend from a broad, fan-shape area and converge on single attachment site where the muscle interacts with a tendon).
- In certain muscles the fasciculi are crossed. These are called cruciate muscles, e.g. sternocleidomastoid, masseter and adductor magnus.

11. Ans. (D) Upper attachment to transverse process of T12

- The iliolumbar ligament is a strong ligament passing from the tip of the transverse process of the fifth lumbar vertebra to the posterior part of the inner lip of the iliac crest (upper margin of ilium).
- It radiates as it passes laterally and is attached by two main bands to the pelvis.
- The lower bands/fibers run to the base of the sacrum; the upper band is attached to the crest of the ilium immediately in the front of the sacroiliac articulation, and is continuous above with the lumbodorsal fascia.
- In front, it is in relation with the Psoas major; behind with the muscles occupying the vertebral groove; above with the quadratus lumborum.
- The ililumbar ligament strengthens the lumbosacral joint.

12. Ans. (A) Greater omentum

- The derivatives of ventral mesentery are lesser omentum, falciform ligament, coronary ligament of liver and triangular ligament of liver.
- The derivatives of dorsal mesentery are greater omentum, gastrosplenic ligament, gastrocolic ligament, lienorenal ligament, mesentery of small intestine, mesoappendix, transverse mesocolon and sigmoid mesocolon.

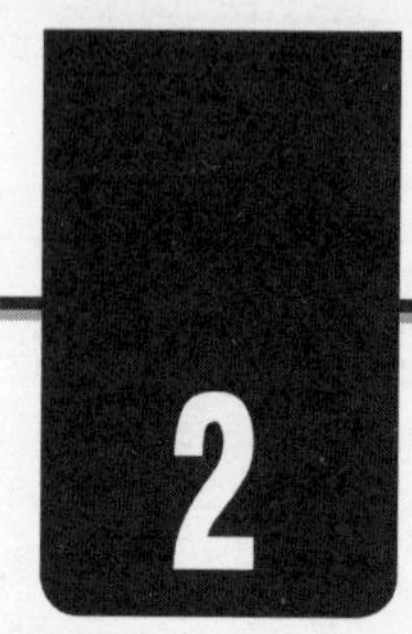

Physiology

1. Export of ions from nucleus to extracellular matrix involve all except:

A. Ran proteins
B. Importins
C. Local signals
D. Caveolins

2. Stimulus for secretion of Müllerian inhibiting substance is present on which chromosome:

A. X chromosome
B. Y chromosome
C. Chromosome 16
D. Chromosome 12

3. In hypovolemic shock what occurs in kidney:

A. Afferent arteriolar resistance increased
B. Urine output increased
C. Efferent arteriolar constriction
D. Increased blood flow to kidney

4. Which of the following is endogenous pyrogen?

A. PGE2
B. PGF1
C. PGI2
D. PGF2 alpha

5. "C" wave in JVP means:

A. Tricuspid valve bulging into right atrium during right ventricular isovolumetric contraction
B. Slow filling at the end of diastole
C. Increasing volume in right atrium during systole
D. At the start of diastole

6. Body fat cannot be measured by?

A. Total body water
B. Body density
C. Total body calcium
D. Waist hip ratio

7. Insulin like growth factors are secreted by:

A. Liver
B. Pancreas
C. Adrenal gland
D. Pituitary gland

8. When Va/Q is infinity means?

A. Partial pressure of O_2 becomes zero
B. No exchange of O_2 and CO_2
C. Partial pressure of CO_2 alone becomes zero
D. Partial pressure of both CO_2 and O_2 remain normal

9. Alpha waves are seen during?

A. Sleep
B. REM movements
C. Relaxed state
D. Active state

10. Components responsible for countercurrent mechanism in kidney are all except:

A. Sodium outflow in thick ascending limb
B. Water outflow in thin descending limb
C. Sodium outflow in thin ascending limb
D. Flow of tubular fluid from PCT to DCT

11. Glucose is absorbed in intestine by?

A. Secondary active transport
B. Facilitated diffusion
C. Simple diffusion
D. Primary active transport

12. Iron is transported from enterocytes through:

A. GLUT1
B. DMT2
C. Ferroprotin 1
D. DMT1

13. In Bartter syndrome defect Is seen in:

A. Defect in PCT
B. Defect in DCT
C. Defect in thick ascending limb of loop of Henle
D. Defect in thick descending limb of loop of Henle

14. Endothelin acts on which receptors?

A. cAMP
B. G proteins
C. Na^+ receptors
D. Calcium receptors

15. Aldosterone synthesis is stimulated by which of the following?

A. ACTH
B. Hyperkalemia
C. Hypernatremia
D. Exogenous steroids

16. ACTH secretion is increased by all except:

A. Metyrapone
B. Na and water retention
C. Aldosterone
D. Adrenal adenoma

Answers with Explanations

1. Ans. (A) Ran proteins

- The basis for selective traffic across the nuclear envelope is best understood for proteins that are imported from the cytoplasm to the nucleus. Such proteins are responsible for all aspects of genome structure and function; they include histones, DNA polymerases, RNA polymerases, transcription factors, splicing factors, and many others. These proteins are targeted to the nucleus by specific amino acid sequences, called nuclear localization signals, that direct their transport through the nuclear pore complex.
- Nuclear localization signals: The T antigen nuclear localization signal is a single stretch of amino acids. In contrast, the nuclear localization signal of nucleoplasmin is bipartite.
- Protein import through the nuclear pore complex can be operationally divided into two steps, distinguished by whether they require energy.
- In the first step, which does not require energy, proteins that contain nuclear localization signals bind to the nuclear pore complex but do not pass through the pore.
- In this initial step, nuclear localization signals are recognized by a cytosolic receptor protein, and the receptor-substrate complex binds to the nuclear pore. The prototype receptor, called importin, consists of two subunits.
  1. One subunit (importin α) binds to the basic amino acid-rich nuclear localization signals of proteins such as T antigen and nucleoplasmin.
  2. The second subunit (importin β) binds to the cytoplasmic filaments of the nuclear pore complex, bringing the target protein to the nuclear pore. Other types of nuclear localization signals, such as those of ribosomal proteins, are recognized by distinct receptors which are related to importin β and function similarly to importin β during the transport of their target proteins into the nucleus.
- The second step in nuclear import, translocation through the nuclear pore complex, is an energy-dependent process that requires GTP hydrolysis. A key player in the translocation process is a small GTP-binding protein called Ran, which is related to the Ras proteins. The conformation and activity of Ran is regulated by GTP binding and hydrolysis, like Ras or several of the translation factors involved in protein synthesis.

Enzymes that stimulate GTP binding to Ran are localized to the nuclear side of the nuclear envelope whereas enzymes that stimulate GTP hydrolysis are localized to the cytoplasmic side. Consequently, there is a gradient of Ran/GTP across the nuclear envelope, with a high concentration of Ran/GTP in the nucleus and a high concentration of Ran/GDP in the cytoplasm.

- This gradient of Ran/GTP is thought to determine the directionality of nuclear transport, and GTP hydrolysis by Ran appears to account for most of the energy required for nuclear import. Importin β forms a complex with importin α and it is associated target protein on the cytoplasmic side of the nuclear pore complex, in the presence of a high concentration of Ran/GDP. This complex is then transported through the nuclear pore to the nucleus, where a high concentration of Ran/GTP is present.
- At the nuclear side of the pore, Ran/GTP binds to importin β, displacing importin α and the target protein. As a result, the target protein is released within the nucleus. The Ran/GTP-importin β complex is then exported to the cytosol, where the bound GTP is hydrolyzed to GDP, releasing importin β to participate in another cycle of nuclear import.
- Some proteins remain within the nucleus following their import from the cytoplasm, but many others shuttle back and forth between the nucleus and the cytoplasm.
- Some of these proteins act as carriers in the transport of other molecules, such as RNAs; others coordinate nuclear and cytoplasmic functions (e.g. by regulating the activities of transcription factors). Proteins are targeted for export from the nucleus by specific amino acid sequences, called nuclear export signals.
- Like nuclear localization signals, nuclear export signals are recognized by receptors within the nucleus that direct protein transport through the nuclear pore complex to the cytoplasm. Interestingly, the nuclear export receptors (called exportins) are related to importin β. Like importin β, the exportins bind to Ran, which is required for nuclear export as well as for nuclear import.
- Thus, exportins form stable complexes with their target proteins in association with Ran/GTP within the nucleus. Following transport to the cytosolic side of the nuclear envelope, GTP hydrolysis leads to dissociation of the target protein, which is released into the cytoplasm.
- Nuclear export. Complexes between target proteins bearing nuclear export signals (NES), exportins, and Ran/GTP form in the nucleus.

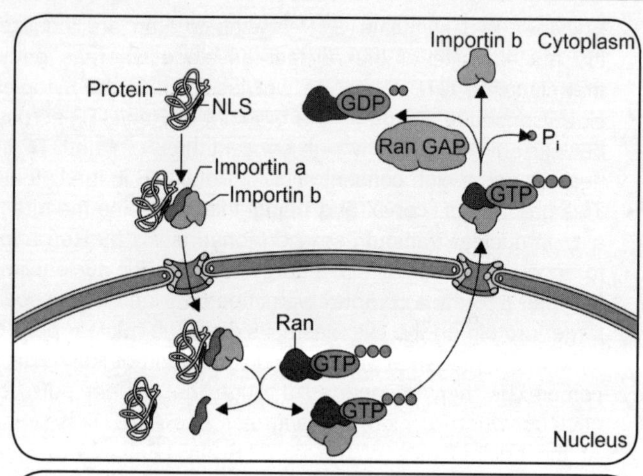

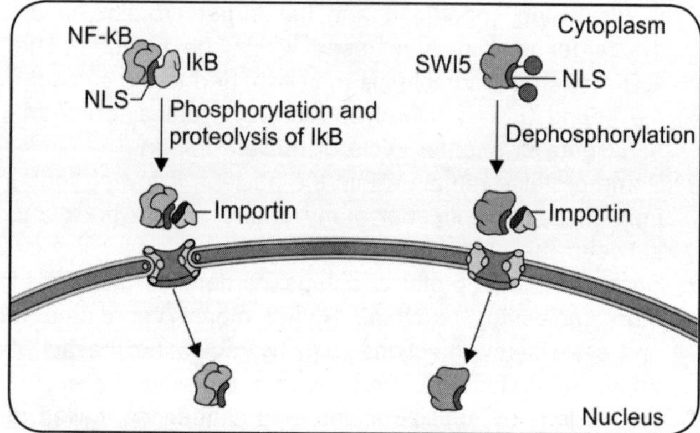

2. **Ans. (B) Y chromosome**
   - Müllerian inhibiting substance (MIS), also called anti-Müllerian hormone (AMH), is a member of the transforming growth factor-β super-family of growth and differentiation response modifiers. It is produced in immature Sertoli cells in male embryos and binds to MIS/AMH receptors in primordial Müllerian ducts to cause regression of female reproductive structures that are the precursors to the fallopian tubes, the surface epithelium of the ovaries, the uterus, the cervix, and the upper third of the vagina.
   - Following the expression of the testis determining factor gene locus, SRY on the Y chromosome, the newly formed testes secrete MIS also known as anti-Müllerian Hormone (AMH) from the Sertoli cells and the Leydig cells produce testosterone. MIS interacts with its cell surface receptors to cause the regression of the female reproductive tract precursor,

the Müllerian duct, and testosterone stimulates the growth of the androgen-dependent male reproductive tract including the external genitalia.

- In the absence the Y chromosome, ovaries will develop and the male genital tract atrophies due to the lack of testosterone. The female tract completes differentiation into the uterus, Fallopian tubes, cervix and upper third of the vagina *in utero* autonomously without sex-hormonal stimulation. Loss of function mutations of either the MIS gene or its cell surface receptor gene leads to the persistence of Müllerian structures in males.

3. **Ans. (A) Afferent arteriolar resistance increased**
   - Hypovolemic shock may occur due to a major hemorrhage or severe dehydration. In either case, the effective circulating volume of the body is severely reduced resulting in inadequate volume to properly perfuse tissues. The systemic nervous system is intensely stimulated in severe hypovolemia and coordinates a number of important compensatory responses which aim to increase cardiac output. These include attempts to increase venous return and thus preload by causing venoconstriction as well as attempts to increase systemic vascular resistance by inducing vasoconstriction. Finally, intense sympathetic stimulation of the kidneys, result in reduced glomerular filtration and increased salt and water resorption of any fluid that is filtered. When such compensatory mechanisms fail, progression to death can be very rapid.
   - A number of endogenous vasoconstrictors are released during hemorrhage. As a direct response to sympathetic nervous system activation, the release of epinephrine and norepinephrine from the adrenal medulla reinforces the actions of direct sympathetic nervous system innervation of the heart and peripheral circulation.
   - Vasopressin, which is a potent vasoconstrictor, is actively secreted by the posterior pituitary gland in response to hemorrhage. Vasopressin release is activated by both the baroreflexes and receptors located in the left atrium. Diminished renal perfusion results in the secretion of renin from the juxtaglomerular apparatus and the subsequent conversion of angiotensinogen to angiotensin, which is also a powerful vasoconstrictor.

4. **Ans. (A) PGE2**
   - Toxins from bacteria such as endotoxin act on monocytes, macrophages, and Kupffer cells to produce cytokines that act as endogenous pyrogens (EPs).

- There is good evidence that IL-1β, IL-6, β-IFN, ϒ-IFN, and TNF–α can act independently to produce fever. These cytokines penetrate the brain. Instead, evidence suggest that they act on the OVLT, one of the circumventricular organs.
- This in turn activates the preoptic area of the hypothalamus. Cytokines are also produced by cells in the central nervous system (CNS) when these are stimulated by infection, and these may act directly on the thermoregulatory centers.
- In addition, the antipyretic affect of aspirin is exerted directly on the hypothalamus, and aspirin inhibits prostaglandin synthesis. PGE2 is one of the prostaglandin that causes fever. It acts on four subtypes of prostaglandins receptors – EP1, EP2, EP3, and EP4, and knockout of the EP3 receptor impairs the febrile response to PGE2, IL-1ß, and bacterial lipopolysaccharide (LPS).

5. Ans. (A) Tricuspid valve bulging into right atrium during right ventricular isovolumetric contraction

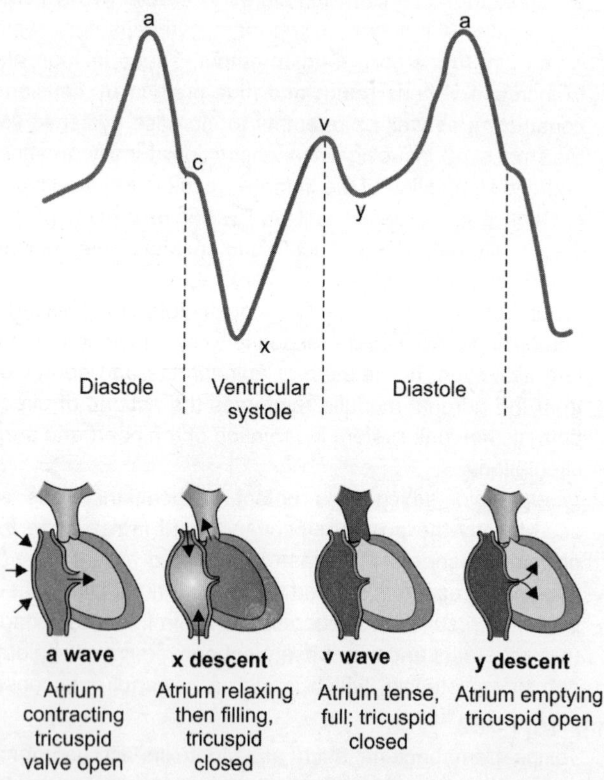

Waveform component	*Phase of cardiac cycle*	*Mechanical event*
a wave	End diastole	Atrial contraction
c wave	Early systole	Tricuspid bulging (IVC)
v wave	Late systole	Systolic filling of the atrium
x descent	Mid systole	Atrial relaxation
y descent	Early diastole	Early ventricular filling

6. **Ans. (B) Body density**
   - Body composition assessments vary in precision and in the target tissue of interest.
   - The most common assessments are anthropometric and include weight, stature, abdominal circumference, and skin-fold measurements.
   - More complex methods include bioelectrical impedance, dual-energy X-ray absorptiometry, body density, and total body water estimates.
   - There is no single universally recommended method for body composition assessment in the obese, but each modality has benefits and drawbacks.

   1. **Indirect methods are:**
      a. Anthropometry
      b. Weight, Stature, and Body Mass Index (BMI)
      c. Abdominal Circumference
      d. Skinfold measurements
      e. Bioelectric impedance analysis: The analysis of body composition by bioelectrical impedance produces estimates of total body water (TBW), fat-free mass (FFM), and fat mass by measuring the resistance of the body as a conductor to a very small alternating electrical current.
   2. **Direct methods are:**
      a. Total Body Water
      b. Total Body Counting and Neutron Activation
   3. **Criterion methods**
      a. Body Density
      b. Dual-Energy X-ray Absorptiometry
      c. Computed Tomography and Magnetic Resonance Imaging
         - Prior to the adoption of DXA, the most accurate method of estimating body fat percentage was to measure that person's average density (total mass divided by total volume) and apply a formula to convert that to body fat percentage.

- Since fat tissue has a lower density than muscles and bones, it is possible to estimate the fat content. This estimate is distorted by the fact that muscles and bones have different densities.

7. Ans. (A) Liver

- The **insulin-like growth factors** (IGFs) are proteins with high sequence similarity to insulin. IGFs are part of a complex system (often referred to as the IGF «axis») consists of two cell-surface receptors (IGF1R and IGF2R), two ligands (Insulin-like growth factor 1 (IGF-1) and Insulin-like growth factor 2 (IGF-2)), a family of six high-affinity IGF-binding proteins (IGFBP-1 to IGFBP-6), as well as associated IGFBP degrading enzymes, referred to collectively as proteases.
- **Insulin-like growth factor** I (IGF-I) is a polypeptide hormone **produced** mainly by the liver in response to the endocrine GH stimulus, but it is also secreted by multiple tissues for autocrine/paracrine purposes.

8. Ans. (B) No exchange of O_2 and CO_2

- V: Ventilation—the air that reaches the alveoli
- Q: Perfusion—the blood that reaches the alveoli via the capillaries

The V/Q ratio can therefore be defined as the ratio of the amount of air reaching the alveoli per minute to the amount of blood reaching the alveoli per minute—a ratio of volumetric flow rates. These two variables, V & Q, constitute the main determinants of the blood oxygen (O_2) and carbon dioxide (CO_2) concentration.

The V/Q ratio can be measured with a ventilation/perfusion scan. AV/Q mismatch can cause a type 1 respiratory failure.

Regional variations in ventilation, perfusion (vent/perf ratio)

- Base of lung: high VA, higher Q, low V A/Q < 1 (wasted perfusion)
- Apex of lung: low VA, lower Q, high V A/Q > 1 (wasted ventilation)
- Middle of lung: moderate VA, moderate Q, ideal VA/Q = 1.

9. Ans. (C) Relaxed state

EEG Wave patterns are:

1. **Delta waves:** It is the frequency range up to 4 Hz. It tends to be the highest in amplitude and the slowest waves. It is seen normally in adults in slow-wave sleep. It is also seen normally in babies. It may occur focally with subcortical lesions and in general distribution with diffuse lesions, metabolic encephalopathy hydrocephalus or deep midline lesions.

2. **Theta waves**: It is the frequency range from 4 to 7 Hz. It is seen normally in young children. It may be seen in drowsiness or arousal in older children and adults; it can also be seen in meditation. Excess theta for age represents abnormal activity. It can be seen as a focal disturbance in focal subcortical lesions. On the contrary this range has been associated with reports of relaxed, meditative, and creative states.
3. **Alpha waves:** It is the frequency range from 7 Hz to 13 Hz. This was the "posterior basic rhythm" seen in the posterior regions of the head on both sides, higher in amplitude on the dominant side. It emerges with closing of the eyes and with relaxation, and attenuates with eye opening or mental exertion.
4. **Beta waves:** It is the frequency range from 14 Hz to about 30 Hz. It is seen usually on both sides in symmetrical distribution and is most evident frontally. Beta activity is closely linked to motor behavior and is generally attenuated during active movements. Low-amplitude beta with multiple and varying frequencies is often associated with active, busy or anxious thinking and active concentration. It may be absent or reduced in areas of cortical damage. It is the dominant rhythm in patients who are alert or anxious or who have their eyes open.

10. Ans. (D) Flow of tubular fluid from PCT to DCT
Countercurrent mechanism

- The concentrating mechanism depends upon the maintenance of gradient of increasing osmolality along the medullary pyramids. This gradient is produced by the operation of the loops of henle as countercurrent multipliers and maintained by the operation of the vasa recta as countercurrent exchanges.
- A countercurrent system is a system in which the inflow runs parallel to, counter to, and in close proximity to the outflow for some distance. This occurs for both loops of Henle and the vasa recta in the renal medulla.
- The operation of each loop of Henle as a countercurrect multiplier depends on the high permeability of the thin descending limb to water (via aquaporin-1), the active transport of Na^+ and Cl^- out of the thick ascending limb, and the inflow of tubular fluid from the proximal tubule, with outflow into the distal tubule.
- The process can be explained using hypothetical steps leading to the normal equilibrium condition, although the steps do not occur in vivo. It is also important to remember that the equilibrium is maintained unless the osmotic gradient is washed out.

- Assume first a condition in which osmolality is 300 mOsm/kg of H_2O throughout the descending and ascending limbs and the medullary interstitium. Assume in addition that the pumps in the thick ascending limb can pump 100 mOsm/kg of Na^+ and Cl^- from the tubular fluid to the interstitium increasing interstitial osmolality 400 mOsm/kg of H_2O. Water then moves out of the thin descending limb, and its contents equilibrate with the interstitium. However, fluid containing 300 mOsm/kg of H_2O is continuously entering this limb from the proximal tubule, so the gradient against which the Na^+ and Cl^- are pumped is reduced and more enters the interstitium. Meanwhile, hypotonic fluid flows into the distal tubule and isotonic and subsequently hypertonic fluid flows into the ascending thick limb. The process keeps repeating, and the final result is a gradient of osmolality from the top to the bottom of the loop.
- In juxtamedullary nephrons with longer loops and thin ascending limbs, the osmotic gradient is spread over a greater distance and the osmolality at the tip of the loop is greater. This is because the thin ascending limb is relatively impermeable to water but permeable to Na^+ and Cl^-. Therefore, Na^+ and Cl^- move down their concentration gradients into the interstitium, and there is additional passive countercurrent multiplication.
- The greater the length of the loop of Henle, the greater the osmolality that can be reached at the tip of the medulla.
- The osmotic gradient in the medullary pyramids would not last long if the Na^+ and urea in the interstitial spaces were removed by the circulation. These solutes remain in the pyramids primarily because the vasa recta operate as countercurrent exchangers. The solutes diffuse of the vessels conducting blood toward the cortex and into the vessels descending into the pyramid. Conversely, water diffuse out of the descending vessels and into the fenestrated ascending vessels. Therefore, the solutes tend to recirculate in the medulla and water tends to bypass it, so that hypertonicity is maintained. The water removed from the collecting ducts in the pyramids is also removed by the vasa recta and enters the general circulation. Countercurrent exchange is a passive process; it depends on movement of water and could not maintain the osmotic gradient along the pyramids if the process of countercurrent multiplication in the loops of henle were to cease.
- It is worth noting that there is a very large osmotic gradient in the loop of henle and, in the presence of vasopressin, in the

collecting ducts. It is the countercurrent system that makes this gradient possible by spreading it along a system of tubules 1 cm or more in length, rather than across a single layer of cells that is only a few micrometers thick. There are other examples of the operation of countercurrent exchangers in animals. One is the heat exchange between the arteries and veane comitantes of the limbs. To a minor degree in humans, but to a major degree in mammals living in cold water, heat is transferred from the arterial blood flowing into the limbs to the adjacent veins draining blood back into the body, making the tips of the limbs cold while conserving body heat.

11. Ans. (A) Secondary active transport

In many situation, the active transport of Na^+ is coupled to the transport of other substances (secondary active transport). For example, the luminal membranes of mucosal cells in the small intestine contains a symport that transports glucose into the cell only if Na^+ binds to the protein and is transported into the cell at the same time. From the cells the about 24% of the energy utilized by cells, and in neurons it accounts for 70%. Thus, it accounts for a large part of the basal metabolism. A major payoff for this energy use is the establishment of the electrochemical gradient in cells.

12. Ans. (D) DMT1

- Most of the iron in the diet is in the ferric (Fe^{3+}) form whereas it is the ferrous (Fe^{2+}) form that is absorbed. Fe^{3+} reductase activity is associated with the iron transporter in the brush borders of the enterocytes.
- Gastric secretions dissolve the iron and permit it to form soluble complexes with ascorbic acid and other substances that aid its reduction to the Fe^{2+} form.
- The importance of this function in humans is indicated by the fact that iron deficiency anemia is a troublesome and relatively frequent complication of partial gastrectomy.
- Almost all iron absorption occurs in the duodenum. Transport of Fe^{2+} into the enterocytes occurs via divalent metal transporter 1 (DMT1). Some is stored in ferritin, and the remainder is transported out of the enterocytes by a basolateral transporter named ferroportin 1. A protein called hephaestin (Hp) is associated with ferrroportin 1. It is not a transporter itself, but it facilitates basolateral transport. In the plasma, Fe^{2+} is converted to Fe^{3+} and bound to the iron transport protein transferrin. This protein has two iron-binding sites. Normally, transferring is about 35% saturated with iron, and the normal

plasma iron level is about 130 µg/dL (23 µmol/L) in men and 110 µg/dL (19 µmol/L) in women.

- Heme binds to an apical transport protein in enterocytes and is carried into the cytoplasm. In the cytoplasm, HO_2, a subtype of heme oxygenase, removes Fe^{2+} from the porphyrin and adds it to the intracellular Fe^{2+} pool.

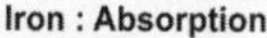

Iron : Absorption

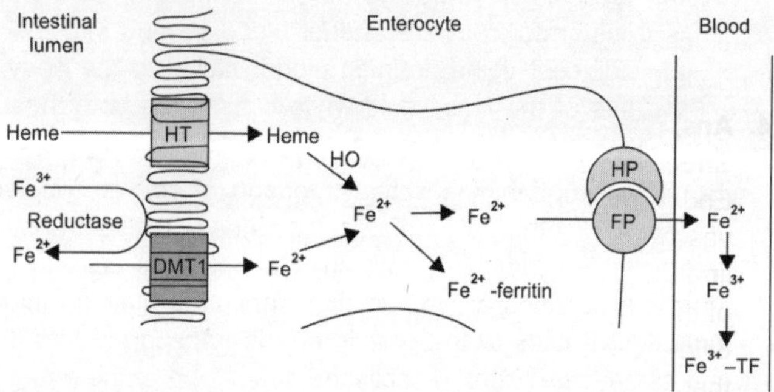

- Inside the enterocyte, iron can either be stored as ferritin or transferred across the basolateral membrane into the plasma, where it is carried by transferrin.

13. Ans. (C) Defect in thick ascending limb of loop of Henle

Genetic mutations in renal transporters

Mutations of individual genes for many renal sodium transporters and channels cause specific syndromes such as Bartter syndrome, Liddle syndrome, and dent diseases. A large number of mutations have been described.

1. Bartter syndrome is a rare but interesting condition that is due to defective transport in the thick ascending limb. It is characterized by chronic Na^+ loss in the urine, with resultant hypovolemia causing stimulation of rennin and aldosterone secretion without hypertension, plus hyperkalemia and alkalosis. The condition can be caused by loss-of-function mutations in the gene for any of four key proteins; the Na^- K^- 2Cl cotransporter, the ROMK K^+ channel, the ClC^- Kb Cl^- channels.

   The stria vascularis in the inner ear is responsible for maintaining the high K^+ concentration in the scala media that is essential for normal hearing. It contains both ClC^- Kb and ClC^- Ka Cl^- channels. Bartter syndrome associated with mutated ClC^- Kb is not associated with deafness because the ClC^- Ka channels can carry the load. However, both type of

Cl^- channels are barttin-dependent, so patients with Bartter syndrome due to mutated barttin are also deaf.

2. Another interesting example involves the proteins polycystin-1 (PKD-1) and polycystin-2 (PKD-2). PKD-1 appears to be a Ca^{2+} receptor that activates a nonspecific ion channel associated with PKD-2. The normal function of this apparent ion channel is unknown, but both proteins are abnormal in autosomal dominant polycystic kidney disease, in which the renal parenchyma is progressively replaced by fluid filled cysts until there is complete renal failure.

14. Ans. (B) G proteins

Endothelins

Endothelial cells also produce endothelin-1, one of the most potent vasoconstrictor agents yet isolated. Endothelin-1 (ET-1), endothlin-2 (ET-2), and endothelin-3 (ET-3) are the members of a family of three similar 21-amino acid polypeptides. Each is encoded by a different gene. The unique structure of the endothelins resembles that of the sarafotoxins, polypeptides found in the venom of a snake, the Israeli burrowing asp.

Endothelins – 1

In endothelial cells, the product of the endothelin-1 gene is processed to a 39 amino acid prohormone, big endothelin-1, which has about 1% of the activity of endothelin-1. The prohormone is cleaved at a tryptophan-valine (Trp–Val) bond to form endothelin-1 by endothelin-converting enzyme. Small amounts of big endothelin-1 and endothelin-1 are secreted into the blood, but for the most part, they are secreted locally and act in a paracrine fashion.

Two different endothelin receptors have been cloned, both of which are coupled via G proteins to phospholipase C. The ETA receptor, which is specific for endothelin-1, is found in many tissues and mediates the vasoconstriction produced by endothelin-1, the ETB receptor responds to all three endothelins, and is coupled to G1. It may mediate vasodilation, and it appears to mediate the developmental effects of the endothelins.

15. Ans. (B) Hyperkalemia

Aldosterone, is the main mineralocorticoid hormone, produced by the zona glomerulosa of the adrenal cortex in the adrenal gland. It plays a central role in the homeostatic regulation of blood pressure, plasma sodium (Na^+), and potassium (K^+) levels.

It has exactly the opposite function of the atrial natriuretic hormone secreted by the heart.

It is part of the renin–angiotensin–aldosterone system.

It has a plasma half-life of under 20 minutes. Drugs that interfere with the secretion or action of aldosterone are in use as antihypertensives, like lisinopril, which lowers blood pressure by blocking the angiotensin-converting enzyme (ACE), leading to lower aldosterone secretion. The net effect of these drugs is to reduce sodium and water retention but increase retention of potassium. Another example is spironolactone, a potassium-sparing diuretic which decreases blood pressure by releasing fluid from the body while retaining potassium.

Stimulation

Aldosterone synthesis is stimulated by several factors:

- Increase in the plasma concentration of angiotensin III, a metabolite of angiotensin II
- Increase in plasma angiotensin II, or potassium levels, which are present in proportion to plasma sodium deficiencies
- Serum potassium concentrations are the most potent stimulator of aldosterone secretion.
- The ACTH stimulation test, which is sometimes used to stimulate the production of aldosterone along with cortisol to determine whether primary or secondary adrenal insufficiency is present. However, ACTH has only a minor role in regulating aldosterone production; with hypopituitarism there is no atrophy of the zona glomerulosa.
- Plasma acidosis
- The stretch receptors located in the atria of the heart. If decreased blood pressure is detected, the adrenal gland is stimulated by these stretch receptors to release aldosterone, which increases sodium reabsorption from the urine, sweat, and the gut.
- Adrenoglomerulotropin, a lipid factor, obtained from pineal extracts. It selectively stimulates secretion of aldosterone.

16. Ans. (C) Aldosterone

Adrenocorticotropic hormone (ACTH, also **adrenocorticotropin, corticotropin)** is a polypeptide tropic hormone produced and secreted by the anterior pituitary gland.

ACTH is an important component of the hypothalamic-pituitary-adrenal axis and is often produced in response to biological stress (along with its precursor corticotropin-releasing hormone from the hypothalamus).

Its principal effects are increased production and release of cortisol by the cortex of the adrenal gland. ACTH is also related to the circadian rhythm.

Deficiency of ACTH is a sign of secondary adrenal insufficiency—suppressed production of ACTH due to an impairment of the pituitary gland or hypothalamus, or tertiary adrenal insufficiency [disease of the hypothalamus, with a decrease in the release of corticotropin releasing hormone (CRH)].

Conversely, chronically elevated ACTH levels occur in primary adrenal insufficiency (e.g. Addison's disease) when adrenal gland production of cortisol is chronically deficient. In Cushing's disease a pituitary tumor is the cause of elevated ACTH (from the anterior pituitary) and an excess of cortisol (hypercortisolism) is known as Cushing's syndrome.

Production and regulation: POMC, ACTH and β-lipotropin are secreted from corticotropes in the anterior lobe (or adenohypophysis) of the pituitary gland in response to the hormone corticotropin-releasing hormone (CRH) released by the hypothalamus. ACTH is synthesized from pre-pro-opiomelanocortin (pre-POMC). The removal of the signal peptide during translation produces the 241-amino acid polypeptide POMC, which undergoes a series of post-translational modifications such as phosphorylation and glycosylation before it is proteolytically cleaved by endopeptidases to yield various polypeptide fragments with varying physiological activity.

Regulation of cortisol Secretion from the Adrenal Cortex

Negative feedback control:

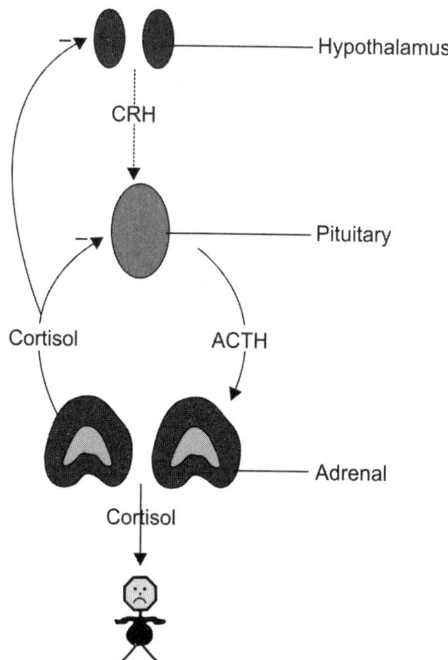

- ACTH release from the anterior pituitary is stimulated by hypothalamic secretion of corticotropin releasing hormone (CRH). CRH →↑ ACTH →↑ Cortisol
- ↑ Cortisol (or synthetic steroids)

  ↓
- Suppress CRH and ACTH secretion.

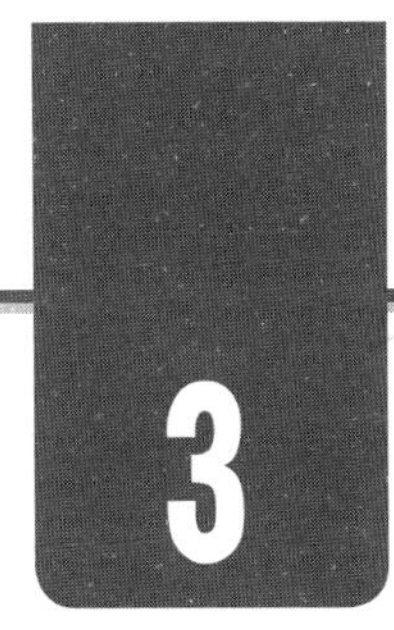

3 Biochemistry

1. Enzyme deficiency in tyrosinosis is:

A. pHPP dehydrogenase
B. Tyrosine ligase
C. Fumarylacetoacetate hydrolase
D. Tyrosine transaminase

2. Which of the following is most abundant end product of fatty acid synthesis?

A. Palmitic acid
B. Arachidonic acid
C. Oleic acid
D. Glutamic acid

3. Lesch-Nyhan syndrome is caused due to deficiency of which enzyme?

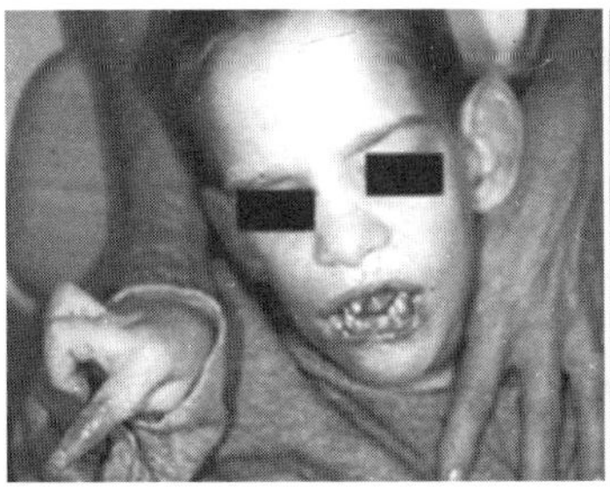

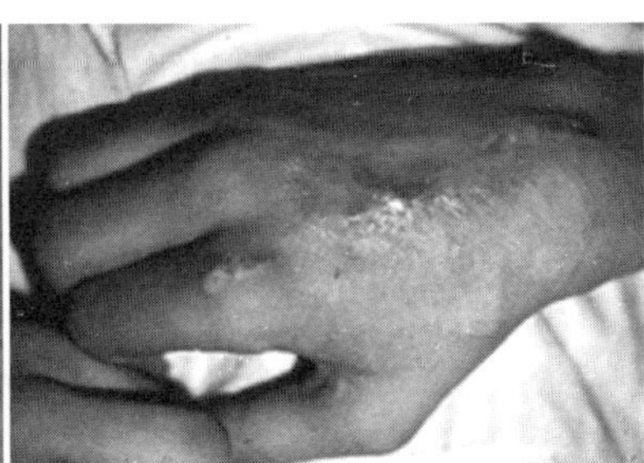

A. HGPRT
B. Tyrosine hydroxylase
C. Xanthine oxidase
D. Uricase

4. To avoid fish odor syndrome, what to be avoided in the food:

A. Pantothenic acid
B. Choline
C. Biotin
D. Pyridoxine

5. VMMA is excreted in urine in which condition?

A. Pheochromocytoma
B. Alkaptonuria
C. Adrenal adenoma
D. Addison's disease

6. Chaperones are helpful in:

A. Folding of proteins
B. Denaturation of proteins
C. Promote aggregation of proteins
D. Protein degradation

7. Galactosemia is possible due to deficiency of the following enzyme except?

A. Galactose-1-phosphate uridylyltransferase
B. HGPRT
C. Galactokinase
D. Epimerase

8. Which of the following is not true about DNA polymerase 1 function?

A. Not required in bacteria
B. Repair any damage with DNA
C. Involved in okazaki fragments
D. Participate in DNA replication

9. Fibrinopeptide A and fibrinopeptide B are acidic due to the presence of which amino acids in its structure:

A. Serine and threonine
B. Glutamate and aspartate
C. Histidine and lysine
D. Glutamine and valine

Answers with Explanations

1. **Ans. (C) Fumarylacetoacetate hydrolase**
   - **Type 1 tyrosinemia** also known as **hepatorenal tyrosinemia** or **tyrosinosis** the most severe form of tyrosinemia, is caused by a deficiency of the enzyme fumarylacetoacetate hydrolase.
   - Type 1 tyrosinemia typically presents in the infancy as failure to thrive and hepatomegaly. The primary effects are progressive liver and kidney dysfunction. The liver disease causes cirrhosis, conjugated hyperbilirubinemia, elevated AFP, hypoglycemia and coagulation abnormalities. This can lead to jaundice, ascites and hemorrhage. There is also an increased risk of hepatocellular carcinoma. The kidney dysfunction presents as Fanconi syndrome: Renal tubular acidosis, hypophosphatemia and aminoaciduria. Cardiomyopathy, neurologic and dermatologic manifestations are also possible. The urine has an odor of boiled cabbage or rancid butter.
   - Type 1 tyrosinemia is inherited in an autosomal recessive pattern.
   - Pathophysiology: Fumarylacetoacetate hydrolase catalyzes the final step in the degradation of tyrosine-fumarylacetoacetate to fumarate, acetoacetate and succinate. Fumarylacetoacetate accumulates in hepatocytes and proximal renal tubal cells and causes oxidative damage and DNA damage leading to cell death and dysfunctional gene expression which alters metabolic processes like protein synthesis and gluconeogenesis. The increase in fumarylacetoacetate inhibits previous steps in tyrosine degradation leading to an accumulation of tyrosine in the body. Tyrosine is not directly toxic to the liver or kidneys but causes dermatologic and neurodevelopmental problems.
   - The primary treatment for type 1 tyrosinemia is nitisinone (Orfadin) (also used for the treatment of alkaptonuria) and restriction of tyrosine in the diet. Nitisinone inhibits the conversion of 4-OH-phenylpyruvate to homogentisic acid by 4-Hydroxyphenylpyruvate dioxygenase, the second step in tyrosine degradation.
   - By inhibiting this enzyme, the accumulation of the fumarylacetoacetate is prevented. Previously, liver transplantation was the primary treatment option and is still used in patients in whom nitisinone fails.

2. Ans. (A) Palmitic acid

- Arachidonic acid is obtained by the conversion of linoleic acid which must be obtained in diet.
- Oleic acid is an ω9 fatty acid which is generated from saturated fatty acids, and is not considered a product of the regular fatty acid syntheis pathway.
- Glutamic acid is not a fatty acid synthesis product.

3. Ans. (A) HGPRT

Slide 1 showing nibbling of lips and fingers; slide 2 showing bite marks on hand inflicted by self. Self mutilation seen in Lesch-Nyhan syndrome; characteristic of the disease in children.

Clinical signs and symptoms seen in Lesch-Nyhan syndrome:

- **Biochemical: Hyperuricemia can result in**
  - Gout (joint pains)
  - Nephrolithiasis (abdominal pain, may be radiating in nature)
  - Tophi
- **Neurological**
  - Mental Retardation (Poor performance in school)
  - Dystonia, variable
- **Neuropsychiatric**
  - Aggressive Behavior (frequent fight, quarreling with siblings)
  - Self-Mutilation Tendency (associated with muscle loss; biting, chewing, etc.)
- Inheritance is **XLR**, enzyme absent is HGPRTase; in some patient where the enzyme is not absent, but only diminished, have a less severe condition called Kelley-Seegmiller Syndrome, where neurological and neuropsychiatric symptoms are either absent or very mild.

4. Ans. (B) Choline

- Fish odor syndrome, more correctly known as Trimethylaminuria, is a metabolic disorder first described in 1970. It is characterized by abnormal excretion of trimethylamine in the urine, breath, sweat and vaginal secretions. It may be primary in origin or secondary to liver or kidney damage, or it may be caused by an increase in the precursors of trimethylamine, such as choline, lecithin or carnitine in the diet.
- The primary syndrome is inherited in an autosomal recessive manner. The defective enzyme is flavin-containing monooxygenase 3, the gene for which (FMO3) is located in chromosome region 1q23–25. Trimethylamine is derived from the intestinal bacterial degradation of foods rich in choline,

lecithin and carnitine. Trimethylamine produced within the intestinal tract is rapidly absorbed and is converted within the liver, by the action of flavin-containing monooxygenase 3, to trimethylamine N-oxide, which is then excreted in the urine. Affected individuals have a reduced capacity to metabolize trimethylamine into trimethylamine N-oxide. Excessive amounts of the volatile molecule are therefore excreted in the body fluids, which give off a strong fishy smell.

- The biochemical diagnosis is established by measuring the ratio of trimethylamine N-oxide to trimethylamine in the urine. Among people without trimethylaminuria, more than 97% of excretion occurs as trimethylamine N-oxide. In patients with the condition, the ratio is reduced.
- Treatment includes counselling and dietary modifications. An explanation of the biochemical nature of the disorder and the exacerbating factors such as menstruation may assist in relieving patients' anxiety. Behavioral counseling may help with depression and other psychological symptoms. Genetic counseling should be considered if the patient has the primary form of the syndrome. Dietary adjustments include avoidance of choline-rich foods such as egg yolk, liver, kidney, peas, soybeans and sea fish.
- Expert opinion suggests that a short course of low-dose neomycin or metronidazole can be used to suppress production of trimethylamine in the gut. The use of mildly acidic soaps may help to reduce the odor in some patients.
- Flavin-containing monooxygenase 3 is known to be involved in the nicotinamide adenine dinucleotide phosphate–dependent oxidation and metabolism of a number of drugs such as tamoxifen, ketoconazole, sulindac sulphide and benzydamine. Given this involvement, case reports of exacerbation of fish odor syndrome in association with these drugs and other medications might be expected, because patients with primary trimethylaminuria may have a reduced ability to metabolize these compounds.
- However, restricting dietary choline can have important repercussions. Choline deficiency may result in hepatocellular injury, neurological disease, and even a predisposition to cancer. Notably, pregnant women have an increased choline requirement so restricting intake may be even less desirable in this demographic.

5. **Ans. (A) Pheochromocytoma**
   - **Vanillylmandelic acid (VMA), a metabolic by-product of norepinephrine and epinephrine, can be used to detect neuroblastoma and other tumors of neural crest origin.**
   - **The reference ranges of vanillylmandelic acid in children are as follows:**
     - Younger than 1 year: < 27 mg/g creatinine
     - Age 1–2 years: < 18 mg/g creatinine
     - Age 2–4 years: < 13 mg/g creatinine
     - Age 5–9 years: < 8.5 mg/g creatinine
     - Age 10–14 years: < 7 mg/g creatinine

   The reference range in persons aged 15 years and older is 2–7 mg/24 hours
   - **Conditions associated with elevations in urinary vanillylmandelic acid include the following:**
     - Neuroblastoma
     - Pheochromocytoma
     - Other neural crest tumors (e.g. ganglioblastoma, ganglioneuroma)
     - Severe anxiety/stress
   - **In the evaluation of pheochromocytoma, vanillylmandelic acid is now considered the least-specific test for catecholamine metabolites with a false-positive rate greater than 15%. Measurement of metanephrine, an intermediate metabolite between epinephrine and vanillylmandelic acid is now considered the most sensitive and specific test for pheochromocytoma. Besides plasma free metanephrines and urine metanephrines, urine or plasma catecholamine tests are also preferred over vanillylmandelic acid testing.**
   - **Foods that can increase urinary catecholamines include the following:**
     - Coffee
     - Tea
     - Bananas
     - Chocolate
     - Cocoa
     - Citrus fruits
     - Vanilla
   - **Drugs that can increase urinary vanillylmandelic acid include the following:**
     - Appetite suppressants
     - Caffeine

- Histamine
- Imipramine
- Insulin
- Epinephrine
- Levodopa
- Lithium
- Morphine
- Nitroglycerin
- Rauwolfia alkaloids
- Isoproterenol
- Methocarbamol
- Sulfonamide
- Chlorpromazine

- **Drugs that can decrease urine vanillylmandelic acid include the following:**
  - Clonidine
  - Disulfiram
  - Guanethidine
  - MAO inhibitors
  - Salicylates
  - Reserpine
  - Methyldopa

6. **Ans. (A) Folding of proteins**

   Auxiliary proteins assisting in folding are:
   - Chaperones
     - Chaperonins
     - Heat shock proteins
   - Protein disulphide isomerase
   - Peptidyl-prolyl cis-trans isomerase
   - Calnexin
   - Calreticulin
   - GRP-94 (glucose regulated protein)
   - BiP (Ig heavy chain binding protein)

7. **Ans. (B) HGPRT**

   (A more than C)
   - **Hypergalactosemia is associated with the following 3 enzyme deficiencies:**
     1. Galactokinase converts galactose to galactose-1-phosphate and is not a common deficiency.
     2. Uridine diphosphate (UDP) galactose-4-epimerase epimerizes UDP galactose to UDP glucose and is also uncommon.

3. Galactose-1-phosphate uridyltransferase (GALT) is responsible for hereditary galactosemia and is the most common deficiency. This enzyme catalyzes conversion of galactose-1-phosphate and UDP glucose to UDP galactose and glucose-1-phosphate. Individuals with GALT deficiency manifest abnormal galactose tolerance.

- **Hereditary galactosemia is among the most common carbohydrate metabolism disorders and can be a life-threatening illness during the newborn period.**
- **Parents often complain to physicians about various feeding difficulties with their newborn, most notably, vomiting. Almost all infants on a lactose-containing diet manifest poor weight gain.**
- **Physical Examination:** Untreated infants with severely deficient galactose-1-phosphate uridylyltransferase (GALT) activity typically present with the following variable findings:
  - Poor growth within the first few weeks of life
  - Jaundice
  - Bleeding from coagulopathy
  - Liver dysfunction and/or hepatomegaly
  - Cataracts (sometimes as early as the first few days of life)
  - Lethargy
  - Hypotonia
  - Sepsis (*E. coli*)
  - Seizures
  - Brain edema
- **Surprisingly, ascites may also be detected during early infancy. In some patients, ascites are detected as early as the first few days of life.**
- **In an infant or child with cataracts, galactosemia must be excluded. If unsure, consult an ophthalmologist because some cataracts, especially congenital cataracts, are visible only by using a slit lamp.**
- **Vitreous hemorrhage is a known complication of galactosemia, although its prevalence is unknown. An enigmatic linkage of *E. coli* sepsis with galactosemia is noted. Galactosemia should be high on the differential diagnosis of term infants with sepsis caused by infection with this pathogen.**
- **Learning problems and speech and language deficits are common; language acquisition may be delayed.**
- **The most common findings in adults include hypergonadotropic hypogonadism or primary ovarian**

insufficiency in women, although some women have become pregnant, most notably blacks who probably have variant disease, but also white women with classic galactosemia. Short stature and neurologic abnormalities (e.g. tremor, ataxia, dystonia) also occur in a minority of patients.

8. **Ans. (A) Not required in bacteria**
   (C more than D)

Prokaryotic DNA Replication: Enzymes and their function.	
Enzyme/protein	*Specific function*
DNA pol I	Exonuclease activity removes RNA primer and replaces with newly synthesized DNA
DNA pol II	Repair function
DNA pol III	Main enzyme that adds nucleotides in the 5'-3' direction
Helicase	Opens the DNA helix by breaking hydrogen bonds between the nitrogenous bases
Ligase	Seals the gaps between the Okazaki fragments to create one continuous DNA strand
Primase	Synthesizes RNA primers needed to start replication
Sliding clamp	Helps to hold the DNA polymerase in place when nucleotides are being added
Topoisomerase	Helps relive the stress on DNA when unwinding by causing breaks and then resealing the DNA
Single-stranded binding proteins (SSB)	Binds to single-stranded DNA to avoid DNA rewinding back

9. **Ans. (B) Glutamate and aspartate**
   - Fibrinogen (340 kDa) is a soluble plasma glycoprotein that consists of three nonidentical pairs of polypeptide chains, covalently linked by disulphide bonds.
   - All three chains are synthesized in the liver, three structural genes involved are on the same chromosome, and their expression is coordinately regulated in humans.
   - The amino terminal regions of the six chains are held in close proximity by a number of disulphide bonds, while the carboxy terminal regions are spread apart, giving rise to a highly asymmetric, elongated molecule.

- The A and B portions of the Aα and Bβ chains, designated fibrinopeptides A and B, respectively, at the amino terminal ends of the chains, bear excess negative charges as a result of the presence of aspartate and glutamate residues, as well as unusual tyrosine-O-sulphate in FPB.
- These negative charges contribute to the solubility of fibrinogen in plasma and also serve to prevent aggregation by causing electrostatic repulsion between fibrinogen molecules.

4 Pathology

1. Section of lung showing what?

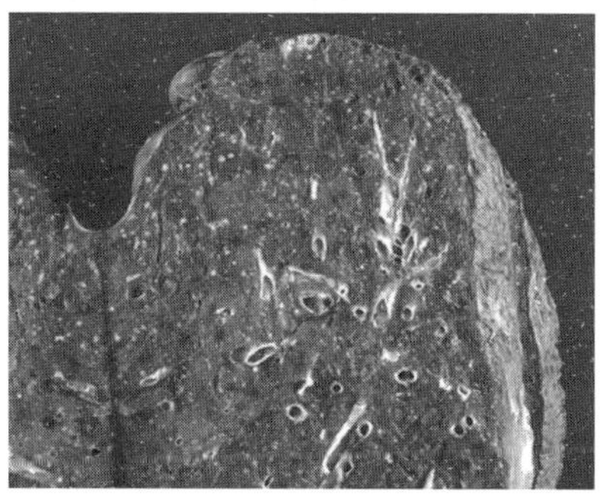

A. Miliary Tb
B. Pneumoconiosis
C. Bronchiectasis
D. Pneumonia

2. A 38-year-old female with neck swelling shown is gross and histology of the tissue, what is the diagnosis?

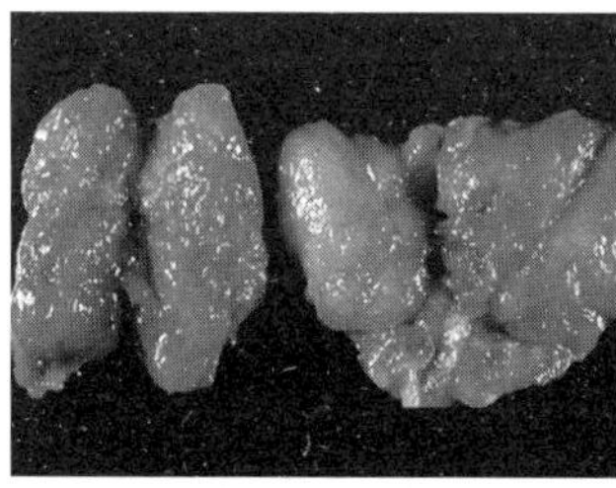

A. NHL
B. MCT
C. Melanoma
D. Hashimoto's thyroiditis

3. CD59 deficiency leads to:

A. Chediak-Higashi syndrome
B. Lysosomal disorders
C. Chronic granulomatous disease
D. Paroxysmal nocturnal hemoglobinuria

4. Which of the following is a epithelial tumor of stomach?

A. Leiomyosarcoma
B. Lymphoma
C. GIST
D. Gastric adenocarcinoma

5. A lady died suddenly with pulmonary thromboembolism. A specimen of liver was given. Most likely finding is:

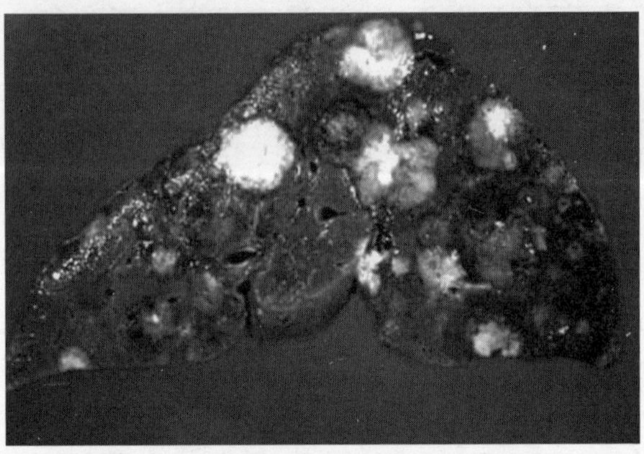

A. Multifocal hepatic adenomas
B. Liver metastasis
C. Invasive angiocarcinoma
D. Metastasis from PE

6. After surgery in Scrotum, tumor specimen obtained is shown below. What is the diagnosis?

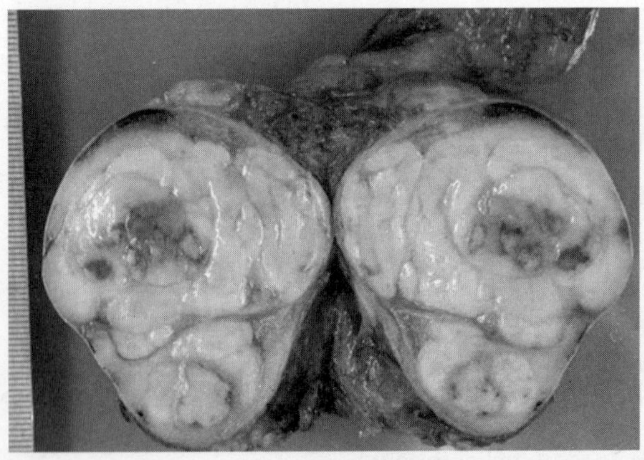

A. Seminoma
B. Teratoma
C. Dysgerminoma
D. Yolk sac tumor

7. Stellate granuloma with necrotic debris with neutrophils is seen in:

A. Crohn's disease
B. Syphilis
C. Sarcoidosis
D. Cat-scratch disease

8. Anaplasia is:

A. Changing one type of epithelium to another
B. Nuclear chromatin changes
C. Lack of differentiation
D. Morphological changes

9. Not commonly seen in anterior mediastinal space is:

A. Thymoma
B. Neural tumors
C. NHL
D. Thyroid carcinoma

10. Hyperacute graft rejection is seen within:

A. 24 hours
B. 2 weeks
C. 1 year
D. In minutes

11. Opsonization is done by:

A. C_{3a}
B. C_{3b}
C. C_{5a}
D. C_{5d}

12. Nude mice can accept xenograft because it lacks which immunal cells?

A. T cells
B. B cells
C. Dendritic cells
D. Memory cells

13. In Alzheimer's what is incorrect?

A. Intracellular neurofibrillary tangles
B. Intracellular neuritic plaques
C. Loss of cholinergic neurons in nucleus basalis of Meynert
D. Loss of recent memory

14. BT is increased in deficiency of:

A. vWF
B. Hemophilia A
C. Hemophilia B
D. HSP

15. Rheumatoid arthritis is associated with all except:

A. Decreased neutrophils
B. Increased macrophages
C. Increased lymphocytes
D. Increased neutrophils

16. DVT is a manifestation of:

A. Hemophilia A
B. Leiden mutation
C. Vitamin K deficiency
D. Chronic liver failure

17. Gene involved in Cowden syndrome is:

A. PTEN
B. Rb
C. P53
D. Ras

18. In 20-year-old girl reddish brown soft to firm nodule seen on the chest not increasing in size, histopathology image is given, what is the diagnosis?

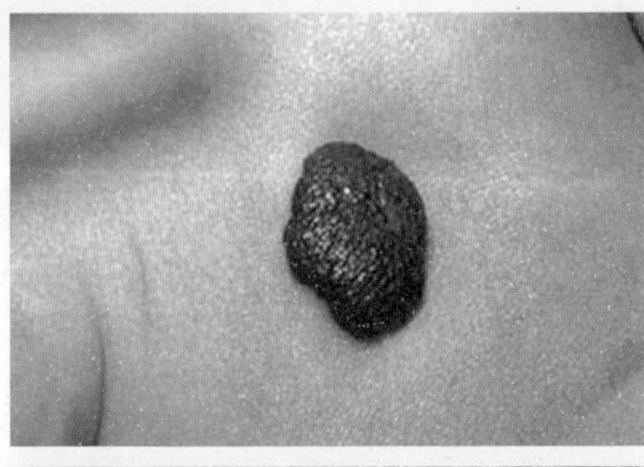

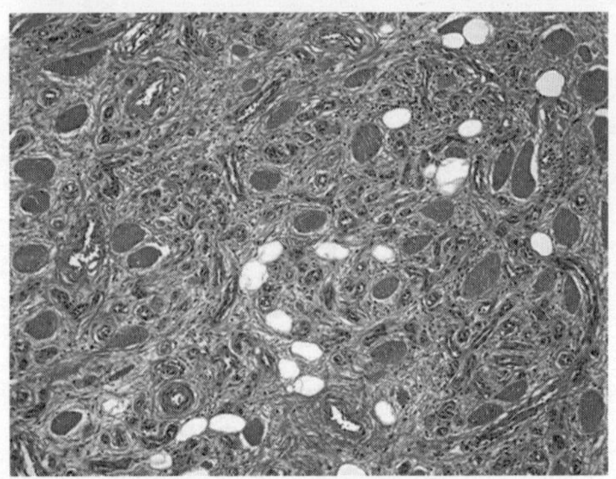

A. Hemangioma
B. Nevus
C. Lipoma
D. Paget's disease

19. Whole blood is used in diagnosis of TB in:

A. Gamma interferon assay
B. Gene expert
C. Bactec test
D. Blood culture

20. Biopsy of small intestine with foamy macrophages are seen. What is the diagnosis?

A. Whipple's disease
B. Abetalipoproteinemia
C. Lysosomal disorder
D. Giardiasis

21. H and L variety of Reed-Sternberg cells are seen in:

A. Lymphocytic predominance
B. Nodular sclerosis
C. Lymphocyte-depleted
D. Mixed cellularity

22. Newly erupted teeth is covered by:

A. Perikymata
B. Nasmyth's membrane
C. Fibrous tissue
D. All of the above

23. Bernard–Soulier syndrome is due to deficiency of:

A. Gp 2b/3a
B. Gp 1b
C. vWF
D. TNF

24. RET proto-oncogene is associated with development of:

A. Medullary carcinoma thyroid
B. Astrocytoma
C. Paraganglioma
D. Hurthle cell tumor thyroid

Answers with Explanations

1. **Ans. (A) Miliary Tb**

   This is a 'miliary pattern' of granulomas because there are a multitude of small tan granulomas about 2 to 4 mm in size, scattered throughout the lung parenchyma. The miliary pattern gets its name from the resemblance of the granulomas to millet seeds.
   - Miliary TB can occur when TB lung lesions erode pulmonary veins or when extrapulmonary TB lesions erode systemic veins.
   - This results in hematogenous dissemination of tubercle bacilli producing myriads of 1–2 mm lesions throughout the body in susceptible hosts.
   - Miliary spread limited to the lungs can occur following erosion of pulmonary arteries by TB lung lesions.

2. **Ans. (D) Hashimoto's thyroiditis**

   Chronic Lymphocytic (Hashimoto) thyroiditis:
   - Hashimoto's thyroiditis is the most common cause of hypothyroidism in areas of the world where iodine levels are sufficient.
   - It is characterized by the gradual thyroid failure secondary to autoimmune destruction of the thyroid gland.
   - It is most prevalent between the ages of 45 and 65 years and is more common in women than in men, with female predominance in a ratio of 10:1 to 20:1.
   - Although it is primarily a disease of older women, it can occur in children and is a major cause of nonendemic goiter in children.

   Pathogenesis
   - It is caused by a breakdown in **self-tolerance** to thyroid autoantigens. Thus, circulating autoantibodies against thyroid antigens are present in the vast majority of patients who demonstrate progressive depletion of thyroid epithelial cells (thyrocytes) and their replacement by mononuclear cell infiltration and fibrosis. The inciting events leading to breakdown in self-tolerance have not been fully elucidated, but multiple immunologic mechanisms that may contribute to thyrocyte damage have been identified including:
     - **CD8+ cytotoxic T cell–mediated cell death:** CD8+ cytotoxic T cells may cause thyrocyte destruction.
     - **Cytokine-mediated cell death:** Excessive T cell activation leads to the production of inflammatory cytokines such as interferon-γ in the thyroid gland with resultant recruitment and activation of macrophages and damage to follicles.

- Binding of **antithyroid antibodies** (antithyroglobulin, and antithyroid peroxidase antibodies) followed by antibody-dependent cell–mediated cytotoxicity.

- A significant genetic component to the disease pathogenesis is supported by the concordance of disease in as many as 40% of monozygotic twins as well as the presence of circulating antithyroid antibodies in approximately 50% of asymptomatic siblings of affected patients. Increased susceptibility to Hashimoto's thyroiditis is associated with polymorphisms in multiple immune regulation–associated genes, the most significant of which is the linkage to **cytotoxic T lymphocyte–associated antigen-4** (CTLA4) gene which codes for a negative regulator of T cell function.

Morphology

- The thyroid usually is diffusely and symmetrically enlarged, although more localized enlargement may be seen in some cases.
- The cut surface is pale and gray-tan in appearance, and the tissue is firm and somewhat friable. Microscopic examination reveals widespread infiltration of the parenchyma by a **mono-nuclear inflammatory infiltrate** containing small lymphocytes, plasma cells, and well-developed **germinal centers**.
- The thyroid follicles are atrophic and are lined in many areas by epithelial cells distinguished by the presence of abundant eosinophilic, granular cytoplasm, termed **Hurthle** or **oxyphil cells.** This is a metaplastic response of the normally low cuboidal follicular epithelium to ongoing injury; on ultrastructural examination, the Hürthle cells are characterized by the numerous prominent mitochondria. Interstitial connective tissue is increased and may be abundant.
- Less commonly, the thyroid is small and atrophic as a result of more extensive fibrosis **(fibrosing variant).** Unlike in Reidel thyroiditis, the fibrosis does not extend beyond the capsule of the gland.

Clinical Features

- It comes to clinical attention as painless enlargement of the thyroid usually associated with some degree of hypothyroidism in a middle-aged woman.
- The enlargement of the gland usually is symmetric and diffuse, but in some cases it may be sufficiently localized to raise suspicion for neoplasm.

- In the usual clinical course, hypothyroidism develops gradually. In some cases, however, it may be preceded by transient thyrotoxicosis caused by disruption of thyroid follicles with secondary release of thyroid hormones (hashitoxicosis). During this phase, free T4 and T3 concentrations are elevated, TSH is diminished, and radioactive iodine uptake is decreased. As hypothyroidism supervenes, T4 and T3 levels progressively fall, accompanied by a compensatory increase in TSH.
- Patients with Hashimoto's thyroiditis often have other autoimmune diseases and are at increased risk for the development of B cell non-Hodgkin lymphomas, which typically arise within the thyroid gland.
- The relationship between Hashimoto disease and thyroid epithelial cancers remains controversial with some morphologic and molecular studies suggesting a predisposition to papillary carcinomas.

3. Ans. (D) Paroxysmal nocturnal hemoglobinuria

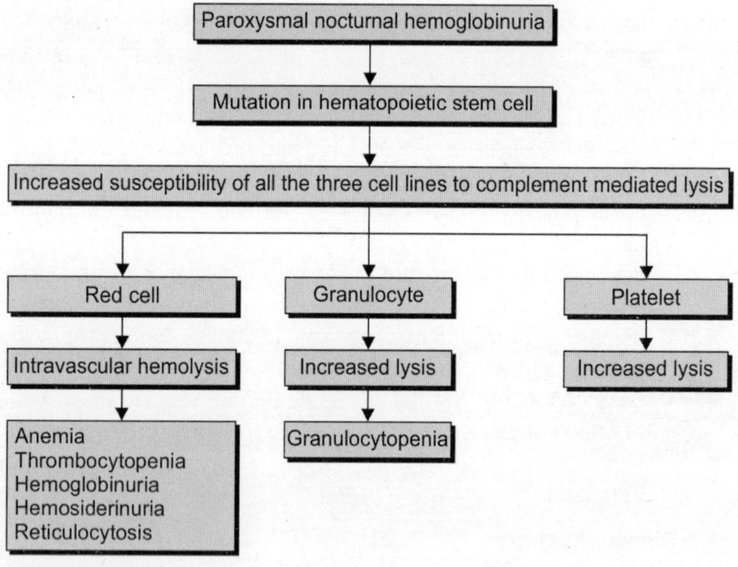

Triad

1. IV hemolysis
2. Pancytopenia
3. Increase risk of venous thrombosis

Pathophysiology

- **PNH** occurs in patients who are unable to bind the regulatory proteins, DAF (CD55), HRF or MIRL (CD59) on their red cell surfaces. Spontaneous complement–mediated lysis of erythrocytes occurs.
- Hemolysis in PNH is due to an intrinsic abnormality of the red cell which makes it exquisitely sensitive to activated complement whether it is activated through the alternative pathway or through an antigen-antibody reaction.
- The former mechanism is mainly responsible for intravascular hemolysis in PNH.
- The latter mechanism explains why the hemolysis can be dramatically exacerbated in the course of a viral or bacterial infection.
- Hypersusceptibility to complement is due to deficiency of several protective membrane proteins, of which CD59 is the most important because it hinders the insertion of C9 polymers into the membrane.
- The molecular basis for the deficiency of these proteins is due to the shortage of a unique glycolipid molecule, GPI, which, through a peptide bond, anchors these proteins to the surface membrane of cells.
- The shortage of GPI is due in turn to a mutation in an X-linked gene called PIG-A required for an early step in GPI biosynthesis.

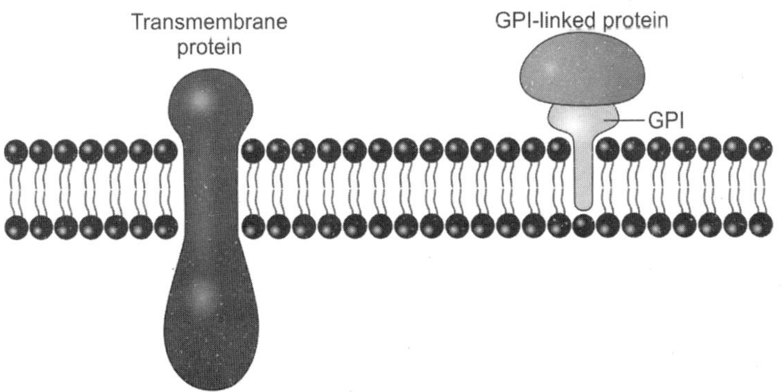

Two kinds of membrane proteins: Transmembrane and glycosylphosphatidylinositol (GPI)-linked. The latter are anchored to cell membranes through a covalent attachment to a glycosylphospatidylinositol moiety. In PNH, GPI cannot be synthesized, leading to a global deficiency of GPI-linked membrane protein.

Clinical Features of PNH

- **Intravascular hemolysis**
  - Most of the clinical features of PNH can be attributed to intravascular hemolysis. The hemolysis is paroxysmal and usually occurs in the night.
  - During sleep at night, we all tend to retain CO_2 leading to mild respiratory acidosis the pH of the blood gets slightly reduced, low pH leads to activation of the complement.
  - Activation of the complement in turn causes intravascular **hemolysis, leukopenia, thrombocytopenia (Pancytopenia)**.
  - This is also the basis for Ham's acidified serum test which is used to diagnose PNH. When the blood is placed in acidic medium, it undergoes hemolysis.
  - Splenomegaly is not a feature.
- **Thrombosis**
  - Platelets are decreased in PNH. But despite the presence of thrombocytopenia, PNH is associated with an increased incidence of thrombosis.
  - **Budd-Chiari syndrome is one** of the common clinical manifestations of thrombosis, it occurs due to hepatic vein thrombosis. Ascites with acute hepatomegaly with pain in abdomen, without previous liver disease.

Diagnosis of PNH Tests

- Ham's test is based upon susceptibility of RBC's to complement mediated lysis in patients with PNH.
- Sucrose lysin test.
- Flow cytometry **is the gold standard in diagnosis. Analysis GPI-linked proteins CD59, DAF.**
- Bone Marrow in PNH
  - Normoblastic hyperplasia is the characteristic finding in PNH (Pancytopenia with normoblastic hypercellular BM).
  - At some stage of disease BM may become hypocellular or **even aplastic** (25% cases – aplastic).
- **Leukocyte alkaline phosphatase in PNH is decreased.**
- **Other:**
  - **Hb↓**
  - **MCV↑**

Complications

- Aplastic anemia can occur
- AML can occur in (10%) cases

Causes of Deaths

- Venous thrombosis (most common cause of death in PNH is cortical vein thrombosis)
- Infection
- Bleeding.

Treatment

- FA, Blood transfusion, BMT.
- **New Drug Eculizumab** is a monoclonal antibody that specifically binds to the complement protein C5, thus inhibiting terminal complement mediated intravascular hemolysis in PNH patients. It is also useful in rheumatoid arthritis and other chronic inflammatory diseases, e.g. nephritis.

4. Ans. (D) Gastric adenocarcinoma

WHO histological classification of gastric tumors:

Intraepithelial neoplasia	*Non-epithelial tumors*
• Adenoma • Carcinoma - Adenocarcinoma - Intestinal type - Diffuse type - Papillary adenocarcinoma - Tubular adenocarcinoma - Mucinous adenocarcinoma potential - Signet-ring cell carcinoma Adenosquamous carcinoma - Squamous cell carcinoma - Small cell carcinoma - Undifferentiated carcinoma - Others • Carcinoid (well differentiated endocrine neoplasm)	• Leiomyoma • Schwannoma • Granular cell tumor • Glomus tumor • Leiomyosarcoma • GI stromal tumor - Benign - Uncertain malignant - Malignant • Kaposi sarcoma • Others • Malignant lymphoma

5. Ans. (D) Metastasis from PE

- A **liver metastasis** is a malignant tumor in the liver that has spread from another organ affected by cancer. The liver is a common site for metastatic disease because of its rich, dual blood supply (the liver receives blood via the hepatic artery and portal vein).
- Metastatic tumors in the liver are 20 times more common than primary tumors. In 50% of all cases the primary tumor is of the gastrointestinal tract, other common sites include the breast, ovaries, bronchus and kidney.

- Tumor emboli entering the sinusoids through the liver blood supply appear to be physically obstructed by the Kupffer cells, but if tumor emboli are larger, they tend to become lodged in the portal venous branches.

Features

- Hepatomegaly - with a nodular free edge of liver
- Tenderness
- Cachexia
- Ascites
- Jaundice
- Pyrexia - up to 10% of patients
- Alkaline Phosphatase (ALP) and gamma-glutamyl transpeptidase (GGT) elevated
- Ultrasound scan and CT scan - multiple filling defects.

Diagnosis

- **Hemoglobin decrease**
- Liver function test: ALP elevated, bilirubin elevated, albumin decrease
- Carcinoembryonic antigen for colorectal secondaries
- Ultrasound scan
- CT scan
- Biopsy under ultrasound control

Treatment

- Treatment consists of surgery (hepatectomy), chemotherapy and/or therapies specifically aimed at the liver like radiofrequency ablation, transcatheter arterial chemoembolization, selective internal radiation therapy and irreversible electroporation.
- For most patients no effective treatment exists because both lobes are usually involved making surgical resection impossible.
- Younger patients with metastases from colorectal cancer confined to one lobe of the liver and up to 4 in number may be treated by partial hepatectomy.
- In selected cases, chemotherapy may be given systemically or via hepatic artery.
- In some tumors, notably those arising from the colon and rectum, apparently solitary metastases or metastases to one or other lobes may be resected.
- A careful search for other metastases is required including local recurrence of the original primary tumor (e.g. via colonoscopy) and dissemination elsewhere (e.g. via CT of the thorax).

- Five year survival rates of 30–40% have been reported following resection.

6. **Ans. (A) Seminoma**

Testicular tumors

- Tumors of the testis are relatively uncommon, although their incidence has increased in recent years.
- They account for less than 1% of all cancer death.
- Testicular tumors are important, however, as many occur in young men and are the most common form of malignancy in males under 35 years.
- Many are highly malignant.

Etiology

- Maldescent of the testis is the only known risk factor for the tumor development.
- An undescended testis is 10 times more likely to develop a tumor than an intrascrotal testis. About 10% of all testicular tumors develop in testes that are, or have been cryptorchid.

Clinical features

Testicular tumors may present with:

- Painless unilateral enlargement of testis
- Secondary hydrocele
- Symptoms from metastases
- Retroperitoneal mass
- Gynecomastia.
- The majority of testicular tumors present as slow, painless enlargement of one testis.
- On examination, there is a smooth or irregular firm enlargement of the testis.
- There may be a loss of testicular sensation on palpation.
- Less often, the patient notices a more rapidly enlarging scrotal swelling due to a secondary hydrocele around the tumor.
- Some of the more malignant tumors may produce symptoms from metastases initially, e.g. hemoptysis from lung deposits, or pain from hepatomegaly.

Classification

- Testicular tumors may be derived from germ cells or non-germ cells; 85–90% are of germ cell origin.
- Germ cell tumors include seminomas, teratomas and their subtypes.
- Non-germ cell tumors include those arising from the Sertoli cells of the seminiferous tubules and the interstitial cells.

The most widely used classification of testicular neoplasms is as follows:

- Seminoma
- Teratoma
- Combined (mixed) germ cell tumor-seminoma and teratoma
- Malignant lymphoma
- Yolk sac tumor
- Interstitial (Leydig) cell tumor
- Sertoli cell tumor
- Metastatic tumors
- Adenomatoid tumor
- Paratesticular sarcoma.

Seminoma

- Most common type of testicular tumor
- Germ cell origin arising in the seminiferous epithelium
- Peak incidence: 30–50 years
- Histological subtypes: Classical-lymphocytic stromal infiltrate; spermatocytic; anaplastic; with syncytiotrophoblast giant cells-contain human chorionic gonadotropin (hCG); combined with other types of tumor
- Five histological subtypes of seminoma are recognized:
  1. Classical
  2. Spermatocytic
  3. Anaplastic
  4. With syncytiotrophoblast giant cells
  5. Combined with other types of germ cell tumor.

Morphology

- The histologic appearances of germ cell tumors may be **pure** (i.e. composed of a single histologic type) or **mixed** (seen in 40% of cases).
- **Seminomas** are soft, well-demarcated, gray-white tumors that bulge from the cut surface of the affected testis.
- Large tumors may contain foci of coagulation necrosis usually without hemorrhage.
- Microscopically, seminomas are composed of **large, uniform cells with distinct cell borders, clear, glycogen-rich cytoplasm, and round nuclei with conspicuous nucleoli.** The cells often are arrayed in small lobules with intervening fibrous septa. A lymphocytic infiltrate usually is present and may, on occasion, overshadow the neoplastic cells.

- Seminomas may also be accompanied by an ill-defined granulomatous reaction. In approximately 15% of cases, syncytiotrophoblasts are present that are the source of the minimally elevated serum hCG concentrations encountered in some males with pure seminoma. Their presence has no bearing on prognosis.

Classical Seminoma

- This is the most common subtype.
- It is composed of uniform cells with well-defined cell borders.
- The cytoplasm is vacuolated and contains glycogen.
- In most of these tumors the stroma contains a variable lymphocytic infiltrate, a favorable prognostic feature.
- Some tumors may have a histiocytic granulomatous response in the stroma with fibrosis which correlates with a better prognosis.

7. **Ans. (D) Cat-scratch disease**
   - **Cat-scratch disease** (**CSD**) is a common and usually benign infectious disease caused by the bacterium *Bartonella-henselae*. It is most commonly found in children following a scratch or bite from a cat within about 1 to 2 weeks.
   - **Signs and symptoms: It commonly presents as tender, swollen lymph nodes near the site of the inoculating bite or scratch or on the neck, and is usually limited to one side (regional lymphadenopathy) and occurs 1–3 weeks after inoculation.**
   - **A vesicle or an erythematous papule may form at the site of initial infection.**
   - **Most patients also develop systemic symptoms such as malaise, decreased appetite, and aches.**
   - **Other associated complaints include headache, chills, muscular pains, joint pains, arthritis, backache, and abdominal pain. It may take 7 to 14 days, or as long as 2 months for symptoms to appear.**
   - **Most cases are benign and self-limiting, but lymphadenopathy may persist for several months after other symptoms disappear.**
   - **The disease usually resolves spontaneously with or without treatment in one month.**
   - In rare situations, CSD can lead to the development of serious neurologic or cardiac sequelae such as meningoencephalitis, encephalopathy, seizures, or endocarditis.

- Endocarditis associated with *Bartonella* infection has a particularly high mortality.
- Parinaud's oculoglandular syndrome is the most common ocular manifestation of CSD, and is a granulomatous conjunctivitis with concurrent swelling of the lymph node near the ear. Optic neuritis or neuroretinitis is one of the atypical presentations.
- Immunocompromised patients are susceptible to other conditions associated with *B. henselae* and *B. quintana*, such as bacillary angiomatosis or bacillary peliosis. Bacillary angiomatosis is primarily a vascular skin lesion that may extend to bone or be present in other areas of the body.
- Bacillary peliosis is caused by *B. henselae* that most often affects patients with HIV and other conditions causing severe immune compromise.
- **Diagnosis:** The Warthin–Starry stain can be helpful to show the presence of *B. henselae*, but is often difficult to interpret. *B. henselae* is difficult to culture and can take 2–6 weeks to incubate. The best diagnostic method currently available is polymerase chain reaction which has a sensitivity of 43–76% and a specificity (in one study) of 100%.
- **Histology**

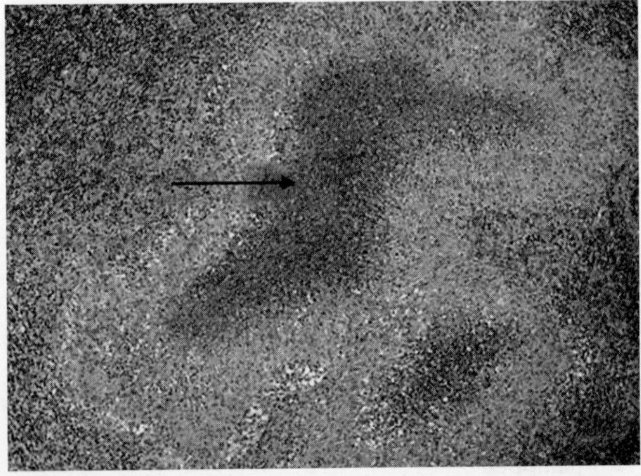

  - High-magnification micrograph of CSD showing a granuloma and a microabscess with neutrophils (H and E stain).
  - It is characterized by granulomatous inflammation on histological examination of the lymph nodes.

- Under the microscope, the skin lesion demonstrates a circumscribed focus of necrosis, surround by histiocytes, often accompanied by multinucleated giant cells, lymphocytes and eosinophils.
- The regional lymph nodes demonstrate follicular hyperplasia with central stellate necrosis with neutrophils, surrounded by palisading histiocytes (suppurative granulomas) and sinuses packed with monocytoid B cells, usually without perifollicular and intrafollicular epithelioid cells.

8. Ans. (C) Lack of differentiation

- Malignant neoplasms that are composed of undifferentiated cells are said to be anaplastic. Lack of differentiation, or anaplasia, is considered a hallmark of malignancy.
- The term anaplasia literally means 'backward formation'—implying dedifferentiation, or loss of the structural and functional differentiation of normal cells. It is now known, however, that at least some cancers arise from stem cells in tissues; in these tumors, failure of differentiation rather than dedifferentiation of specialized cells accounts for their undifferentiated appearance.
- Recent studies also indicate that in some cases, dedifferentiation of apparently mature cells does occur during carcinogenesis.
- Anaplastic cells display marked pleomorphism (i.e. variation In size and shape). Often the nuclei are extremely hyperchromatic (dark-staining) and large resulting in an increased nuclear-to-cytoplasmic ratio that may approach 1:1 instead of the normal 1:4 or 1:6.
- Giant cells that are considerably larger than their neighbors may be formed and possess either one enormous nucleus or several nuclei.
- Anaplastic nuclei are variable and bizarre in size and shape. The chromatin is coarse and clumped, and nucleoli may be of astounding size. More important, mitoses often are numerous and distinctly atypical; anarchic multiple spindles may produce tripolar or quadripolar mitotic figures.
- Also anaplastic cells usually fail to develop recognizable patterns of orientation to one another (i.e. they lose normal polarity). They may grow in sheets with total loss of communal structures such as glands or stratified squamous architecture.

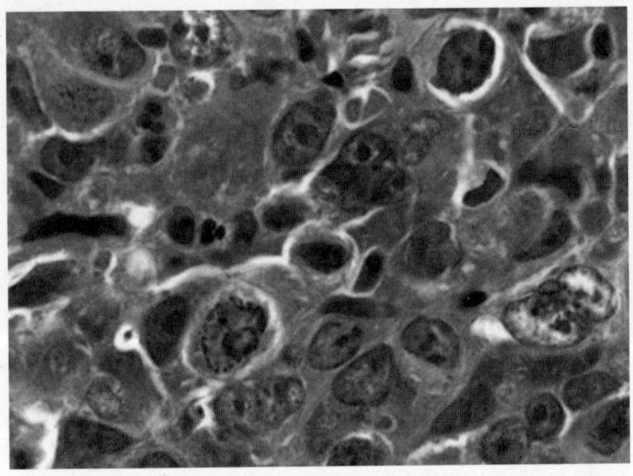

9. **Ans. (B) Neural tumors**

Summary of mediastinal tumors by compartment		
Anterior mediastinum	*Middle mediastinum*	*Posterior mediastinum*
Thymoma	Esophageal tumor	Neurogenic tumors
Thymic carcinoma	Parathyroid adenoma	Neuroendocrine tumors
Thymolipoma	Bronchogenic cyst	
Thymic cyst	Esophageal ductal cyst	
Hodgkins lymphoma	Tracheal tumors	
Non-Hodgkin's lymphoma	Pericardiac cyst	
Germ cell tumors/ teratoma		
Thyroid/substernal goiter		

10. **Ans. (D) In minutes**

- Hyperacute rejection occurs within minutes to a few hours after transplantation in a presensitized host and typically is recognized by the surgeon just after the vascular anastomosis is completed. In contrast with a nonrejecting kidney graft which regains a normal pink color and tissue turgor and promptly excretes urine, a hyperacutely rejecting kidney rapidly becomes cyanotic, mottled, and flaccid and may excrete only a few drops of bloody fluid. The histologic picture is characterized by widespread acute arteritis and arteriolitis, vessel thrombosis, and ischemic necrosis, all resulting from the binding of preformed antibodies to graft endothelium. Virtually all arterioles and arteries exhibit characteristic acute fibrinoid necrosis of their walls with narrowing or complete occlusion of the lumens by precipitated fibrin and cellular debris.

- Acute rejection may occur within days to weeks of transplantation in a nonimmunosuppressed host or may appear months or even years later, even in the presence of adequate immunosuppression. It is caused by both cellular and humoral immune mechanisms, and in any one patient, one or the other may predominate, or both may be present. On histologic examination, cellular rejection is marked by an interstitial mononuclear cell infiltrate with associated edema and parenchymal injury, whereas humoral rejection is associated with vasculitis.
  - **Acute cellular rejection** most commonly is seen within the first month after transplantation and typically is accompanied by clinical signs of renal failure. Histologic examination usually shows extensive interstitial CD4+ and CD8+ T cell infiltration with edema and mild interstitial hemorrhage. Glomerular and peritubular capillaries contain large numbers of mononuclear cells which also may invade the tubules leading to focal tubular necrosis. In addition to tubular injury, CD8+ T cells also may injure the endothelium causing an endothelitis. Cyclosporine (a widely used immunosuppressive agent) is also nephrotoxic and induces so called arteriolar hyaline deposits. Renal biopsy is used to distinguish rejection from drug toxicity. Accurate recognition of cellular rejection is important because patients typically respond promptly to increased immunosuppressive therapy.
  - **Acute humoral rejection** (rejection vasculitis) caused by antidonor antibodies also may participate in acute graft rejection. The histologic lesions may take the form of necrotizing vasculitis with endothelial cell necrosis; neutrophilic infiltration; deposition of antibody, complement, and fibrin; and thrombosis. Such lesions may be associated with ischemic necrosis of the renal parenchyma. Somewhat older subacute lesions are characterized by marked thickening of the intima by proliferating fibroblasts, myocytes, and foamy macrophages. The resultant narrowing of the arterioles may

cause infarction or renal cortical atrophy. The proliferative vascular lesions mimic arteriosclerotic thickening and are believed to be caused by cytokines that stimulate proliferation of vascular smooth muscle cells. Local deposition of complement breakdown products (specifically C4d) is used to detect antibody-mediated rejection of kidney allografts.

- **Chronic rejection:** Patients present with chronic rejection late after transplantation (months to years) with a progressive rise in serum creatinine levels (an index of renal function) over a period of 4 to 6 months. Chronic rejection is dominated by vascular changes, interstitial fibrosis, and loss of renal parenchyma; there are typically only mild or no ongoing cellular parenchymal infiltrates. The vascular changes occur predominantly in the arteries and arterioles which exhibit intimal smooth muscle cell proliferation and extracellular matrix synthesis. These lesions ultimately compromise vascular perfusion and result in renal ischemia manifested by the loss or hyalinization of glomeruli, interstitial fibrosis, and tubular atrophy. The vascular lesion may be caused by cytokines released by activated T cells that act on the cells of the vascular wall, and it may be the end stage of the proliferative arteritis.

11. Ans. (B) C_{3b}

- Opsonization involves the binding of an opsonin, e.g. antibody, to an epitope on an antigen. After opsonin binds to the membrane, phagocytes are attracted to the pathogen.
- The Fab portion of the antibody binds to the antigen, whereas the Fc portion of the antibody binds to an Fc receptor on the phagocyte, facilitating phagocytosis.
- The core receptor + opsonin complex also creates byproducts like C3b and C4b which are important components for the efficient function of the complement system. These components are deposited on the cell surface of the pathogen and aid in its destruction.
- The cell can also be destroyed by a process called antiphagocytic cell-mediated cytotoxicity in which the pathogen does not need to be phagocytosed to be destroyed. During this process, the pathogen is opsonized and bound with the antibody IgG via its Fab domain. This allows the antibody binding of an immune effector cell via its Fc domain.
- Antibody-dependent cell-mediated inherent mediation then triggers a release of lysis products from the bound immune effector cell (monocytes, neutrophils, eosinophils and NK cells).

Lack of mediation can cause inflammation of surrounding tissues and damage to healthy cells.

12. Ans. (A) T cells

Transplants (Allografts)

- The graft rejection response is initiated mainly by host T cells that recognize the foreign HLA antigens of the graft, either directly (on APCs in the graft) or indirectly (after uptake and presentation by host APCs).
- Types and mechanisms of rejection comprise the following:
  - **Hyperacute rejection:** Pre-formed antidonor antibodies bind to graft endothelium immediately after transplantation, leading to thrombosis, ischemic damage, and rapid graft failure.
  - **Acute cellular rejection:** T cells destroy graft parenchyma (and vessels) by cytotoxicity and inflammatory reactions.
  - **Acute humoral rejection:** Antibodies damage graft vasculature.
  - **Chronic rejection:** Dominated by arteriosclerosis, this type is probably caused by T cell reaction and secretion of cytokines that induce proliferation of vascular smooth muscle cells associated with parenchymal fibrosis.

13. Ans. (D) Loss of recent memory

Alzheimer disease (AD) is the most common cause of dementia in the elderly population.

- The disease usually manifests with the insidious onset of impaired higher intellectual function and altered mood and behavior.
- Later, this progresses to disorientation, memory loss and aphasia, findings indicative of severe cortical dysfunction and over another 5 to 10 years, the patient becomes profoundly disabled, mute and immobile.
- Death usually occurs from intercurrent pneumonia or other infections.
- Age is an important risk factor for AD; the incidence is about 3% in persons 65 to 74 years old, 19% in those 75 to 84 years old, and 47% in those older than 84 years.
- Most cases of AD are sporadic, but at least 5% to 10% are familial. Sporadic cases rarely present before 50 years of age, but early onset is seen with some heritable forms.

Pathogenesis

Study of the familial forms of AD supports a model in which a peptide called beta amyloid, or Aβ accumulates in the brain over time initiating a chain of events that result in AD.

- Aβ is created when the transmembrane protein amyloid precursor protein (APP) is sequentially cleaved by the enzymes β-amyloid converting enzyme (BACE) and γ-secretase .
- APP also can be cleaved by α-secretase and γ-secretase, which liberates a different peptide that is nonpathogenic. Mutations in APP or in components of γ-secretase (presenilin-1 or presenilin-2) lead to familial AD by increasing the rate at which Aβ is generated.
- The APP gene is located on chromosome 21, and the risk of AD is also higher in those with an extra copy of the APP gene, such as patients with trisomy 21 (Down syndrome) and persons with small interstitial duplications of APP, presumably because this too leads to greater Aβ generation.
- The other major genetic risk factor is a variant of apolipoprotein E called ε4 (ApoE4). Each ApoE4 allele that is present increases the risk of AD by approximately 4 fold and also appears to lower the age of onset. How ApoE4 influences Aβ accumulation is unknown; it may increase Aβ aggregation or deposition, or decrease Aβ clearance.
- While large deposits of Aβ are a feature of end-stage AD,small aggregates of Aβ may also be pathogenic, as they alter neurotransmission and are toxic to neurons and synaptic endings. Large deposits in the form of plaques also lead to neuronal death, elicit a local inflammatory response that can result in further cell injury, and may cause altered region-to region communication through mechanical effects on axons and dendrites.
- The presence of Aβ also leads to hyperphosphorylation of the neuronal microtubule binding protein tau. This increased level of phosphorylation causes tau to redistribute from axons into dendrites and cell bodies, where it aggregates into tangles which also contribute to neuronal dysfunction and cell death.

Morphology

Macroscopic examination of the brain shows a variable degree of cortical atrophy resulting in a widening of the cerebral sulci that is most pronounced in the frontal, temporal, and parietal lobes. With significant atrophy, there is compensatory ventricular enlargement (hydrocephalus ex vacuo).

- At the microscopic level, AD is diagnosed by the presence of **plaques** (an extracellular lesion); and **neurofibrillary tangles** (an intracellular lesion). Because these may also be present to a lesser extent in the brains of elderly nondemented persons, the current criteria for a diagnosis of AD are based on a combination of clinical and pathologic features.
- There is a fairly constant progressive involvement of different parts of the brain: Pathologic changes (specifically plaques, tangles, and the associated neuronal loss and glial reaction) are first evident in the entorhinal cortex, then in the hippocampal formation and isocortex, and finally in the neocortex. Silver staining or immunohistochemistry methods are extremely helpful in assessing the true lesional burden.
- **Neuritic plaques** are focal, spherical collections of dilated, tortuous, silver-staining neuritic processes (dystrophic neurites), often around a central amyloid core.
- Neuritic plaques range in size from 20 to 200 μm in diameter; microglial cells and reactive astrocytes are present at their periphery. Plaques can be found in the hippocampus and amygdala as well as in the neocortex, although there usually is relative sparing of primary motor and sensory cortices until late in the disease course.
- The amyloid core contains Aβ. Aβ deposits can also be found that lack the surrounding neuritic reaction, termed **diffuse plaques**; these typically are found in the superficial cerebral cortex, the basal ganglia, and the cerebellar cortex and may represent an early stage of plaque development.
- A major component of paired helical filaments is abnormally hyperphosphorylated **tau**. Tangles are not specific to AD, being found in other degenerative diseases as well.

14. Ans. (A) vWF

von Willebrand's disease

- von Willebrand's disease (vWD) is a common hereditary bleeding disorder.
- It is characterized by a prolonged BT and reduced factor VIII – C levels between about 10–40%.
- Joint bleeding is rare.
- The gene for von Willebrand factor (vWF) is located on chromosome 12 and is inherited as an autosomal disorder.
- Type I, II and IIB are autosomal dominant type. IIC and III are autosomal recessive. (Autosomal hemophilia–New Name)

- **Clinical features:** Superficial bruising, epistaxis, menorrhagia and GI bleeding are common especially after trauma or surgery.
- The diagnostic pattern consist of:
  - Prolonged bleeding time and prolonged clotting time.
  - Reduced plasma vWF concentrations
  - Reduction in **biological activity as measured by ristocetin cofactor assay (P) aggregation in response to ristocetin is ↓**
  - Reduced factor VIII activity.
  - **Von Willebrand's Disease PT is normal but PTT is prolonged.**
- **Management**
  - Desmopressin.
  - Factor VIII—C concentrates (contain adequate vWF also)
  - Cryoprecipitate: It contains all of the vWF multimers. It is the safest and most cost–effective modality of treatment.
  - Platelet transfusions for cases with uncontrolled bleeding.
  - Fresh frozen plasma (FFP) can be given for mild disease.

Property	*VWF*	*Factor VIII*
Gene	Located on chromosome XII	Located on X chromosome
Inheritance	Autosomal dominant	Sex linked
Synthesis	Endothelial cells, megakaryocytes platelets (not in liver cells)	In liver cells
Function	Facilitate the adhesion of platelets to subendothelial collagen	Activation of factor X in coagulation cascade
Disease	vWD	Hemophilia

Features of vWF and differences with hemophilia A

Feature	*Hemophilia A*	*Von Willebrand disease*
Inheritance	X-linked recessive	Autosomal dominant
Factor VIIIc	Decreased	Normal
VWF	Normal	Decreased
Common presentation	Features of clotting disorder	Features of bleeding disorder ± clotting disorder
	Skin/Mucosal bleeding -	Skin/Mucosal bleeding +
	Hemarthrosis ++	Hemarthrosis+

Contd...

Contd...

Feature	*Hemophilia A*	*Von Willebrand disease*
Bleeding Time	Normal	Prolonged
APTT	Prolonged	Prolonged (may be normal)
PT	Normal	Normal
Thrombin time	Normal	Normal
Fibrinogen	Normal	Normal
Platelet aggregation in response to Ristocetin	Normal	Decreased

15. Ans. (D) Increased neutrophils

Clinical examples of leukocyte-induced injury	
Disorder	*Cells and molecules involved in injury*
Acute	
Acute respiratory distress syndrome	Neutrophils
Acute transplant rejection	Lymphocytes; antibodies and complement
Asthma	Eosinophils; IgE antibodies
Glomerulonephritis	Antibodies and complement: Neutrophils, monocytes
Septic shock	Cytokines
Chronic	
Rheumatoid arthritis	Lymphocytes, macrophages; antibodies
Asthma	Eosinophils; IgE antibodies
Atherosclerosis	Macrophages; lymphocytes
Chronic transplant rejection	Lymphocytes, macrophages: Cytokines
Pulmonary fibrosis	Macrophages; fibroblasts

16. Ans. (B) Leiden mutation

Primary (inherited) hypercoagulability most often is caused by mutations in the factor V and prothrombin genes:

- Approximately 2 to 15% of whites carry a specific factor V mutation (called the Leiden mutation, after the Dutch city where it was first described).The mutation alters an amino acid residue in factor V and renders it resistant to protein C. Thus, an important antithrombotic counter-regulatory mechanism is lost.

Heterozygotes carry a 5-fold increased risk for venous thrombosis, while homozygotes having a 50-fold increased risk.

- A single-nucleotide substitution (G to A) in the 3′-untranslated region of the prothrombin gene is a fairly common allele (found in 1 to 2% of the general population). This variant results in increased prothrombin transcription and is associated with a nearly three-fold increased risk for venous thromboses.
- Less common primary hypercoagulable states include inherited deficiencies of anticoagulants such as antithrombin III, protein C, or protein S; affected patients typically present with venous thrombosis and recurrent thromboembolism in adolescence or early adult life. Congenitally elevated levels of homocysteine contribute to arterial and venous thromboses (and indeed to the development of atherosclerosis).

17. Ans. (A) PTEN

Syndrome	*Mean age at presentation (years)*	*Mutated gene(s)*	*GI lesions*	*Selected extragastrointestinal manifestations*
Peutz-Jeghers syndrome	10–15	LKB1/ STK11	Arborizing polyps-small intestine > colon > stomach; colonic adenocarcinoma	Mucocutaneous pigmentation; increased risk of thyroid, breast, lung, pancreas, gonadal and bladder cancers
Juvenile polyposis	< 5	SMAD4, BMPR1A	Juvenile polyps; increased risk of gastric, small intestinal, colonic and pancreatic adenocarcinoma	Pulmonary arteriovenous malformations, digital clubbing
Cowden syndrome, Bannayan-Riley-Ruvalcaba syndrome	< 15	PTEN	Hamartomatous polyps, lipomas, ganglioneuromas, inflammatory polyps; increased risk of colon cancer	Benign skin tumors, benign and malignant thyroid and breast lesions

Contd...

Contd...

Syndrome	*Mean age at presentation (years)*	*Mutated gene(s)*	*GI lesions*	*Selected extragastrointestinal manifestations*
Cronkhite-Canada syndrome	> 50	Non-hereditary	Hamartomatous colon polyps, crypt dilatation and edema in nonpolypoid mucosa	Nail atrophy, hair loss, abnormal skin pigmentation, cachexia, anemia
Tuberous sclerosis	Infancy to adulthood	TSC1, TSC2	Hamartomatous polyps (rectal)	Facial angiofibroma, cortical tubers, renal angiomyolipoma
Familial adenomatous polyposis (FAP)				
Classic FAP	10–15	APC, MUTYH	Multiple adenomas	Congenital RPE hypertrophy
Attenuated FAP	40–50	APC, MUTYH	Multiple adenomas	
Gardner syndrome	10–15	APC, MUTYH	Multiple adenomas	Osteomas, desmoids, skin cysts
Turcot syndrome	10–15	APC, MUTYH	Multiple adenomas	CNS tumors, medulloblastoma

18. Ans. (A) Hemangioma

- Hemangiomas are the most common tumors of infancy. Both cavernous and capillary hemangiomas may be encountered, although the latter often are more cellular than in adults and thus may be deceptively worrisome-appearing.
  - In children, most hemangiomas are located in the skin, particularly on the face and scalp where they produce flat to elevated, irregular, red-blue masses; the flat, larger lesions are referred to as port wine stains. They may enlarge as the child gets older, but in many instances they spontaneously regress.
  - The vast majority of superficial hemangiomas have no more than a cosmetic significance; rarely, they may be the manifestation of a hereditary disorder associated with disease

within internal organs, such as the von Hippel-Lindau and Sturge-Weber syndromes.

- A subset of CNS cavernous hemangiomas can occur in the familial setting; affected families harbor mutations in one of three cerebral cavernous malformation (CCM) genes.

19. Ans. (A) Gamma interferon assay

Tuberculosis: It is the classic granulomatous infection. The disease is divided into primary and secondary (or reactivation) tuberculosis.

- **Primary tuberculosis:** The disease is acquired from the initial exposure to *M. tuberculosis*, most commonly as a result of inhaling infected aerosols generated when a person with cavitary tuberculosis coughs.

  Pathology

  - The Ghon complex is the first lesion of primary tuberculosis and consists of a peripheral parenchymal granuloma, often in the upper lobes.
  - When it is associated with an enlarged mediastinal lymph node a Ranke complex is formed.
  - Microscopically, a granuloma with central caseous necrosis shows varying degrees of fibrosis.
    - Apical scarring with the appearance of a fibronodular patch or ill-defined reticular shadow in the upper lung fields on chest X-ray is known as '**Simon's focus**'.
    - **Purl's lesion:** Lesion at **the apex of lung in chronic cases.**
    - **Assmann's focus**: Typically apical (site of highest oxygen tension)
    - **TB Simon's focus:** Early hematogenous seedling in apex of lungs.
    - **Ghon's complex:** Parenchymal subpleural lesion + draining lymphatics + enlarged caseous lymph nodes in primary tuberculosis
    - **Ranke complex:** Healed lesions in lung parenchyma and hilar lymph nodes undergoing calcification due to TB
    - **Rich focus:** Tuberculous caseous foci in brain, meninges and spinal cord.
- **Secondary tuberculosis:** This stage represents either reactivation of primary pulmonary tuberculosis or a new infection in a host previously sensitized by primary tuberculosis.

Pathology

- A cellular immune response occurs after a latent interval and leads to formation of many granulomas and extensive tissue necrosis.
- The apical and posterior segments of the upper lobes are most commonly involved.
- A diffuse, fibrotic, poorly defined lesion develops. Some erode into a bronchus creates a tuberculous cavity.
- Tuberculous cavities range in size from under 1 cm in diameter to large cystic areas.
- The tuberculous cavity often communicates freely with a bronchus, and spreads the infection within the lung.

Secondary tuberculosis is associated with a number of complications:

- Miliary tuberculosis refers to the presence of multiple, small (size of millet seeds), tuberculous granulomas in many organs.
- Hemoptysis
- Bronchopleural fistula occurs when a subpleural cavity ruptures into the pleural space. In turn, tuberculous empyema and pneumothorax result.
- Tuberculous laryngitis
- Intestinal tuberculosis.

Testing for Latent Tuberculosis Infection

- The goal of testing for LTBI is to identify individuals who are at increased risk for the development of active TB; these individuals would benefit most from treatment of LTBI (also termed preventive therapy or prophylaxis). Thus, only those who would benefit from treatment should be tested; a decision to test should presuppose a decision to treat if the test is positive.
- In general, testing for LTBI is indicated when the risk of development of disease from latent infection (if present) is increased; examples include likely recent infection (e.g. close contact of a person with TB) or a decreased capacity to contain latent infection (e.g. because of immunosuppression, as in the case of young children in contact with those with active TB, people living with human immunodeficiency virus (HIV) infection, or otherwise immunosuppressed persons because of medications or conditions such as uncontrolled diabetes).
- In contrast, screening for LTBI in persons or groups who are healthy and have a low risk of progressing to active disease is not appropriate, since the positive predictive value of LTBI

testing is low and the risks of treatment can outweigh the potential benefits. The balance of risk and benefit is also different in high-burden settings, where the risk of reinfection may be high and screening for LTBI will have a low negative predictive value. For children, the risk-to-benefit ratio is more favorable than for adults.

- There is no diagnostic gold standard for LTBI, and all existing tests are indirect approaches which provide immunological evidence of host sensitization to TB antigens. There are two accepted but imperfect tests for identification of LTBI: The tuberculin skin test (TST) and the interferon-gamma (IFNγ) release assay (IGRA). Both tests depend on cell-mediated immunity (memory T-cell response) and neither test can accurately distinguish between LTBI and active TB disease.

IGRA: Assay principles

- IGRAs are in vitro blood tests of cell-mediated immune response; they measure T-cell release of IFN-γ following stimulation by antigens specific to the *M. tuberculosis* complex (with the exception of BCG substrains), i.e. early secreted antigenic target 6 (ESAT-6) and culture filtrate protein 10 (CFP-10). These antigens are encoded by genes located within the region of difference 1 (RD1) locus of the *M. tuberculosis* genome. They are more specific than PPD for *M. tuberculosis* because they are not encoded in the genomes of any BCG vaccine strains or most species of NTM, other than *M. marinum, M. kansasii, M. szulgai, and M. flavescens*. However, not all NTMs have been studied for cross-reactivity. There is some evidence of cross-reactivity between ESAT-6 and CFP-10 of *M. tuberculosis* and *M. leprae*, but the clinical significance of this in settings where leprosy and TB are endemic (e.g. India and Brazil) is poorly characterized.
- Two commercial IGRA are available in many countries: the QuantiFERON-TB Gold in tube (QFT) assay (Cellestis/Qiagen, Carnegie, Australia) and the T-SPOT.TB assay (Oxford Immunotec, Abingdon, UK). Both tests are approved by the US food and drug administration (FDA) and Health Canada and are Conformité Européenne (CE) marked for use in Europe.
- The QFT assay is an enzyme-linked immunosorbent assay (ELISA)-based, whole-blood test that uses peptides from the RD1 antigens ESAT-6 and CFP-10 as well as peptides from one additional antigen (TB7.7 [Rv2654c] which is not an RD1 antigen) in an in-tube format. The result is reported as quantification

of IFN-γ in international units (IU) per milliliter. An individual is considered positive for *M. tuberculosis* infection if the IFN-γ response to TB antigens is above the test cutoff (after subtracting the background IFN-γ response of the negative control).

- The T-SPOT. TB assay is an enzyme-linked immunosorbent spot (ELISPOT) assay performed on separated and counted peripheral blood mononuclear cells (PBMCs) that are incubated with ESAT-6 and CFP-10 peptides. The result is reported as the number of IFN-γ-producing T cells (spot-forming cells). An individual is considered positive for *M. tuberculosis* infection if the spot counts in the TB antigen wells exceed a specific threshold relative to the negative control wells. Indeterminate IGRA results can occur due to a low IFN-γ response to the positive (mitogen) control or a high background response to the negative control.

20. Ans. (a) Whipple's disease

Microscopic (histologic) appearance in Whipple's disease

- Noncaseating granulomas
- Numerous foamy macrophages in lamina propria containing PAS+ (diastase resistant) granules and rod shaped bacilli by EM
- Dilated lymphatics or fat vacuoles
- Often multinucleated giant cells; rarely epithelioid granulomas in minority
- In mesentery or retroperitoneal nodes, resembles lipogranulomatous inflammation with round empty spaces.

21. Ans. (A) Lymphocytic predominance

Nodular Lymphocyte-Predominant Hodgkin lymphoma

- This subtype accounting for about 5% of Hodgkin lymphoma is characterized by the presence of lymphocytic and histiocytic (L&H) variant RS cells that have a delicate multilobed, puffy nucleus resembling popped corn ('popcorn cell').
- L&H variants usually are found within large nodules containing mainly small resting B cells admixed with a variable number of macrophages. Other types of reactive cells such as eosinophils, neutrophils, and plasma cells are scanty or absent and typical RS cells are rare.
- Unlike the Reed-Sternberg variants in 'classical' forms of Hodgkin lymphoma, L&H variants express B cell markers (e.g. CD20) and usually fail to express CD15 and CD30. Most patients with this subtype present with isolated cervical or axillary lymphadenopathy and the prognosis typically is excellent.

22. Ans. (B) Nasmyth's membrane

- Primary enamel cuticle also called Nasmyth's membrane is thin membrane of tissue also known as reduced enamel epithelium (REE) produced by the ameloblast that covers the tooth once it has erupted.
- This tissue is primarily basal lamina.
- It is usually worn away by mastication and cleaning.
- It protects enamel from resorption by cells of the dental sac and also secretes desmolytic enzymes for the elimination of the dental sac allowing fusion between reduced enamel epithelium and oral epithelium.
- This process allows eruption of the tooth without bleeding.

23. Ans. (B) Gp 1b

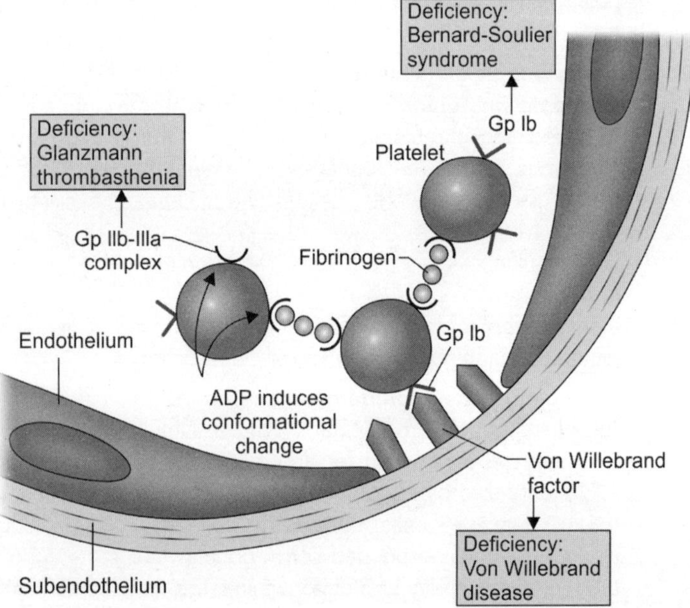

Fig.: Platelet adhesion and aggregation. Von willebrand factor functions as an adhesion bridge between subendothelial collagen and the glycoprotein Ib (Gp Ib) platelet receptor. Platelet aggregation is accomplished by fibrinogen binding to platelet Gp IIb-IIIa receptors on different platelets. Congenital deficiencies in the various receptors or bridging molecules lead to the diseases indicated in the colored boxes. (ADP, adenosine disphosphate).

24. Ans. (A) Medullary carcinoma thyroid

- Medullary thyroid carcinomas: In contrast with the other subtypes of thyroid carcinomas, these neoplasms arise from the parafollicular C cells rather than the follicular epithelium.
- Familial medullary thyroid carcinomas occur in multiple endocrine neoplasia type 2 (MEN-2) and are associated with germline RET proto-oncogene mutations that lead to constitutive activation of the receptor.
- RET mutations are also seen in approximately one half of nonfamilial (sporadic) medullary thyroid cancers.
- Chromosomal rearrangements involving RET such as the RET/PTC translocations reported in papillary cancers are not seen in medullary carcinomas.

5 Pharmacology

1. Amphotericin B acts on:

A. Cell wall
B. Cell membrane
C. Ribosome
D. mRNA

2. Alternative to epinephrine for pulseless arrest according to advanced cardiac life support is which drug?

A. Vasopressin
B. Amiodarone
C. Low dose dopamine
D. Low dose atropine

3. Anaerobic bacteria are intrinsically resistant to:

A. Beta lactam antibiotics
B. Aminoglycosides
C. Metronidazole
D. Meropenem

4. Niacin is given caustiously in insulin resistant diabetic patients because:

A. It hinders metabolism of diabetic drugs
B. It causes scleroderma hindering administration of insulin
C. It causes hyperglycemia
D. It causes insulin resistance

5. Sacubitril is a:

A. Renin antagonist
B. Neprilysin inhibitor
C. Neuropeptidase inhibitor
D. ACE inhibitor

6. Antihypertensive contraindicated in PIH:

A. Alpha methyldopa
B. Labetalol
C. Hydralazine
D. Atenolol

7. Tadalafil should not be given with:

A. Vasodilators
B. Antibiotics
C. Vasoconstrictors
D. Valproate

8. Which of these need regular monitoring?

A. Enoxaparin
B. Lepirudin
C. Dabigatran
D. Fondaparinux

9. Apixaban's mechanism of action is?

A. Xa inhibitor
B. Antithrombin
C. V inhibitor
D. Thrombin inhibitor

10. Mechanism of action of Colchicine used in acute gout is:

A. Mobilization of uric acid
B. Inhibit migration of lymphocytes
C. Increase in lymphocytes
D. Affects purine metabolic pathway

11. Which of the following prolong Q-T interval?

A. Quinidine
B. Lignocaine
C. Ciprofloxacin
D. Propranolol

12. pKa is the pH at which?

A. 10 percent of the drug is ionized and 90 percent is nonionized
B. 50 percent of the drug is ionized and 50 percent is nonionized
C. 90 percent of the drug is ionized and 10 percent is nonionized
D. 100 percent of the drug is ionized

13. Mechanism of action of curare like drugs is?

A. Persistently depolarizing at neuromuscular junction
B. Act competitively on Ach receptors blocking post-synaptically
C. Repetitive stimulation of Ach receptors on muscle end plate
D. Inhibiting the calcium channel on presynaptic membrane

14. Centrally acting muscle relaxant with alpha 2 adrenergic agonist activity is?

A. Chlorzoxazone
B. Baclofen
C. Tizanidine
D. Pirenzepine

15. Which of the following drug is a corticosteroid inhibitor?

A. Metyrapone
B. Finasteride
C. Flutamide
D. Mifepristone

16. All of the following drugs are bacteriostatic except?

A. Vancomycin
B. Clindamycin
C. Tetracycline
D. Linezolid

17. Which of the following statements about prasugrel is true as compared to clopidogrel?

A. It is slower acting than clopidogrel
B. It is contraindicated in stroke
C. It is a reversible antagonist of ADP receptors
D. Decrease the risk of bleeding

18. Serotonin is chemically?

A. 5-hydroxytryptamine
B. 5-hydroxyphenethylamine
C. N-methyl-N-phenylamine
D. 3-Methoxytyramine

19. Physiological dose of hydrocortisone (mg/kg/day) is:

A. 5 mg/kg/day
B. 10 mg/kg/day
C. 15 mg/kg/day
D. 20 mg/kg/day

20. Pirenzepine is used for:

A. Gastric ulcer
B. Glaucoma
C. Hypertension
D. Congestive cardiac failure

21. Which of the following causes melanosis coli?

A. Senna
B. Sorbitol
C. Magnesium sulphate
D. Bisacodyl

22. Which among the following will be the choice of antibiotic for a bedridden patient with catheter-related UTI and pneumonia?

A. Amoxicillin
B. Beta-lactam antibiotics with beta-lactamase
C. 3rd generation cephalosporins
D. 2nd generation cephalosporins

23. Nitric oxide acts by increasing?

A. BRCA 1
B. cAMP
C. Interleukin
D. cGMP

Answers with Explanations

1. **Ans. (B) Cell membrane**

   Mechanism of action of different drugs:
   - **Inhibit cell wall synthesis:** Penicillins, cephalosporins, cycloserine, vancomycin, bacitracin.
   - **Cause leakage from cell membranes:** Polypeptides—polymyxins, colistin, bacitracin. Polyenes amphotericin B, nystatin, hamycin.
   - **Inhibit protein synthesis:** Tetracyclines, chloramphenicol, erythromycin, clindamycin, linezolid.
   - **Cause misreading of m-RNA code and affect permeability:** Aminoglycosides—streptomycin, gentamicin, etc.
   - **Inhibit DNA gyrase:** Fluoroquinolones—ciprofloxacin and others.
   - **Interfere with DNA function:** Rifampin.
   - **Interfere with DNA synthesis:** Acyclovir, zidovudine.
   - **Interfere with intermediary metabolism:** Sulfonamides, sulfones, PAS, trimethoprim, pyrimethamine, metronidazole.

2. **Ans. (A) Vasopressin**

   An individual who collapses suddenly is managed in five stages:
   1. Initial evaluation and basic life support if cardiac arrest is confirmed
   2. Public access defibrillation (when available)
   3. Advanced life support
   4. Post-resuscitation care
   5. Long-term management.

   The initial response, including confirmation of loss of circulation, followed by basic life support and public access defibrillation, can be carried out by physicians, nurses, paramedical personnel and trained lay persons.
   - **Vasopressin** (antidiuretic hormone or ADH) is often used as an adjunctive therapy to catecholamine vasopressors in the treatment of **distributive or vasodilatory shock**. It causes peripheral vasoconstriction via V1 receptors located in smooth muscle cells and attenuation of nitric oxide (NO) synthesis and GMP, the second messenger of NO. The rationale for using low dose vasopressin in the management of septic shock includes the relative deficiency of vasopressin in late shock. It also potentiates the effects of catecholamines in the vascu-

Ventricular fibrillation or pulseless ventricular tachycardia

Immediate defibrillation within 5 minutes of onset; 60–90 seconds of CPR before defibrillation for delay ≥ 5 minutes

↓ **If return of circulation fails**

2 Minutes of chest compressions at >100/min followed by repeat shock; repeat sequence twice if needed

↓ **If return of circulation fails**

Continue chest compressions, intubate, IV access

↓

Epinephrine, 1 mg IV - or - vasopressin, 40 units IV; follow with repeat defibrillation at maximum energy within 30–60 seconds as required; repeat epinephrine

↓ **If return of circulation fails**

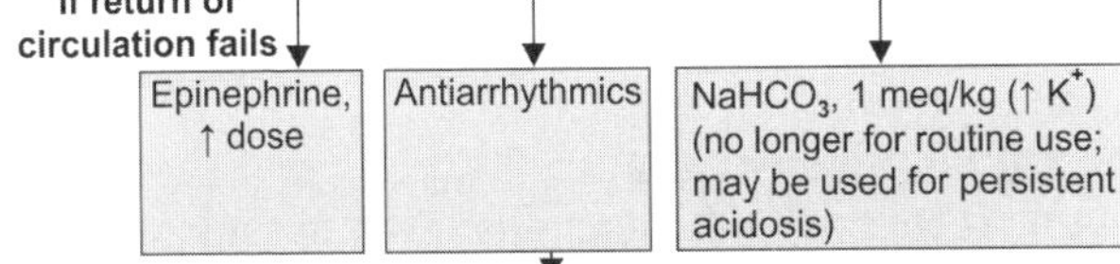

↓

Amiodarone: 150 mg over 10 min, 1 mg/min
Lidocaine: 1.5 mg/kg repeat in 3–5 min
Magnesium sulfate: 1–2 gm IV (polymorphic VT)
Procainamide: 30 mg/min, to 17 mg/kg [monomorphic VT]

↓ **If return of circulation fails**

Defibrillate, CPR: Drug - Shock - Drug - Shock

Bradyarrhythmia/asystole | **Pulseless electrical activity**

↓

CPR, intubate, IV access

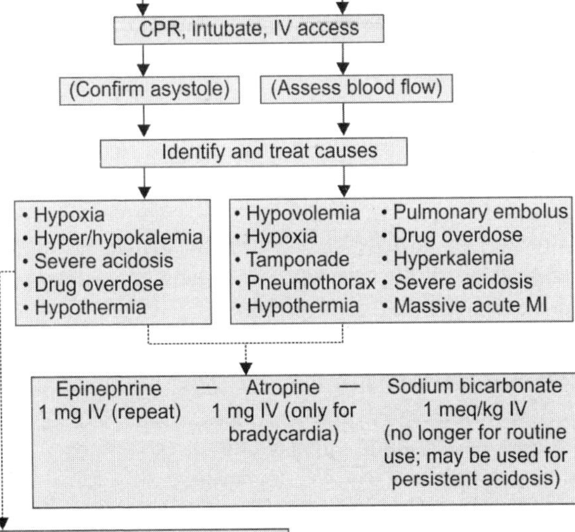

Pacing—External or pacing wire

lature and stimulates cortisol production. Some studies have reported reduced catecholamine requirements with vasopressin administration.

- Intravenous infusion of vasopressin at a low dose (0.01–0.04 units/min) may be safe and beneficial in septic patients with hypertension that is refractory to fluid resuscitation and conventional catecholamine vasopressors. Higher doses of vaospressin decrease cardiac output and may put patients at greater risk for splanchnic and coronary artery ischemia. Studies do not favor the use of vasopressin as first-line therapy. In the Vasopressin and Septic Shock Trial (VASST), low doses of vasopressin did not reduce mortality compared with norepinephrine in patients with septic shock who were being treated with catecholamine vasopressors.

3. Ans. (B) Aminoglycosides

- **Anaerobic bacterial infections:** They occur mostly after colorectal or pelvic surgery, appendicectomy, etc. Brain abscesses and endocarditis may be caused by anaerobic organisms. Metronidazole is an effective drug for these and is generally used in combination with gentamicin or cephalosporins (many are mixed infections). For serious cases IV administration is recommended: 15 mg/kg infused over 1 hr followed by 7.5 mg/kg every 6 hrs till oral therapy can be instituted with 400–800 mg TDS. *Prophylactic use* in high risk situations (colorectal/biliary surgery) is recommended. Other drugs effective in anaerobic infections are clindamycin and chloramphenicol.
- **Natural resistance:** Some microbes have always been resistant to certain AMAs. They lack the metabolic process or the target site which is affected by the particular drug. This is generally a group or species characteristic, e.g. gram-negative bacilli are normally unaffected by penicillin G; aerobic organisms are not affected by metronidazole; while anaerobic bacteria are not inhibited by aminoglycoside antibiotics or *M. tuberculosis* is insensitive to tetracyclines. This type of resistance does not pose a significant clinical problem.

4. Ans. (C) It causes hyperglycemia

Nicotinic Acid (Niacin): It is a B group vitamin which in much higher doses reduces plasma lipids. This action is unrelated to its vitamin activity and not present in nicotinamide. When nicotinic acid is given, TGs and VLDL decrease rapidly, followed by a modest fall in LDL-CH and total CH. A 20–50% reduction in plasma TGs and 15–25% reduction in CH levels has been recorded.

Nicotinic acid is the most effective drug to raise HDL-CH, probably by decreasing rate of HDL destruction; a 20–35% increase is generally obtained.

Adverse effects:

- The large doses needed for hypolipidemic action are poorly tolerated. Only about half of the patients are able to take the full doses. It is a cutaneous vasodilator: marked flushing, heat and itching (especially in the blush area) occur after every dose. This is associated with release of PGD2 in the skin, and can be minimized by starting with a low dose taken with meals and gradually increasing as tolerance develops. Use of sustained release (SR/ER) tablet also subdues flushing. Aspirin taken before niacin substantially attenuates flushing by inhibiting PG synthesis. *Laropiprant* is a specific antiflushing drug with no hypolipidemic action of its own, that has been combined with nicotinic acid to minimize flushing.
- Dyspepsia is very common; vomiting and diarrhea occur when full doses are given. Peptic ulcer may be activated.
- Dryness and hyperpigmentation of skin can be troublesome.
- Other long-term effects are—liver dysfunction and jaundice. Serious liver damage is the most important risk.
- Hyperglycemia, precipitation of diabetes (should not be used in diabetics).
- Hyperuricemia and gout, atrial arrhythmias.
- It is contraindicated during pregnancy and in children.
- Postural hypotension may occur in patients on antihypertensives when they take nicotinic acid.
- Risk of myopathy due to statins is increased.

5. **Ans. (B) Neprilysin inhibitor**
   - **Sacubitril** is an antihypertensive drug used in combination with valsartan. The combination drug sacubitril/valsartan is also used for the treatment of heart failure.
   - It is a prodrug that is activated to sacubitrilat (LBQ657) by deethylation via esterases.
   - It inhibits the enzyme neprilysin, which is responsible for the degradation of atrial and brain natriuretic peptide, two blood pressure-lowering peptides that work mainly by reducing blood volume.
   - In addition, neprilysin degrades a variety of peptides including bradykinin, an inflammatory mediator exerting potent vasodilatory action.

6. **Ans. (D) Atenolol**

Hypertension in pregnancy: A sustained BP reading above 140/90 mm Hg during pregnancy has implications both for the mother and the fetus—reduction of BP clearly reduces risks. Two types of situations are possible:

1. A woman with preexisting essential hypertension becomes pregnant.
2. Pregnancy induced hypertension; as in toxemia of pregnancy—preeclampsia.

- Toxemic hypertension is associated with a hyperadrenergic state, decrease in plasma volume (despite edema) and increase in vascular resistance.
- In the first category the same therapy instituted before pregnancy may be continued.
- **Antihypertensives to be avoided during pregnancy are:**
  - **ACE inhibitors, ARBs:** Risk of fetal damage, growth retardation.
  - **Diuretics:** Tend to reduce blood volume accentuate uteroplacental perfusion deficit (of toxemia)—increase risk of fetal wastage, placental infarcts, miscarriage, stillbirth.
  - **Nonselective blockers:** Propranolol has been implicated to cause low birth weight, decreased placental size, neonatal bradycardia and hypoglycemia.
  - **Sodium nitroprusside:** Contraindicated in eclampsia.
- **Antihypertensives found safer during pregnancy are:**
  - Hydralazine
  - Methyldopa (a positive Coombs' test occurs, but has no adverse implication).
  - **Dihydropyridine CCBs:** if used, they should be continued before labor as they weaken uterine contractions.
  - Cardioselective β blockers and those with ISA, e.g. atenolol, metoprolol, pindolol, acebutolol—may be used if no other choice.
  - Prazosin and clonidine—provided that postural hypotension can be avoided.

7. **Ans. (A) Vasodilators**

- **Tadalafil:**
- It is a more potent and longer acting congener of sildenafil.
- t½ 18 hours and duration of action 24–36 hours.
- Peak plasma levels are attained between 30–120 min; time to onset of action may be longer.

- Side effects, risks, contraindications and drug interactions are similar to sildenafil.
- In addition, back pain is reported, which has been ascribed to some degree of PDE II inhibition by tadalafil.
- Because of its longer lasting action, nitrates are contraindicated for upto 3 days after tadalafil.
- Due to its lower affinity for PDE-6, visual disturbances occur less frequently.
- **Dose:** 10 mg at least 30 min before intercourse (max 20 mg).

8. Ans. (B) Lepirudin

A. Direct thrombin inhibitors: Unlike heparin, these recently developed anticoagulants bind directly to thrombin and inactivate it without the need to combine with and activate AT III.

- **Lepirudin:** This recombinant preparation of hirudin (a polypeptide anticoagulant secreted by salivary glands of leech) binds firmly to the catalytic as well as the substrate recognition sites of thrombin and inhibits it directly. Injected IV, it is indicated only in patients who are at risk of heparin induced thrombocytopenia. On repeated/prolonged administration, antibodies against the lepirudin-thrombin complex may develop resulting in prolonged anticoagulant effect and possibility of anaphylaxis. Its action cannot be reversed by protamine or any other antidote.
- **Bivalirudin:** It is a smaller peptide prepared synthetically which has actions and uses similar to lepirudin. However, its action is slowly reversible due to cleavage of its peptide bonds by thrombin itself.
- **Argatroban:** This is a synthetic nonpeptide compound which binds reversibly to the catalytic site of thrombin, but not to the substrate recognition site. As such, it produces a rapid and short-lasting antithrombin action. Administered by IV infusion, it can be used in place of lepirudin for short-term indications in patients with heparin induced thrombocytopenia.

B. Fondaparinux: The pentasaccharide with specific sequence that binds to AT III with high affinity to selectively inactivate factor Xa without binding thrombin (factor IIa), has been recently produced synthetically and given the name *fondaparinux.* It is being increasingly used and has been marketed in India as well. The bioavailability of fondaparinux injected SC is 100% and it is longer acting (t½ 17 hours). Metabolism is minimal, and it is largely excreted unchanged by the kidney. As such, it is not to be used in renal failure patients. It is less likely to cause thrombocytopenia compared to even LMW heparins. Risk of osteoporosis after prolonged use is also minimal. It does not require laboratory monitoring of aPTT, and is a longer acting alternative to LMW heparins with the above advantages. *Dose:* 5–10 mg SC once daily.

C. **Dabigatran etexilate:** It is a prodrug which after oral administration is rapidly hydrolysed to *dabigatran*, a direct thrombin inhibitor which reversibly blocks the catalytic site of thrombin and produces a rapid (within 2 hours) anticoagulant action. Though oral bioavailability is low, the anticoagulant effect is consistent, and no laboratory monitoring is required. The plasma t½ is 12–14 hours and duration of action 24 hours. In the UK, Canada and Europe it is approved for prevention of venous thromboembolism following hip/knee joint replacement surgery. Administered in a dose of 110 mg (75 mg for elderly > 75 years) once daily, it has been found comparable to warfarin. In another large trial dabigatran etexilate 150 mg twice daily has yielded superior results to warfarin for prevention of embolism and stroke in patients of atrial fibrillation. In the USA it is approved for this indication. Adverse effects are bleeding and less commonly hepatobiliary disorders.

9. **Ans. (A) Xa inhibitor**
   - Four new oral anticoagulants are—dabigatran, rivaroxaban, apixaban and edoxaban.
   - **Apixaban** is more efective than warfarin at stroke prevention while having a substantially lower risk of major bleeding and a lower risk of all-cause mortality. Its dosage is 5 mg twice daily or 2.5 mg twice daily for patients with two or three high-risk criteria (age 80 years or older, body weight 60 kg or less, and serum creatinine 1.5 mg/dL or more). It is associated with less intracranial hemorrhage and is well tolerated. It was shown as to be superior to aspirin (and better tolerated) in the AVERROES trial of patients deemed not suitable for warfarin.
   - These NOACs have important advantages over warfarin, and therefore they are recommended preferentially over VKAs in the European guidelines.

10. **Ans. (B) Inhibit migration of lymphocytes**

    Colchicine:
    - It is an alkaloid from *Colchicum autumnale* which was used in gout since 1763. The pure alkaloid was isolated in 1820. It is

neither analgesic nor antiinflammatory, but it specifically suppresses gouty inflammation. It does not inhibit the synthesis or promote the excretion of uric acid. Thus, it has no effect on blood uric acid levels.

- An acute attack of gout is started by the precipitation of urate crystals in the synovial fluid. On being engulfed by the synovial cells, they release mediators and start an inflammatory response. Chemotactic factors are produced → granulocyte migration into the joint; they phagocytose urate crystals and release a glycoprotein which aggravates the inflammation by:
  - Increasing lactic acid production from inflammatory cells → local pH is reduced → more urate crystals are precipitated in the affected joint.
  - Releasing lysosomal enzymes which cause joint destruction.
- Colchicine does not affect phagocytosis of urate crystals, but inhibits release of chemotactic factors and of the glycoprotein, thus suppressing the subsequent events. By binding to fibrillar protein tubulin, it inhibits granulocyte migration into the inflamed joint and thus interrupts the vicious cycle.
- Other actions of colchicine are:
  - **Antimitotic:** Causes metaphase arrest by binding to microtubules of mitotic spindle. It was tried for cancer chemotherapy but abandoned due to toxicity. It is used to produce polyploidy in plants.
  - Increases gut motility through neural mechanisms.
- **Pharmacokinetics:** It is rapidly absorbed orally, partly metabolized in liver and excreted in bile, undergoes enterohepatic circulation ultimate disposal occurs in urine and feces over many days. Binding of colchicine to intracellular tubulin contributes to its large volume of distribution and slow elimination. Inhibitors of CYP3A4 retard colchicine metabolism and enhance its toxicity.
- **Toxicity** is high and dose related. Nausea, vomiting, watery or bloody diarrhea and abdominal cramps occur as dose limiting adverse effects. Accumulation of the drug in intestine and inhibition of mitosis in its rapid turnover mucosa is responsible for the toxicity. In overdose, colchicines produces kidney damage, CNS depression, intestinal bleeding; death is due to muscular paralysis and respiratory failure. Chronic therapy with colchicine is not recommended because it causes aplastic anemia, agranulocytosis, myopathy and loss of hair.

- **Uses:**
  - **Treatment of acute gout:** Colchicine is the fastest acting drug to control an acute attack of gout; 0.5 mg 1–3 hourly with a total of 3 doses in a day; maximum 6.0 mg in a course spread over 3–4 days. Control of attack is usually achieved in 4–12 hours. A second course should not be started before 3–7 days. The response is dramatic, so much so that it may be considered diagnostic. However, because of higher toxicity, it is used only when NSAIDs are ineffective or cannot be used. Maintenance doses (0.5–1 mg/day) may be given for 4–8 weeks in which time control of hyperuricemia is achieved with other drugs.
  - **Prophylaxis:** Colchicine 0.5–1 mg/day can prevent further attacks of acute gout, but NSAIDs are generally preferred. Taken at the first symptom of an attack, small doses (0.5–1.5 mg) of colchicine abort it.

11. Ans. (A) Quinidine

Drugs that prolong Q-T interval (have potential to precipitate Torsades de pointers)		
1	Antiarrhythmics	Quinidine, procainamide, disopyramide, propafenone, amiodarone
2	Antimalarials	Quinine, mefloquine, artemisinin, halofantrine
3	Antibacterials	Sparfloxacin, moxifloxacin
4	Antihistaminics	Terfenadine, astemizole, ebastine
5	Antidepressants	Amitryptyline and other tricyclics
6	Antipsychotics	Thioridazine, pimozide, aripiprazole, ziprasidone
7	Prokinetic	Cisapride

12. Ans. (B) 50 percent of the drug is ionized and 50 percent is nonionized

Most drugs are weak electrolytes, i.e. their ionization is pH dependent (contrast strong electrolytes that are nearly completely ionized at acidic as well as alkaline pH). The ionization of a weak acid HA is given by the equation:

- $pH = pKa + \log \frac{[A^-]}{[HA]}$

pKa is the negative logarithm of acidic dissociation constant of the weak electrolyte. If the concentration of ionized drug $[A^-]$ is equal to concentration of unionized drug [HA], then

- $\frac{[A^-]}{[HA]} = 1$

Since log 1 is 0, under this condition

- *pH = pKa*

Thus, *pKa* is numerically equal to the pH at which the drug is 50% ionized.

13. **Ans. (B) Act competitively on ACh receptors blocking post-synaptically**
    - Curare is an example of a non-depolarizing muscle relaxant that blocks the nicotinic acetylcholine receptor (nAChR), one of the two types of acetylcholine (ACh) receptors, at the neuromuscular junction.
    - The main toxin of curare, d-tubocurarine, occupies the same position on the receptor as ACh with an equal or greater affinity, and elicits no response, making it a competitive antagonist.
    - The antidote for curare poisoning is an acetylcholinesterase (AChE) inhibitor (anti-cholinesterase), such as physostigmine or neostigmine. By blocking ACh degradation, AChE inhibitors raise the amount of ACh in the neuromuscular junction; the accumulated ACh will then correct for the effect of the curare by activating the receptors not blocked by toxin at a higher rate.
    - The time of onset varies from within one minute (for tubocurarine in intravenous administration), to between 15 and 25 minutes (for intramuscular administration).
14. **Ans. (C) Tizanidine**
    - **Tizanidine:** This clonidine congener is a central α 2 adrenergic agonist—inhibits release of excitatory amino acids in the spinal interneurones. It may facilitate the inhibitory transmitter glycine as well. Polysynaptic reflexes are inhibited resulting in decreased muscle tone and frequency of muscle spasms without reducing muscle strength. Efficacy similar to baclofen or diazepam has been noted in multiple sclerosis, spinal injury and stroke, with fewer side effects.
    - It is absorbed orally, undergoes first pass metabolism and is excreted by the kidney.
    - t½ 2–3 hours.
    - It is indicated in spasticity due to neurological disorders and in painful muscle spasms of spinal origin.
    - Side effects are dry mouth, drowsiness, night-time insomnia and hallucinations. Dose-dependent elevation of liver enzymes

occurs. Though no consistent effect on BP has been observed, it should be avoided in patients receiving antihypertensives, especially clonidine.

- **Dose:** 2 mg TDS; max 24 mg/day.

15. **Ans. (A) Metyrapone**

Metyrapone: Inhibits 11-b hydroxylase in adrenal cortex and prevents synthesis of hydrocortisone so that its blood level falls → increased ACTH release → increased synthesis, release and excretion of 11-desoxycortisol in urine.

- It (2–4 g/d) inhibits 11β-hydroxylase activity and normalizes plasma cortisol in up to 75% of patients.
- Side effects include nausea and vomiting, rash and exacerbation of acne or hirsutism.
- Thus, it is used to test the responsiveness of pituitary and its ACTH producing capacity.

16. **Ans. (A) Vancomycin**

A. Primarily bacteriostatic are:

1. Sulfonamides
2. Erythromycin
3. Tetracyclines
4. Clindamycin
5. Chloramphenicol
6. Linezolid
7. Ethambutol

B. Primarily bactericidal are:

1. Penicillins
2. Cephalosporins
3. Aminoglycosides
4. Vancomycin
5. Polypeptides
6. Ciprofloxacin
7. Rifampin
8. Metronidazole
9. Isoniazid
10. Cotrimoxazole
11. Pyrazinamide

- Some primarily static drugs may become cidal at higher concentrations (as attained in the urinary tract), e.g. erythromycin, nitrofurantoin.
- On the other hand, some cidal drugs, e.g. cotrimoxazole, streptomycin may only be static under certain circumstances.

17. **Ans. (B) It is contraindicated in stroke**

- **ADP receptor antagonists:** These include the thienopyridines (clopidogrel and prasugrel) and ticagrelor. All of these drugs target P2Y12, the key ADP receptor on platelets.
- **Mechanism of action:** The thienopyridines are structurally related drugs that selectively inhibit ADP-induced platelet aggregation by irreversibly blocking P2Y12.
- Clopidogrel and prasugrel are prodrugs that require metabolic activation by the hepatic cytochrome P450 (CYP) enzyme system.
- Prasugrel is about 10-fold more potent than clopidogrel and has a more rapid onset of action because of better absorption and more streamlined metabolic activation.
- Prasugrel was compared with clopidogrel in 13,608 patients with acute coronary syndromes who were scheduled to undergo percutaneous coronary intervention. The incidence of the primary efficacy endpoint, a composite of cardiovascular death, MI or stroke, was significantly lower with prasugrel than with clopidogrel (9.9% and 12.1%, respectively), mainly reflecting a reduction in the incidence of nonfatal MI.
- The incidence of stent thrombosis also was significantly lower with prasugrel (1.1% and 2.4%, respectively). However, these advantages were at the expense of significantly higher rates of fatal bleeding (0.4% and 0.1%, respectively) and life-threatening bleeding (1.4% and 0.9%, respectively) with prasugrel. Because patients older than age 75 years and those with a history of prior stroke or transient ischemic attack have a particularly high-risk of bleeding, prasugrel should generally be avoided in older patients, and the drug is contraindicated in those with a history of cerebrovascular disease.
- Caution is required if prasugrel is used in patients weighing less than 60 kg or in those with renal impairment.
- Because of the negative results of this study, prasugrel is reserved for patients undergoing percutaneous coronary intervention. In this setting, prasugrel is usually given in conjunction with aspirin. To reduce the risk of bleeding, the daily aspirin dose should be ≤100 mg.
- **Dosing:** Clopidogrel is given once daily at a dose of 75 mg. Loading doses of clopidogrel are given when rapid ADP receptor blockade is desired. For example, patients undergoing coronary stenting are often given a loading dose of 300 mg, which produces inhibition of ADP-induced platelet aggregation

in about 6 h; loading doses of 600 or 900 mg produce an even more rapid effect. After a loading dose of 60 mg, prasugrel is given once daily at a dose of 10 mg. Patients older than age 75 years or weighing less than 60 kg should receive a lower daily prasugrel dose of 5 mg.

- **Side effects:** The most common side effect of clopidogrel and prasugrel is bleeding. Because of its greater potency, bleeding is more common with prasugrel than clopidogrel. To reduce the risk of bleeding, clopidogrel and prasugrel should be stopped 5–7 days before major surgery. In patients taking clopidogrel or prasugrel who present with serious bleeding, platelet transfusion may be helpful. Hematologic side effects, including neutropenia, thrombocytopenia, and thrombotic thrombocytopenic purpura (TTP) are rare.

18. Ans. (A) 5-hydroxytryptamine

5-hydroxytryptamine (5-HT, Serotonin): *Serotonin* was the name given to the vasoconstrictor substance which appeared in the serum when blood clotted and *Enteramine* to the smooth muscle contracting substance present in enterochromaffin cells of gut mucosa. In the early 1950s both were shown to be *5-hydroxytryptamine* (5-HT).

- About 90% of body's content of 5-HT is localized in the intestines; most of the rest is in platelets and brain. It is also found in wasp and scorpion sting, and is widely distributed in invertebrates and plants (banana, pear, pineapple, tomato, stinging nettle, cowhage).
- 5-HT is a potent depolarizer of nerve endings. It thus exerts direct as well as reflex and indirect effects. Tachyphylaxis is common with repeated doses of 5-HT.

19. Ans. (A) 5 mg/kg/day

Hydrocortisone (cortisol): Acts rapidly but has short duration of action. In addition to primary glucocorticoid, it has significant mineralocorticoid activity as well. Used for:

- Replacement therapy—20 mg morning + 10 mg afternoon orally.
- Shock, status asthmaticus, acute adrenal insufficiency—100 mg IV bolus + 100 mg 8 hourly IV infusion.
- Topically and as suspension for enema in ulcerative colitis.
- *Congenital adrenal hyperplasia (adrenogenital syndrome)*: Hydrocortisone 0.6 mg/kg daily given in divided doses round the clock to maintain feedback suppression of pituitary.

- If a patient on corticosteroids is to be anesthetized, give 100 mg hydrocortisone intraoperatively because anesthesia is a stressful state—can precipitate adrenal insufficiency and cardiovascular collapse.
- **Hormone replacement therapy for adult hypopituitarism:**
    - Hydrocortisone (10–20 mg am; 5–10 mg pm)
    - Cortisone acetate (25 mg am; 12.5 mg pm)
    - Prednisone (5 mg am)

20. Ans. (A) Gastric ulcer

- **Pirenzepine** (**Gastrozepin**), an M_1 selective antagonist, is used in the treatment of peptic ulcers, as it reduces gastric acid secretion and reduces muscle spasm.
- It causes decreased gastric motility leading to delayed gastric emptying and constipation.
- It has no effects on the brain and spinal cord as it cannot diffuse through the blood–brain barrier.
- It has been investigated for use in myopia control.
- It promotes the homodimerization or oligomerization of M_1 receptors.

21. Ans. (A) Senna

- Senna is a purgative obtained from leaves and pods of certain *Cassia sp.*, while *Cascara sagrada* is the powdered bark of the buck-thorn tree.
- Unabsorbed in the small intestine, they are passed to the colon where bacteria liberate the active *anthrol* form, which either acts locally or is absorbed into circulation—excreted in bile to act on small intestine. Thus, they take 6–8 hours to produce action.
- Taken by lactating mothers, the amount secreted in milk is sufficient to cause purgation in the suckling infant.
- The purgative action and uses of anthraquinones are quite similar to those of diphenylmethane.
- Taken at bedtime—a single, soft but formed evacuation generally occurs in the morning. Cramps and excessive purging occur in some individuals.
- The active principle of these drugs acts on the myenteric plexus to increase peristalsis and decrease segmentation.
- They also promote secretion and inhibit salt and water absorption in the colon.
- Senna anthraquinone has been found to stimulate PGE2 production in rat intestine. This is prevented by indomethacin and the purgative action is reduced.

- Skin rashes, fixed drug eruption are the occasional adverse effects.
- Regular use for 4–12 months causes colonic atony and mucosal pigmentation (melanosis).

22. Ans. (B) Beta-lactam antibiotics with beta-lactamase

- **Catheter-associated UTI:** It is defined by bacteriuria and symptoms in a catheterized patient. The signs and symptoms either are localized to the urinary tract or can include otherwise unexplained systemic manifestations, such as fever. The accepted threshold for bacteriuria to meet the definition of CAUTI is ≥103 CFU/mL, while the threshold for bacteriuria to meet the definition of ASB is ≥105 CFU/mL.
- The formation of biofilm (a living layer of uropathogens) on the urinary catheter is central to the pathogenesis of CAUTI and affects both therapeutic and preventive strategies. Organisms in a biofilm are relatively resistant to killing by antibiotics, and eradication of a catheter-associated biofilm is difficult without removal of the device itself.
- Furthermore, because catheters provide a conduit for bacteria to enter the bladder, bacteriuria is inevitable with long-term catheter use.
- The typical signs and symptoms of UTI, including pain, urgency, dysuria, fever, peripheral leukocytosis, and pyuria, have less predictive value for the diagnosis of infection in catheterized patients.
- Furthermore, the presence of bacteria in the urine of a patient who is febrile and catheterized does not necessarily predict CAUTI, and other explanations for the fever should be considered.
- The etiology of CAUTI is diverse, and urine culture results are essential to guide treatment. Fairly good evidence supports the practice of catheter change during treatment for CAUTI. The goal is to remove biofilm-associated organisms that could serve as a nidus for reinfection.
- Pathology studies reveal that many patients with long-term catheters have occult pyelonephritis.
- In general, a 7- to 14-day course of antibiotics is recommended, but further studies on the optimal duration of therapy are needed. In the setting of long-term catheter use, systemic antibiotics, bladder-acidifying agents, antimicrobial bladder washes, topical disinfectants, and antimicrobial drainage-bag solutions have all been ineffective at preventing the onset of

bacteriuria and have been associated with the emergence of resistant organisms.

- The best strategy for prevention of CAUTI is to avoid insertion of unnecessary catheters and to remove catheters once they are no longer necessary. However, intermittent catheterization may be preferable to long-term indwelling urethral catheterization in certain populations (e.g. spinal cord–injured persons) to prevent both infectious and anatomic complications.
- Antimicrobial catheters impregnated with silver or nitrofurazone have not been shown to provide significant clinical benefit in terms of reducing rates of symptomatic UTI.
- Cystitis is a risk factor for recurrent cystitis and pyelonephritis. ASB is common among elderly and catheterized patients but does not in itself increase the risk of death. The relationships among recurrent UTI, chronic pyelonephritis, and renal insufficiency have been widely studied. In spinal cord–injured patients, use of a long-term indwelling bladder catheter is a well-documented risk factor for bladder cancer. Chronic bacteriuria resulting in chronic inflammation is one possible explanation for this observation.
- Most common pathogens involved were *Escherichia coli* and *Klebsiella pneumoniae* which produce the enzymes Extended Spectrum β-Lactamases (ESBLs).

23. Ans. (D) cGMP

- Nitric oxide causes smooth muscle relaxation by generating cGMP intracellularly which then promotes dephosphorylation of myosin light chain kinase (MLCK) so that myosin fails to interact with actin. Inhibition of PDE-5, the cGMP degrading isoenzyme in cavernosal and vascular smooth muscle, results in accumulation of cGMP and marked potentiation of NO action.
- Estrogens induce nitric oxide synthase and PGI2 production in vascular endothelium. The increased availability of NO and PGI2 could promote vasodilatation.
- Organic nitrates are rapidly denitrated enzymatically in the smooth muscle cell to release the reactive free radical *nitric oxide (NO)* which activates cytosolic guanylyl cyclase → increased cGMP→ causes dephosphorylation of myosin light chain kinase (MLCK) through a cGMP dependent protein kinase (See Figure on next page). Reduced availability of phosphorylated (active) MLCK interferes with activation of myosin → it fails to interact with actin to cause contraction.

Consequently relaxation occurs. Raised intracellular cGMP may also reduce Ca^{2+} entry—contributing to relaxation.

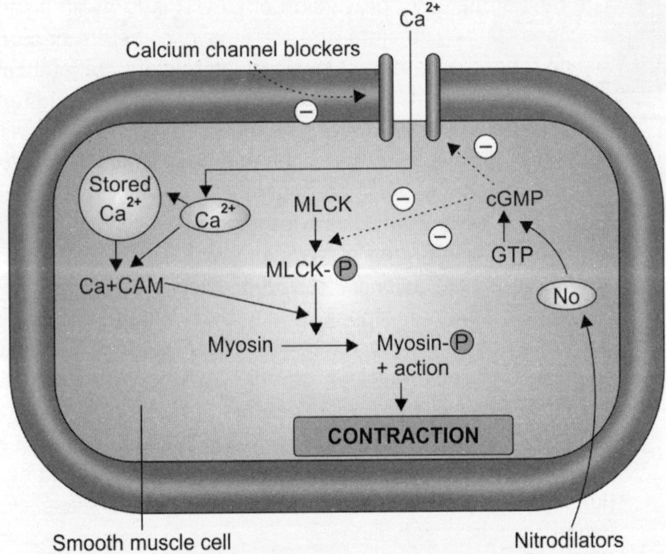

Mechanism of vascular smooth muscle relaxant action of nitrodilators like glyceryl trinitrate and calcium channel blockers; (---→) Inhibition. CAM—Calmodulin; NO—Nitric oxide; MLCK—Myosin light chain kinase; MLCK-P—Phosphorylated MLCK; GTP—Guanosine triphosphate; cGMP—Cyclic guanosine monophosphate

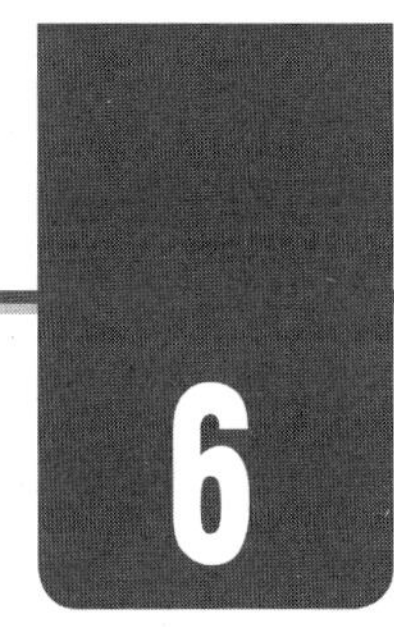

6 Microbiology

1. Cutaneous larva migrans caused by:

A. *Nector americanus* B. *Ancylostoma duodenale*
C. *Ancylostoma brazilense* D. *Ancylostoma caninum*

2. Adult form of echinococcus granulosus has definite host as:

A. Dog B. Cat
C. Cattle D. Pig

3. Slide of peripheral blood smear of a patient suffering with fever and chills is shown. Vector for the disease shown in the image is:

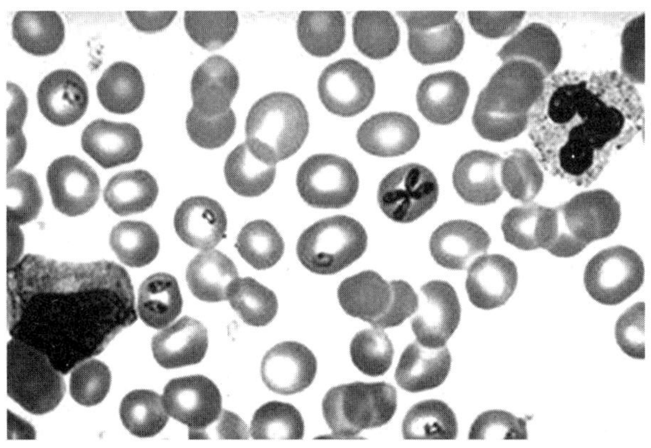

A. Hard tick B. Anopheles
C. Culex D. Tsetse fly

4. Which can grow in acidic medium?

A. *Lactobacillus* B. *Peptostreptococcus*
C. *Staphylococcus* D. *Streptococcus*

5. What is Dane particle?

A. HBV DNA B. HBsAg
C. HCV D. HBeAg

6. Burkholderia cepacia is intrinsically resistant to:

A. Ceftazidime
B. Trimethoprim/sulfamethoxazole
C. Temocillin
D. Cefotetan

7. Acute hemorrhagic conjunctivitis is caused by which enterovirus?

A. Enterovirus 70
B. Enterovirus 71
C. Adenovirus
D. Enterovirus 69

8. Transduction is mediated by:

A. Bacteriophage
B. Plasmid
C. Metaphage
D. Cosmids

9. Scromboid fish poisoning is due to which of the following Gram-negative bacteria?

A. *E. coli*
B. *Salmonella*
C. *Proteus*
D. *Shigella*

10. Mycoplasma is inherently resistant to:

A. Doxycycline
B. Azithromycin
C. Ceftriaxone
D. Ciprofloxacin

11. Sabin-Feldman dye test is done for:

A. Toxoplasmosis
B. Echinococcosis
C. Chagas disease
D. Sleeping sickness

Answers with Explanations

1. **Ans. (C) Ancylostoma brasilense**
   Non-human *Ancylostoma* species cause cutaneous larvae migrans. It is a serpiginous skin eruption caused by burrowing larvae of animal hookworms (usually the cat and the cat hook worm). The larvae hatch from eggs passed in dog and cat feces and mature in the soil. Humans become infected after skin contact with contaminated soil. After larvae penetrate the skin, erythematous lesions form along the tortuous tracks of their migration. It is also known as creeping eruption.
   - **Cutaneous larva migrans (creeping eruption),** common causes are:
     - **Ancylostoma brasiliense (most common)**
     - *A. caninum*
     - *Uncinaria stenocephala*
     - *Gnathostoma spinigerum*
     - *Bunostomum phlebotomum*
   - **Visceral larva migrans**, common causes are:
     - **Toxocara canis** (most common)
     - *T. cati*
     - *Angiostrongylus cantonensis*
     - *Angiostrongylus costaricensis*
     - *Anisakis* spp.
2. **Ans. (A) Dog**
   Habitat of echinococcus granulosus: The adult worm lives in the jejunum and duodenum of dogs and other canine carnivora (wolf and fox). The larval stage (hydatid cyst) is found in humans and herbivorus animals (sheep, goat, cattle and horse). Intermediate host: Sheep, pig, goat, cattle, **man (dead end host)**.
3. **Ans. (A) Hard tick**
   - Ticks transmit the human strain of babesiosis.
   - **Definitive host:** Ixodid ticks.
     - **Intermediate host:** Man or other mammals.
     - **Infective form:** Sporozoites are the infective form for humans.
     - **Mode of transmission:** Infection in vertebrate occurs through bite of the nymphal stage of Ixodid ticks.
   - *Babesia* parasites reproduce in red blood cells where they can be seen as cross-shaped inclusions (four merozoites asexually budding, but attached together forming a structure looking like a 'Maltese cross') and cause hemolytic anemia, quite similar to malaria.

- 'Maltese cross formations' on the blood film are diagnostic (pathognomonic) of babesiosis, since they are not seen in malaria, the primary differential diagnosis.
- Rings of *Babesia* spp. have delicate cytoplasm and are often pleomorphic. Infected red blood cells (RBCs) are not enlarged; multiple infection of RBCs can be common. Rings are usually vacuolated and do not produce pigment.
- Careful examination of multiple smears may be necessary, since *Babesia* may infect less than 1% of circulating red blood cells, thus be easily overlooked.
- Serologic testing for antibodies against *Babesia* (both IgG and IgM) can detect low-level infection in cases with a high clinical suspicion, but negative blood film examinations. Serology is also useful for differentiating babesiosis from malaria in cases where people are at risk for both infections.
- Since detectable antibody responses require about a week after infection to develop, serologic testing may be falsely negative early in the disease course.
- A polymerase chain reaction (PCR) test has been developed for the detection of *Babesia* from the peripheral blood. PCR may be at least as sensitive and specific as blood-film examination in diagnosing babesiosis, though it is also significantly more expensive. Most often, PCR testing is used in conjunction with blood film examination and possibly serologic testing.

4. Ans. (A) Lactobacillus

- **Lactobacillus** is a genus of gram-positive, facultative anaerobic or microaerophilic, rod-shaped, non-spore-forming bacteria. They are a major part of the lactic acid bacteria group (i.e. they convert sugars to lactic acid). They are normally a major part of the vaginal microbiota.
- **Acidophiles:** Organisms that grow best at low pH are called acidiophiles. The cytoplasm of these organisms is acidic in nature. Some acidophiles are also thermophiles in nature. Many fungi grow optimum pH 5 or below and few grow well at pH values as level as 2. However, a few bacteria prefer to grow at more extreme pH values, e.g. thiobacillus, thioxydents has an optimum pH of 2-3.5.
- **Neutrophils:** Most microorganism whose optimum pH for growth is between pH 6 and 8 are refer to as neutrophils. Most bacteria grow best at the neutral pH 7 with a normal range between 6 and 8, e.g. *E. coli*, *Klebsiella*, *Salmonella,* etc.

- **Alkaliphiles:** Some organisms which have very optimum PH for growth. Sometimes as high as PH 10–12 are called alkaliphiles. Alkaliphilic microorganisms are usually found in highly basic habited such as soda lakes and high carbonate soil. Some alkaliphiles have been found to be industrial importance because they produce hydrolytic enzymes such as proteases and lipases which function well at alkaline and are used as supplements for household detergents, e.g. bacillus alkaliphile, *vibrio*.

5. Ans. (B) HBsAg

- Hepatitis B virus (HBV) is a member of the hepadnavirus family. The virus particle (virion) consists of an outer lipid envelope and an icosahedral nucleocapsid core composed of protein. These virions are 30–42 nm in diameter.
- The nucleocapsid encloses the viral DNA and a DNA polymerase that has reverse transcriptase activity. The outer envelope contains embedded proteins that are involved in viral binding of, and entry into susceptible cells. The virus is one of the smallest enveloped animal viruses.
- The 42 nm virions, which are capable of infecting liver cells known as hepatocytes are referred to as 'Dane particles'. In addition to the Dane particles, filamentous and spherical bodies lacking a core can be found in the serum of infected individuals. These particles are not infectious and are composed of the lipid and protein that forms part of the surface of the virion which is called the surface antigens (HBsAg) and is produced in excess during the life cycle of the virus.
- The virion is a double-walled, spherical structure and measures 42 nm in diameter. It was first demonstrated by Dane in 1970 and so is known as Dane particle.
- By electron microscopy three types of particles can be seen in the serum from patients with hepatitis B. These are:
  1. Spherical particles measuring 22 nm in diameter
  2. Filamentous or tubular particles with a diameter of 22 nm and of varying length
  3. Double-walled, spherical structures measuring 42 nm in diameter. The former two particles are antigenically identical and are known as hepatitis B surface antigen, or HBsAg. The latter particle is the complete hepatitis viral particle known as Dane particle.

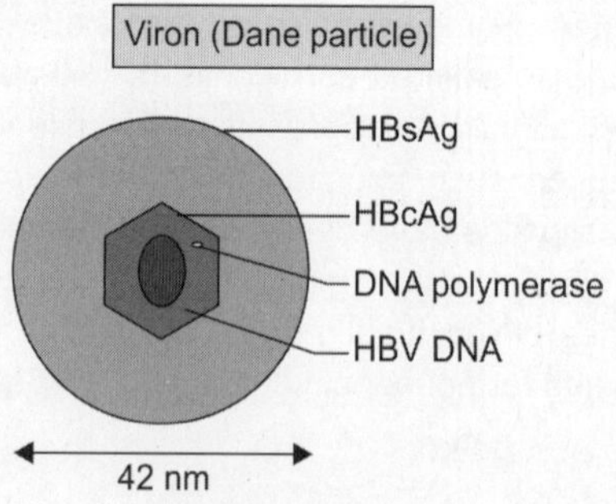

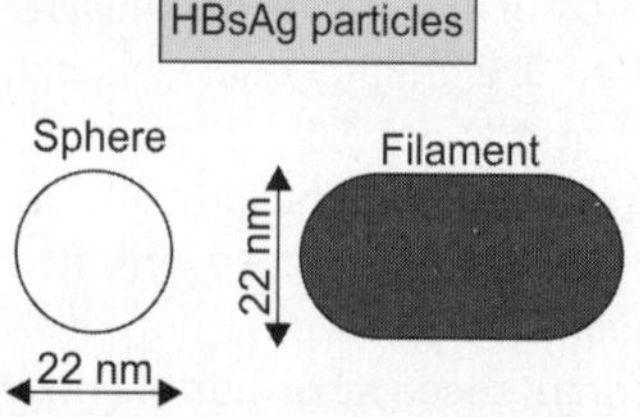

6. **Ans. (D) Cefotetan**
   - *B. Cepacia Complex* strains are intrinsically resistant to a wide range of antimicrobial agents including aminoglycoside, polymyxin, first and second generation cephalosporins and carboxypenicillins.
   - Antimicrobial agents that are effective against *B. Cepacia Complex* in vitro include trimethoprim/sulfamethoxazole, ceftazidime, carbapenems, ureidopenicillin, fluoroquinolone, minocyline and chloramphenicol.
   - *B. cepacia* is a Gram-negative, motile bacillus and stains irregularly with Gram-staining. It is an aerobe, grows well on nutrient agar at 25–30°C. On nutrient agar, the bacteria produce non-diffusible reddish purple pigmented colonies on prolonged incubation. They grow on blood agar.

7. **Ans. (A) Enterovirus 70**

   Acute hemorrhagic conjunctivitis (AHC) is caused by *Coxsackievirus* group A24 and Enterovirus 70. AHC is a highly contagious ocular infection which can cause large-scale epidemics. Transmission is facilitated by overcrowding and unsanitary conditions. The infection is transmitted directly from finger or fomite to eye. The condition is most prevalent in adults between 20 and 50 years.

Enterovirus 70

It is a member of the genus of viruses called Enterovirus and family of the viruses Picornaviridae. Usually very small (about 30 nm in diameter), it is non-enveloped (meaning it only has a nucleic acid core and protein capsid) and has a single-stranded positive-sense RNA genome; the protein capsid the virus itself is surrounded by icosahedral. It is known as one of the more new enteroviruses within this category. It spreads easily from one person's eyes to another's through contact with infected objects like fingers, or through the eye secretion itself. It infrequently causes polio-like permanent paralysis.

Coxsakievirus A24 variant

It is another member of the genus of viruses called Enterovirus and family of the viruses Picornaviridae. Its isolation host is human. It is an antigenic variant of the Coxsakievirus A24. It was studied independently for the first time in Singapore in 1970.

Adenovirus 11

They are medium-sized variant that are nonenveloped like Enterovirus 70. They have a double-stranded linear DNA genome. There are 57 variants of this virus that each cause 5–10% of upper respiratory infections in humans. These viruses are some of the largest nonenveloped viruses in existence, and because of this they can pass through the endosome without any necessary envelope fusion.

8. **Ans. (A) Bacteriophage**
   - **Transduction** is the process by which foreign DNA is introduced into a cell by a virus or viral vector. An example is the viral transfer of DNA from one bacterium to another. It does not require physical contact between the cell donating the DNA and the cell receiving the DNA (which occurs in conjugation), and it is DNase resistant (transformation is susceptible to DNase).
   - The transfer of a portion of DNA from one bacterium to another mediated by a bacteriophage is known as transduction.
   - Conjugation is a process of transfer of DNA from the donor bacterium to the recipient bacterium during the mating of two bacterial cells with the help of plasmids.

9. **Ans. (C) Proteus**
   - **Scombroid fish poisoning** is a food borne illness that results from eating spoiled (decayed) fish. Along with ciguatera, it is listed as a common type of seafood poisoning. The toxin believed to be responsible is histamine formed as the flesh

of the fish begins to decay. As histamine is also the natural agent involved in allergic reactions, scombroid food poisoning often gets misidentified as a food allergy.

- Histidine is an amino acid that exists naturally in many types of food (including fish) and at temperatures above 16°C/60°F it is converted to the biogenic amine histamine via the enzyme histidine decarboxylase produced by symbiotic bacteria such as *Morganella morganii* (this is one reason why fish should be stored in the freezer).
- Scombroid poisoning occurs after the ingestion of fresh, canned or smoked fish with high histamine levels due to improper processing or storage. The decarboxylation process is induced by enzymes produced by primarily enteric Gram-negative bacteria (e.g. *Morganella morganii, Escherichia coli, Klebsiella species* and *Pseudomonas aeruginosa*) found in the fish's cutis and intestines.

10. Ans. (C) Ceftriaxone

Mycoplasma is a genus of bacteria that lack a cell wall around their cell membrane. Without a cell wall, they are unaffected by many common antibiotics such as penicillin or other β-lactam antibiotics that target cell wall synthesis.

They are resistant to penicillins and cephalosporins because these antibiotics act on the cell wall which is lacking in mycoplasmas. *M. pneumoniae* remains susceptible to tetracyclines and erythromycin because these antibiotics act on the mycoplasmas by inhibiting synthesis of protein.

11. Ans. (A) Toxoplasmosis

- A **Sabin–Feldman dye test** is a serologic test to diagnose for toxoplasmosis.
- The test is based on the presence of certain antibodies that prevent methylene blue dye from entering the cytoplasm of Toxoplasma organisms.
- Patient serum is treated with toxoplasma trophozoites and complements as activator and then incubated. After incubation, methylene blue is added.
- If anti-Toxo antibodies are present in the serum, because these antibodies are activated by the complements and lyse the parasite membrane, Toxoplasma trophozoites are not stained (positive result); if there are no antibodies, trophozoites with intact membrane are stained and appear blue under microscope (negative result).

7 Forensic Medicine and Toxicology

1. According to Indian Penal Code, McNaughton's rule is adopted under which section?

A. CrPC 84 B. IPC 84
C. CrPC 48 D. IPC 48

2. Basisphenoid fuses with basioccipital at what age?

A. 16–18 years B. 12–15 years
C. 18–25 years D. 9–12 years

3. Posthumous child means?

A. Child born after father death
B. Child born after mother death
C. Child born before father death
D. Child born out of marriage

4. Which is the first organ to putrefy?

A. Brain B. Kidney
C. Heart D. Prostrate

5. Mummified body smells like:

A. Odorless B. Fishy
C. Putrid D. Rancid

6. Blue colored gastric mucosa on autopsy is due to poisoning by:

A. Arsenic B. Mercury
C. Sodium amytal D. Copper

7. Muscle pain, nephropathy caused by which metal poisoning:

A. Arsenic B. Cadmium
C. Mercury D. Lead

8. Locard is famous for?

A. Theory of exchange
B. Fingerprint study
C. Formula for estimation of stature
D. System of personal identification using the body measurement

9. In Maastricht classification of donation after cardiac death which category is stage 3?

A. Awaiting cardiac arrest
B. Brought in dead
C. Unsuccessful resuscitation
D. Cardiac arrest after brainstem death

Answers with Explanations

1. **Ans. (B) IPC 84**
   - **Section 84 in the Indian Penal Code**
     84. Act of a person of unsound mind—nothing is an offence which is done by a person who, at the time of doing it, by reason of unsoundness of mind, is incapable of knowing the nature of the act, or that he is doing what is either wrong or contrary to law.
   - **Section 83 in the Indian Penal Code**
     83. Act of a child above seven and under twelve of immature understanding—nothing is an offence which is done by a child above seven years of age and under twelve, who has not attained sufficient maturity of understanding to judge of the nature and consequences of his conduct on that occasion.

2. **Ans. (C) 18–25 years**

   The **basilar part** of the occipital bone (also **basioccipital**) extends forward and upward from the foramen magnum, and presents in front an area more or less quadrilateral in outline.

   In the young skull this area is rough and uneven, and is joined to the body of the sphenoid by a plate of cartilage.

   By the twenty-fifth year this cartilaginous plate is ossified, and the occipital and sphenoid form a continuous bone.

   Age from skull sutures–closure can be estimated as:
   - Metopic suture: 3 years/may remain unfused
   - 20 years: Basiocciput fuses and basisphenoid
   - 30 to 40 years: Sagittal suture–post one-third
   - 40 to 50 years: Anterior one-third of sagittal suture + lower half of coronal suture
   - 50 to 60 years: Middle sagittal + upper coronal suture
   - Lambdoid suture: Starts closing near lambda and completed around 45 years
   - Most reliable: Sagittal > Lambdoid > Coronal

3. **Ans. (A) Child born after father death**

   Legitimacy: Section 112 IEA

   A child is presumed to be legitimate if born during:
   - Continuance of a valid marriage
   - Within 280 days after its dissolution–mother remained unmarried.

   Posthumous child–born after death of his father-mother being conceived by said father.

4. Ans. (A) Brain

Putrefaction

- Two factors are responsible for that:
  1. **Bacterial enzymes**: From colon. Chief destructive bacterial agent is *Cl. Welchii*, which produces *lecithinase*—most important enzyme for decomposition causing post-mortem hemolysis, hydrolysis and hydrogenation of body fat.
  2. **Autolysis:** Release of cytoplasm enzymes.
- **Characteristic features**: Color changes + development of foul smelling gases.
- **Color changes:** First visible external evidence of putrefaction - greenish discoloration of the skin over right iliac fossa, due to formation of *Sulphmethemoglobin (green)* (Hb + H_2S)
- Appears in 12 to 18 hours in summer and 1 or 2 days in winter.
- **Marbling:** Staining of the wall of the superficial veins following hemolysis of red cells-prominent in 36 to 48 hours.
- **Organs show putrefactive changes in the following order**:
  - Larynx and trachea
  - Stomach and intestines
  - Spleen
  - Liver: *Honeycomb appearance* ('foamy *liver*')
  - Brain (brains of infants putrefies early)
  - Heart and lungs
  - Kidneys and bladder
  - Blood vessels
  - Uterus—last organ to putrefy in females. A gravid uterus decomposes earlier than a non-gravid uterus
  - Prostate–last to decompose in males
  - Followed by skin, muscle and tendon
    - **Rate of decomposition in different media: Casper's dictum:** A body decomposes in air twice as rapidly as in water and eight times as rapidly as in earth (1:2:8).
- **Putrefaction delayed in:**
  - Death due to wasting diseases, anemia
  - **Poisoning by:**
    - Carbolic acid
    - Zinc chloride
    - Strychnine
    - Chronic heavy metal poisoning, e.g. arsenic

5. **Ans. (A) Odorless**

   Mummification

   - Hot and dry climate favors it sandy, shallow graves
   - Mech: Drying and shrinkage of cadaver due to evaporation of water
   - Features of the body are preserved
   - A mummified body is odorless
   - Time taken: 3 months – 1 year
   - Arsenic and antimony, poisoning favors it.

   Medicolegal importance of adipocere and mummification

   - Face can be identified
   - The cause of death can be determined because injuries are recognized
   - The time since death can be estimated.

6. **Ans. D. Copper**

   - Blue discoloration is also commonly seen with poisonings with copper sulphate, copper succinate, dyes such as methylene blue, toluidine blue and food coloring agents.
   - **Copper:**
     - Common toxic compounds are—Cu sulphate (blue vitriol)-emetic
     - PM findings are:
       - Greenish-blue–froth at mouth/nostril
       - Gastric mucosa and content–greenish/bluish
   - **Chronic Cu poisoning:**
     - Wilson's disease–associated with copper toxicity
     - Vineyard sprayer's lung–chronic inhalation of copper sulphate spray
     - Green or purple line on the gums (as in chronic lead poisoning)
     - Hair, skin and perspiration may become green (golden hair).

7. **Ans. (C) Mercury**

   Mercury poisoning

   - If survive initial stage has glossitis and ulcerative gingivitis which appear in 24 to 36 hours followed by loosening of teeth and necrosis of jaw.
   - Renal tubular necrosis and gangrenous colitis may appear.
   - Chronic Hg poisoning–Hydrargyrism
   - Hatter's shake or Glass blower's shakes:
     - First involves hands than lips and tongue finally involves arms and legs
     - Coarse with jerky movements

- Other features are:
  - **Mercurial erethism:** Excitability, memory loss, insomnia, timidity, sudden attacks of anger and later delusions and hallucinations–mad as a hatter.
  - **Mercuria lentis:** Deposition of Hg on the anterior lens capsule, bilateral and has no effect on visual acuity.
  - **Acrodynia:** Pink disease or Swift's disease.
  - **Minamata Bay epidemic:** Due to chronic organic Hg poisoning (1955).
  - **Treatment:** N-acetyl D-penicillamine/BAL.

8. Ans. (A) Theory of exchange

Locard exchange principle

- 'Whenever 2 objects come in contact with each other, there is a mutual transfer of material from one object to the other'.
- Basis of all crime detection.

9. Ans. (A) Awaiting cardiac arrest

Maastricht classification: Non-heart beating donors are grouped by the Maastricht classification.

I	Brought in dead
II	Unsuccessful resuscitation
III	Awaiting cardiac arrest
IV	Cardiac arrest after brainstem death
V	Cardiac arrest in a hospital inpatient

- Categories I, II, IV and V are termed *uncontrolled* and category III is *controlled*.
- As of yet, only tissues such as heart valves, skin and corneas can be taken from category I donors.
- Category II donors are patients who have had a witnessed cardiac arrest outside hospital, have cardiopulmonary resuscitation by CPR-trained providers commenced within 10 minutes but who cannot be successfully resuscitated.
- Category III donors are patients on intensive care units with non-survivable injuries who have treatment withdrawn; where such patients wished in life to be organ donors, the transplant team can attend at the time of treatment withdrawal and retrieve organs after cardiac arrest has occurred.

8 Orthopedics

1. Non-articular bone pain differentiated from articular bone pain by:

A. Pain in both active and passive movements
B. Pain in only active movements
C. Crepitus
D. Swelling

2. Fallen fragment sign is characteristic of:

A. Aneurysmal bone cyst
B. Simple bone cyst
C. Giant cell tumor
D. Ewing's sarcoma

3. De quervains tenosynovitis involve inflammation of which of these tendons?

A. Extensor pollicis brevis and abductor pollicis longus
B. Adductor pollicis longus and extensor pollicis longus
C. Abductor pollicis longus and extensor pollicis longus
D. Adductor pollicis longus and extensor pollicis brevis

4. A patient present with injury in casualty and you as an intern evaluate this patient and felt the need to be evaluated by the orthopedician by which of the following reason?

A. Increase capillary refilling time in the fingers of the patient
B. Fracture with intra-articular extension
C. Patient with weakness of wrist extensors
D. Patient with wound >10 cm over the fracture site.

5. A patient with history of fall on outstretched hand will most probably have injury to which of the following marked areas in the image?

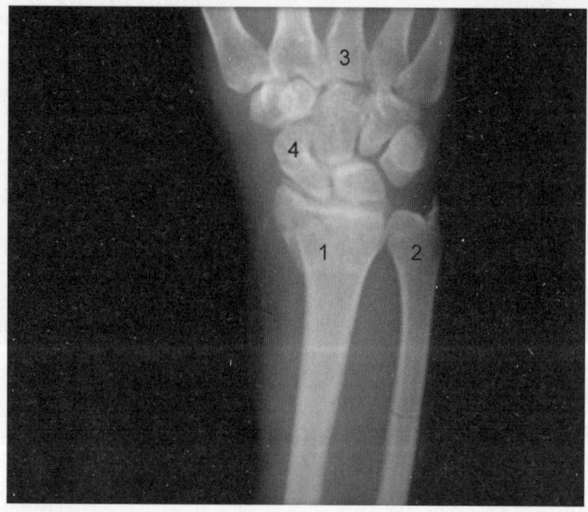

A. 1
B. 2
C. 3
D. 4

6. All of these drug inhibit resorption of bone except:

A. Reloxifene
B. Risedronate
C. Strontium ranelate
D. Teriparatide

7. Tom Smith arthritis most commonly affects:

A. Capital epiphysis of femur
B. Acetabulum
C. Neck of femur
D. Greater trochanter

8. Multifocal osteomyelitis is associated with:

A. SAPHO syndrome
B. Sickle cell anemia
C. Thalassemia
D. Salmonella infection

9. A 25 years old male having pain and deformity of the tibia as shown in X-ray. He had history of trauma 2 years back. What is the most probable diagnosis?

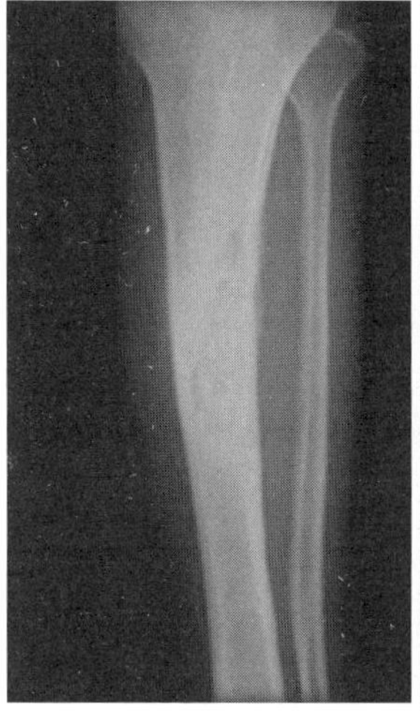
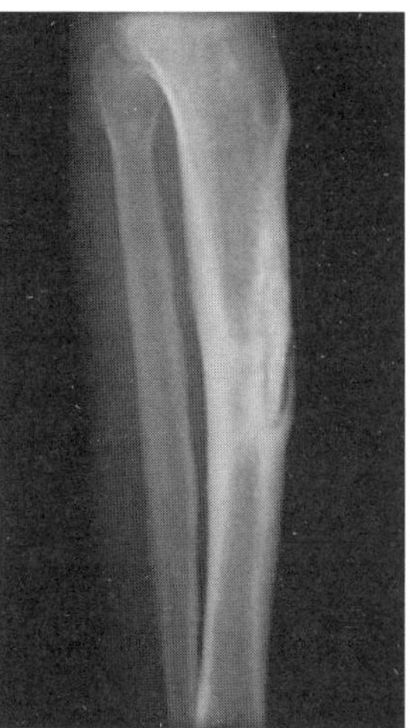

A. Ewing's Sarcoma
B. Chronic osteomyelitis
C. Osteosarcoma
D. Stess fracture tibia

10. In fasciotomy for compartment syndrome which structures are released?

A. Skin
B. Skin, subcutaneous tissue
C. Skin, subcutaneous tissue, superficial fascia, deep fascia
D. Skin, subcutaneous tissue, superficial fascia

11. 8th and 9th coastal cartilages are joined by which joint?

A. Fibrous joint
B. Plane synovial joint
C. Cartilaginous joint
D. Synchondrosis

12. Perilunate dislocation is defined as:

A. Lunate at place while others dislocate
B. Lunate is displaced while other are at place
C. Capitate dislocates volarly
D. Lunate is displaced volarly while carpus dislocate dorsally

13. A boy presented with multiple nonsuppurative osteomyelitis with sickle cell anemia. What will be the causative organism?

A. *Salmonella*
B. *S. aureus*
C. *H. influenzae*
D. Enterobacter species

Answers with Explanations

1. Ans. (B) Pain in only active movements

Articular	*Non-articular*
• Deep or diffuse pain. • Painful or limited range of movement–both active and passive • Swelling of joint • Crepitation • Joint instability • Locking of joint • Deformity	• Localised pain • Point or local tenderness • Painful active movements but not on passive • Physical findings are remote from joint capsule • Swelling, crepitation, joint instability, deformity are rare

2. Ans. (B) Simple bone cyst

Solitary Bone Cyst is also called a simple or unicameral bone cyst and affects children in the first and second decade. They arise in the metaphyses and are central or medullary. The proximal humerus and proximal femur are common sites. An SBC contains serous or serosanguinous fluid. They are seen as osteolytic, expansile lesions causing thinning of the cortex. Often with a fracture in the SBC, a "fallen-fragment" sign is commonly seen.

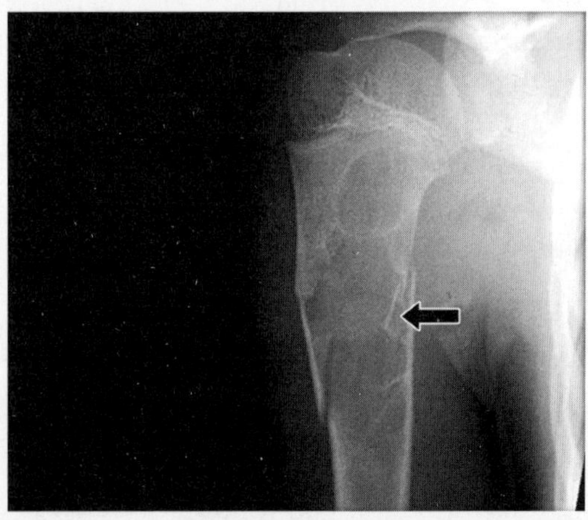

Fallen fragment sign

3. Ans. (A) Extensor pollicis brevis and abductor pollicis longus

- A fibrous extensor retinaculum lies on the dorsum of the wrist, which extends obliquely from the radial styloid process to the ulnar edge of the distal ulna. This extensor retinaculum has six compartments through which the extensor tendons pass. These compartments prevent bowstringing of the extensor tendons and provide reliable landmark for surgical approaches.

- The first compartment contains the tendons of abductor pollicis longus (APL) and extensor pollicis brevis (EPB). These two tendons constitute the radial border of the anatomical snuffbox. Stenosing tenosynovitis of these tendons is common in this compartment and is known as de Quervain's disease.
- The second compartment is located on the radial side of the Lister's tubercle and it contains the tendon of extensor carpi radialis longus and brevis (ECRL and ECRB).Tenosynovitis is also common in this region and is known as intersection syndrome.
- The third compartment contains the tendon of extensor pollicis longus (EPL). EPL forms the ulnar boarder of the anatomical snuffbox. Rupture of the EPL tendon may occur occasionally following fracture of the distal radius or a fracture of the distal radius treated by plating. Attrition of this tendon is also common in rheumatoid arthritis (RA).
- The fourth compartment contains the tendons of extensor digitorum communis and extensor indicis proprius. Tenosynovitis and spontaneous rupture of the tendons of this compartment due to rheumatoid arthritis is commonly seen.
- The fifth compartment contains the tendons of extensor digiti minimi (EDM) and extensor digiti quinti (EDQ). Attritional rupture occurs due to dorsally displaced ulnar head or due to synovitis of rheumatoid arthritis. The sixth compartment contains the tendon of extensor carpi ulnaris (ECU).

4. Ans. (A) Increase capillary refilling time in the fingers of the patient

Tests for Impending/Threatening Volkmann's Ischemic Contracture: Following any injury in and around the elbow and the upper forearm (e.g. war injuries, missile or high velocity injuries, side sweep injury or bullet injury), any tight bandage/plaster in this area, after reducing any fracture or dislocation in this area, or after operating in this area—always apprehend threatened vascular insufficiency and look for:

- Pain—believe your patient if he complains of pain (moderate to severe) especially in the forearm;
- Passive stretching of the fingers aggravates the pain which is progressive;

- Puffiness—swelling of the fingers, dorsum of the hand and palm;
- Pallor—earlier, there is cyanotic hue and then increasing pallor may develop;
- Pressing the nail bed—delayed capillary refilling;
- Pulse (radial) may be feeble, to absent;
- Paraesthesia—in the hand and fingers;
- Power—ask the patient to move the fingers. Earlier pain may have been the preventing factor in moving the fingers, but later actual neurogenic paresis supervenes;
- Perception of temperature—ischemic hand and fingers are comparatively colder.

5. Ans. (A) 1

There are a variety of wrist injuries that can occur from a traumatic fall on an outstretched hand. These injuries are termed FOOSH (fall on an outstretched hand) injuries. Probably the most well-known FOOSH is a distal radius fracture.

In the X-ray labeling is:

1 = Radius
2 = Ulna
3 = 3rd metacarpal
4 = Scaphoid

6. Ans. (D) Teriparatide

- **Teriparatide:** Intermittent administration of low-dose PTH enhances osteoblast activity and bone formation. Two PTH peptides have been approved for the treatment of osteoporosis: teriparatide (PTH 1-34) and PTH 1-84. Teriparatide is reserved for treating women at high-risk for fracture, including those with very low BMD and with a previous vertebral fracture. 20 mcg/day SC is given for 18 months.
- Serum calcium and serum uric acid are monitored at 1, 6, and 12 months. The concomitant use of bisphosphonates may attenuate bone mass improvement seen with PTH alone, but the administration of an antiresorptive agent has to be considered after the treatment in order to maintain the bone gain achieved.

7. Ans. (A) Capital epiphysis of femur

Tom Smith Arthritis:

- Septic arthritis of the hip
- Seen in infants
- Head of femur is completely destroyed by the pyogenic process

- Transphyseal vessels are present in early infancy before the formation of the growth plate. This may account for the frequency of septic arthritis of the hip in the neonate.
- In children, about a third of long-bone osteomyelitis is associated with septic arthritis of the adjacent joint.

Clinical features:

- Onset is acute with rapid abscess formation
- Can be mistaken for a superficial infection
- Can present later with complaints of limp without any pain
- O/E: Affected leg is shorter and hip movements are increased in all directions
- Telescopy test—positive
- X-ray complete absence of the head and neck of femur.
- Condition resembles DDH; complete absence of head and neck and normally developed round acetabulum.

Treatment:

- Acute surgical emergency
- Open drainage of hip joint is the most effective method of treatment in septic arthritis of the hip.
- Arthroscopic drainage can also be attempted.

8. **Ans. (B) Sickle cell anemia**
   - **Chronic recurrent multifocal osteomyelitis:** It was described primarily in children and adolescents. Mean age at CRMO onset is approximately 10 years, with a range of 4–14 years, mean disease duration is approximately 5 years, and the mean number of flares per patient was approximately 6. Most studies reported a predominance in female patients, which is as high as up to 85%, or female to male ratio of 5:1.
   - The etiology of most CRMO cases is not known. The episodes of systemic inflammation occur due to immune dysregulation without autoantibodies, pathogens or antigen-specific T cells. The infantile onset of CRMO is connected with a genetic mutation in Majeed syndrome and the deficiency of interleukin 1 receptor antagonist (DIRA).
   - It is characterized by the non-specific onset of pain with swelling and tenderness over the affected bone or joint, worsening at night. In long bones the metaphyseal regions are affected. The most common locations of osteomyelitis are: distal femur, proximal tibia, distal tibia, and distal fibula – 34%, followed by the clavicle – 24%, chest wall – 13%, vertebral bodies from 2 to 8%, mandible, pelvis – 14%, shoulder girdle, and small bones of the hands.

- Laboratory tests, such as white blood cell (WBC) count, erythrocyte sedimentation rate (ESR) and tumor necrosis factor α (TNF-α) levels may be mildly elevated.
- Differential diagnosis should include acute hematogenous osteomyelitis (CRMO represents 2–5% of all osteomyelitis cases in children and adolescents), neoplasms, especially Ewing sarcoma, eosinophilic granuloma, osteoblastoma, osteoid osteoma as well as Langerhans cell histiocytosis or insufficiency fractures. The diagnosis is based on clinical criteria.
- Early osteomyelitis as well as multifocal osteomyelitis is best demonstrated by a whole body three-phase technetium pyrophosphate bone scan which is highly sensitive to bony involvement.

9. Ans. (B) Chronic osteomyelitis

- Diagnosis of chronic osteomyelitis is based on history, careful physical examinations, routine laboratory profile, radiographic findings and finally confirmed by operative findings when material is recovered for culture, sensitivity tests and histological examination to confirm the diagnosis and to exclude other types of infection. Three types are encountered:
  1. Active infection with swelling and continuous discharge from one or more sinuses.
  2. Controlled infection with frequent attacks of flare up of the infection when both general and local features of subacute infection appear and sinuses with purulent discharge reappear.
  3. Presence of a sinus with minimal discharge from time to time. Changes are evident in the radiograph of the subjacent bone. Patients are worried about the recurrent discharge but otherwise the patient is in good health, and no other local symptoms or signs are present. The culture from discharge usually shows a mixed flora. They are *S. aureus, E. coli, Streptococcus pyogenes, Proteus, Pseudomonas* and other secondary contaminants.
- Treatment should be guided by cultures obtained from bone and usually requires long-term antibiotics. If the infected metaphyseal region is intracapsular, or if blood vessels traverse the physis, may spread to a joint. A large subperiosteal abscess may elevate the periosteum completely from the shaft of the bone, causing occlusion of the main nutrient vessels and death of the cortical bone leading to sequestrum formation. In such situation, the stripped periosteum, provided with its

own blood supply from muscle attachments, lays down new bone (involucrum) in a shell around the old shaft (sequestrum). At the opposite extreme, there are occasionally cases where the blood supply of the whole bone has been lost, the entire diaphysis has sequestrated, and yet very little surrounding subperiosteal bone may be seen.

- Dead bone can be absorbed by granulation tissue. This is only possible when active infection has been controlled, and some blood supply to the bone and surrounding soft tissues is retained. Modern investigations like radionuclide imaging, CT scan or MRI can help to provide detailed information about the bone and surrounding soft tissues, but as these are not widely available and are expensive.
- Where local pain, swelling, irregular fever, raised local temperature, areas of redness, tenderness over the surface on palpation, purulent discharge through sinus or sinuses and thickening of the bone are present, as the infection is active, even though the general symptoms are minimal, with variable thickening of bone and radiographs show presence of sequestra and bone abscess, operative debridement becomes mandatory.

10. Ans. (C) Skin, subcutaneous tissue, superficial fascia, deep fascia

- **Compartment syndrome** is a special entity; common in leg, forearm, thigh and arm; is a syndrome due to increased intra-compartmental pressure within a limited space area.
- *Causes are:* Narrowed space due to tight dressings/plaster cast, lying on one limb in comatous patient; increased content within the compartment due to trauma like fractures, edema, ischemic injury, hematoma, positioning after trauma, burn injury, etc.; high pressure injection injuries like gun injury, oil based material injury, extravasation of chemotherapeutic drugs; snake bite.
- It compromises circulation and function mainly of muscles and nerves. It often maintains the normal colour and temperature of the fingers and distal pulses may not be obliterated in spite of severe muscle ischaemia. Muscle ischemia *more than 4 hours* causes muscle death and myoglobinuria. Irreversible nerve damage develops if ischemia persists for 8 hours.
- Progressive, persistent severe pain which is aggravated by passive muscle stretching is the diagnostic sign. Tense tender regional lymph node is typical. Pulse will be usually normally

felt in compartment syndrome; but may become absent if there is associated arterial injury. Compartment pressure more than 30 mm Hg is an indication for *fasciotomy*.

- It is common in calf and forearm. Closed injuries cause hematoma leading to increased pressure. It is often associated with fracture of the underlying bone which in turn compresses the major vessel further aggravating the ischemia causing ***pallor, pulselessness, pain, paraesthesia, diffuse swelling*** and ***cold limb***.
- If allowed to progress it may eventually lead to ***gangrene*** or ***chronic ischemic contracture*** with deformed, disabled limb.
- ***Muscle necrosis*** releases myoglobulin which is excreted in the urine, damages the kidneys leading into renal failure.
- Affected muscle when passively stretched worsens the pain—the most reliable clinical sign.
- **Problems with the compartment syndrome:**
  - Infection, septicemia and abscess formation
  - Renal failure
  - Gangrene of the limb
  - Chronic ischaemic contracture
  - Disabled limb, Volkmann's ischemic contracture
- **Treatment:** Adequate lengthy incision involving skin, fat and deep fascia should be done until underneath muscle bulges out properly. Multiple incisions should be made if needed. Separate incision in each compartment should be done.
- **Fasciotomy** done in forearm anterior compartment is a specific method. Carpal tunnel *should be released by cutting flexor retinaculum.* Incision begins at the junction of the thenar and hypothenar area; extends proximally initially transverse across flexion crease of the wrist at the ulnar border; then across forearm towards radial side of forearm; then in proximal forearm towards medial side creating convex flap towards lateral side. In the elbow it crosses along the medial border to reach the arm where it runs in arm along the medial part of the anterior arm. Injury to major nerves, palmar cutaneous branch of median nerve should be avoided while placing the incision. Incision should be deepened by cutting the deep fascia along the entire length of the incision.
- *Dorsal fasciotomy* should be added by placing longitudinal lengthy incision in the midline. Two longitudinal incisions on the dorsum of the hand also should be made:

- Antibiotics.
- Catheterisation.
- Mannitol or diuretics to cause diuresis, so as to flush the kidney.
- Fresh blood transfusion.
- Hyperbaric oxygen.

11. **Ans. (B) Plane synovial joint**

Plane synovial joints: Articular surfaces are more or less flat (plane). They permit gliding movements (translations) in various directions.

Examples:

- Intercarpal joints
- Intertarsal joints
- Joints between articular processes of vertebrae
- Cricothyroid joint
- Cricoarytenoid joint
- Superior tibiofibular
- Interchondral joint (5–9 ribs)
- Costovertebral
- Costotransverse
- Acromioclavicular with intra-articular disc
- Carpometacarpal (except first)
- Tarsometatarsal
- Intermetacarpal
- Intermetatarsal
- Chondrosternal (except first)
- Sacroiliac

12. **Ans. (A) Lunate at place while others dislocate**

- **Perilunate dislocations** and **perilunate fracture dislocations** involve dislocation of the carpus relative to the lunate which remains in normal alignment with the distal radius. They should not be confused with lunate dislocations where the lunate is dislocated in a volar direction and no longer has normal radiolunate articulation.
- Overall, carpal dislocations account for less than 10% of all wrist injuries.
- Perilunate dislocations typically occur in young adults with high energy trauma resulting in loading of a hyperextended,

ulnarly deviated hand. Around 60% of perilunate dislocations are associated with a scaphoid fracture which is then termed a **trans-scaphoid perilunate dislocation**.

- Typical history is of a fall onto a dorsiflexed wrist. There may or may not be obvious clinical deformity. Occasionally median nerve injury, arterial compromise or compartment syndrome may be evident due to the dislocation.
- Perilunate dislocation involves traumatic rupture of the radiscaphocapitate, scapholunate interosseous and lunotriquetral interosseous ligaments. Mayfield et. al. have proposed a four stage process to describe perilunar wrist instability where perilunate dislocation represents stage II.
- **Radiographic features:** The majority of cases involve dorsal dislocation of the capitate and carpus relative to the lunate which remains in near-normal alignment with the radius. Volar perilunate dislocation is rare.
- In a trans-scaphoid perilunate dislocation the proximal scaphoid maintains its lunate relationship, and the distal scaphoid and remainder of the carpal bones displace dorsally.
- CT plays an important role in assessing for associated occult fractures; the most common and important being scaphoid fracture.
- **Treatment and prognosis:** Untreated there is a high-risk of median nerve palsy, pressure necrosis, compartment syndrome and long-term wrist dysfunction. As with other dislocations, perilunate dislocation should be reduced as soon as possible. Prompt open reduction with ligamentous repair is necessary.
- Despite treatment, long-term risk of degenerative arthritis is high (~60%).
- Also, there is a higher rate of nonunion of scaphoid fractures when associated with perilunate dislocation than with isolated scaphoid fractures.
- **Differential diagnosis:** The most important differential diagnosis is that of a lunate dislocation which can mimic a perilunate dislocation, especially on AP projection. The key to not confusing the two is the lateral projection.
- In a lunate dislocation, the radiolunate articulation is disrupted and the lunate is dislocated in a palmar direction in a perilunate dislocation, the radiolunate articulation is maintained.

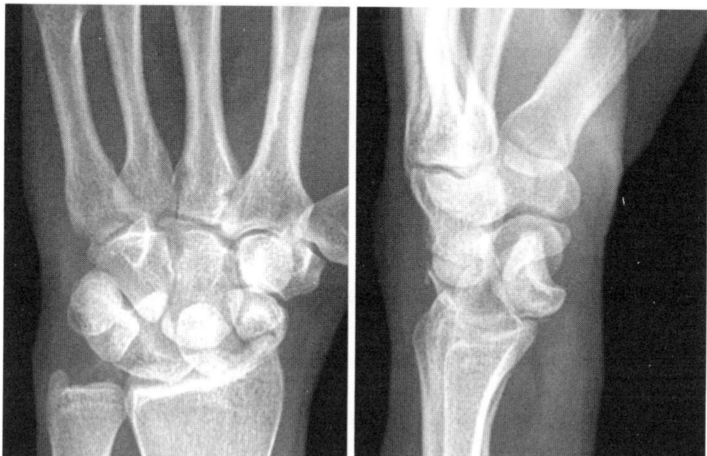

Posteroanterior (PA) and lateral radiographs demonstrating trans-scaphoid perilunate dislocation

13. Ans. (A) Salmonella

- *Salmonella* bacteria infection usually causes diarrhea, fever, vomiting and abdominal cramps after 12–72 hours of infection which recovers within 4–7 days. In severe cases, salmonella infection may spread from the intestine to bloodstream and then other body sites which is known as typhoid fever, which is treated with higher antibiotics. The elderly, infants and those with impaired immune systems are likely to develop severe illness.
- There are two species of *Salmonella*, *Salmonella bongori* and *Salmonella enterica*, later is divided in six subspecies, *enterica, salmae, arizonae, diazonae, houtenase* and *indica*.
- These subspecies are further divided into numerous serovars. The species *Salmonella enteric* contains 60% of the total number of the serovars and 99% of the servoars that are capable of infecting cold and warm blooded animals as well as humans. The sources of infections are usually poultry, pork, beef and fish, infected eggs, milk, tainted fruits and vegetables.
- **Clinical features:** *Salmonella* bacteria infection usually causes diarrhea, fever, vomiting and abdominal cramps after 12–72 hours of infection which recovers within 4–7 days.
- In severe cases, salmonella infection may spread from the intestine to bloodstream and then other body sites which is known as typhoid fever which is treated with higher antibiotics.

- Smaller number of people affected with salmonellosis experience reactive arthritis which can last months or years and can lead to chronic arthritis.
- Salmonella osteomyelitis is common in sickle cell anemia.
- Typhoid fever occurs when bacteria enters the lymphatic system and cause systemic form of salmonellosis. In severe form, patient may land up into hypovolemic shock and also septic shock.
- **Prevention:** Food must be cooked to 68–72°F and liquids such as soups, gravies must be boiled to reduce the chance of food-borne salmonellosis. Freezing kills some *Salmonella*.
- **Treatment:** Antibiotics such as ceftriaxone are given to kill bacteria. Azithromycin is used in resistant bacteria. Antibiotic resistance is increasing throughout the world.

9

Ophthalmology

1. 70 years old lady 2 days following cataract surgery presents with eye complaints as shown in the image. Next step in its management is?

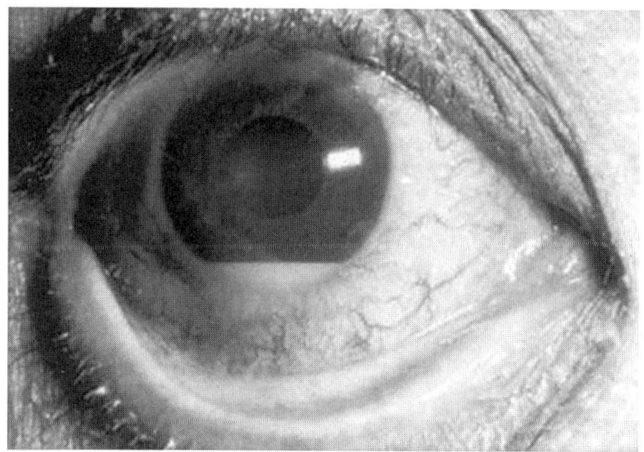

A. Intravitreal antibiotic B. Intravitreal steroids
C. Eye patch and dressing D. Intravitreal mannitol

2. Yoke muscle for right lateral rectus in dextroversion movement of eye is:

A. Left medial rectus B. Left superior rectus
C. Left superior oblique D. Left inferior oblique

3. Last vision to go in glaucoma is:

a. Temporal b. Superior
c. Inferior d. Nasal

4. A 50-year-old emmetropic patient, presbyopic correction needed is?

A. +2D B. +4D
C. +3D D. +1D

5. 3rd nerve palsy in diabetes mellitus characteristically shows?

A. Absent light reflex, accommodation is present
B. Intact light reflex, accommodation is absent
C. Both light and accommodation reflex is absent
D. Both are normal

6. 100 day glaucoma is seen in?

A. Central retinal vein occlusion (CRVO)
B. Central retinal artery occlusion (CRAO)
C. Diabetic retinopathy
D. After injury

7. What is the most serious cause of conjunctivitis that cause blindness in children?

A. *N. gonococcus*
B. *Streptococus*
C. *Staphylococus*
D. *Chlamydia*

8. Most common wall of orbit involved in a blowout fracture is:

A. Medial
B. Floor
C. Lateral
D. Roof

9. Most common cause of neonatal eye infection is?

A. *Staphylococus*
B. *Streptococus*
C. *N. gonorrhoeae*
D. *Chlamydia*

10. Cause of given retina image is:

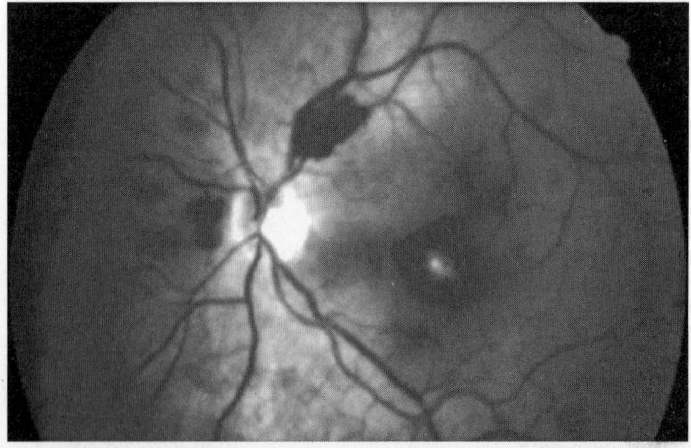

A. Acute leukemia
B. Sickle cell anemia
C. Beta thalassemia
D. Uveal melanoma

11. Which is an example of the simple myopic astigmatism among the prescriptions given below?

A. Treatment with (+) spherical lens
B. Treatment will be cylindrical/plano (-) lens
C. Treatment will be (-) spherical lens
D. (-)(+) (+)(-) on both 90 and 180 degree axis

Answers with Explanations

1. **Ans. (A) Intravitreal antibiotic**
   - The image shows hypopyon indicator of suppuration of cystic spaces, i.e. endophthalmitis. The immediate step in management is Intravitreal antibiotic (cocktail regime) with topical steroids and cycloplegics.
   - Lets discuss the postoperative complications of cataract so that any question asked in future will be covered.

Early postoperative complications after cataract surgery are:

1. ***Hyphema:*** Collection of blood in the anterior chamber may occur from conjunctival or sclera vessels due to minor ocular trauma or otherwise. *Treatment:* Most hyphemas absorb spontaneously and thus need no treatment. Sometimes hyphema may be large and associated with rise in IOP. In such cases, IOP should be lowered by acetazolamide and hyperosmotic agents. If the blood does not get absorbed in a week's time, then a paracentesis should be done to drain the blood.
2. ***Iris prolapse:*** It is usually caused by inadequate suturing of the incision after ICCE and conventional ECCE and occurs during first or second postoperative day. This complication is not known with manual SICS and phacoemulsification technique. *Management:* A small prolapse of less than 24 hours duration may be reposited back and wound sutured. A large prolapse of long duration needs abscission and suturing of wound.
3. ***Striate keratopathy:*** Characterised by mild corneal edema with Descemet's folds is a common complication observed during immediate postoperative period. This occurs due to endothelial damage during surgery. *Management:* Mild striate keratopathy usually disappears spontaneously within a week. Moderate to severe keratopathy may be treated by instillation of hypertonic saline drops (5% sodium chloride) along with steroids.
4. ***Flat (shallow or nonformed) anterior chamber:*** It has become a relatively rare complication due to improved wound closure. It may be due to wound leak, ciliochoroidal detachment or pupil block.
   i. ***Flat anterior chamber with wound leak*** is associated with hypotony. It is diagnosed by Seidel's test. In this test,

a drop of fluorescein is instilled into the lower fornix and patient is asked to blink to spread the dye evenly. The incision is then examined with slit lamp using cobalt-blue filter. At the site of leakage, fluorescein will be diluted by aqueous. In most cases wound leak is cured within 4 days with pressure bandage and oral acetazolamide. If the condition persists, injection of air in the anterior chamber and resuturing of the leaking wound should be carried out.

ii. ***Ciliochoroidal detachment:*** It may or may not be associated with wound leak. Detached ciliochoroid presents as a convex brownish mass in the involved quadrant with shallow anterior chamber. In most cases choroidal detachment is cured within 4 days with pressure bandage and use of oral acetazolamide. If the condition persists, suprachoroidal drainage with injection of air in the anterior chamber is indicated.

iii. ***Pupil block due to vitreous bulge*** after ICCE leads to formation of iris bombe and shallowing of anterior chamber. If the condition persists for 5-7 days, permanent peripheral anterior synechiae (PAS) may be formed leading to secondary angle closure glaucoma. Pupil block is managed initially with mydriatic, hyperosmotic agents (e.g. 20% mannitol) and acetazolamide. If not relieved, then laser or surgical peripheral iridectomy should be performed to bypass the pupillary block.

5. ***Postoperative anterior uveitis*** can be induced by instrumental trauma, undue handling of uveal tissue, reaction to residual cortex or chemical reaction induced by viscoelastics, pilocarpine, etc. *Management:* Includes more aggressive use of topical steroids, cycloplegics and NSAIDs. Rarely systemic steroids may be required in cases with severe fibrinous reaction.
6. ***Bacterial endophthalmitis:*** This is one of the most dreaded complications with an incidence of 0.2 to 0.5 percent. The principal sources of infection are contaminated solutions, instruments, surgeon's hands, patient's own flora from conjunctiva, eyelids and airborne bacteria. *Symptoms and signs* of bacterial endophthalmitis are generally present between 48 and 72 hours after surgery and include: Ocular pain, diminshed vision, eyelid edema, conjunctival chemosis and marked circumciliary congestion, corneal edema, exudates in pupillary

area, hypopyon and diminished or absent red pupillary glow. *Management:* It is an emergency and should be managed energetically. An early diagnosis and vigorous therapy is the hallmark of the treatment of endophthalmitis. Following therapeutic regime is recommended for suspected bacterial endophthalmitis.

A. Antibiotic therapy:

- ***Intravitreal antibiotics and diagnostic tap*** should be made as early as possible. It is performed transconjunctivally under topical anesthesia from the area of pars plana (4–5 mm from the limbus). The vitreous tap is made using 23-gauge needle followed by the intravitreal injection using a disposable tuberculin syringe and 30-gauge needle. The mainstay of treatment of acute bacterial endophthalmitis is intravitreal injection of antibiotics at the earliest possible. Usually a combination of two antibiotics–one effective against Gram-positive coagulase negative staphylococci and the other against Gram-negative bacilli is used as below:
    - ***First choice:*** Vancomycin 1 mg in 0.1 ml plus ceftazidime 2.25 mg in 0.1 ml.
    - ***Second choice:*** Vancomycin 1 mg in 0.1 ml plus amikacin 0.4 mg in 0.1 ml.
    - ***Third choice:*** Vancomycin 1 mg in 0.1 ml plus gentamycin 0.2 mg in 0.1 ml.
        - Some surgeons prefer to add dexamethasone 0.4 mg in 0.1 ml to limit postinflammatory consequences.
        - Gentamycin is 4 times more retinotoxic (causes macular infarction) than amikacin. Preferably the aminoglycosides should be avoided.
        - The aspirated fluid sample should be used for bacterial culture and smear examination. If vitreous aspirate is collected in an emergency when immediate facilities for culture are not available, it should be stored promptly in refrigerator at 4°C.
        - If there is no improvement, a repeat intravitreal injection should be given after 48 hours taking into consideration the reports of bacteriological examination.
- ***Subconjunctival injections*** of antibiotics should be given daily for 5–7 days to maintain therapeutic intraocular concentration:
    - ***First choice:*** Vancomycin 25 mg in 0.5 ml plus ceftazidime 100 mg in 0.5 ml

    - ***Second choice:*** Vancomycin 25 mg in 0.5 ml plus cefuroxime 125 mg in 0.5 ml.
- ***Topical concentrated antibiotics*** should be started immediately and used frequently (every 30 minute to 1 hourly). To begin with a combination of two drugs should be preferred, one having a predominant effect on the Gram-positive organisms and the other against Gram-negative organisms is used as here:
    - Vancomycin (50 mg/ml) or cefazoline (50 mg/ml) plus.
    - Amikacin (20 mg/ml) or tobramycin (15 mg%).
- ***Systemic antibiotics*** have limited role in the management of endophthalmitis, but most of the surgeons do use them.
    - *Ciprofloxacin* intravenous infusion 200 mg BD for 3-4 days followed by orally 500 mg BD for 6-7 days, or
    - *Vancomycin* 1 g IV BD and *ceftazidime* 2 g IV 8 hourly, or
    - *Cefazoline* 1.5 g IV 6 hourly and *amikacin* 1 g IV three times a day.

B. Steroid therapy: Steroids limit the tissue damage caused by inflammatory process. Most surgeons recommend their use after 24 to 48 hours of control of infection by intensive antibiotic therapy. However, some surgeons recommend their immediate use (controversial). Routes of administration and doses are:

- *Intravitreal injection* of dexamethasone 0.4 mg in 0.1ml.
- *Subconjunctival injection* of dexamethasone 4 mg (1ml) OD for 5-7 days.
- *Topical* dexamethasone (0.1%) or pred acetate (1%) used frequently.
- *Systemic steroids.* Oral corticosteroids should preferably be started after 24 hours of intensive antibiotic therapy. A daily therapy regime with 60 mg prednisolone to be followed by 50, 40, 30, 20 and 10 mg for 2 days each may be adopted.

C. Supportive therapy:

- **Cycloplegics:** Preferably 1% atropine or alternatively 2% homatropine eyedrops should be instilled TDS or QID.
- **Antiglaucoma drugs:** In patients with raised intraocular pressure drugs such as oral acetazolamide (250 mg TDS) and timolol (0.5% BD) may be prescribed.

D. Vitrectomy operation: It should be performed if the patient does not improve with the above intensive therapy for 48 to 72 hours or when the patient presents with severe infection with visual acuity reduced to light perception. Vitrectomy helps in removal of infecting organisms, toxins and enzymes present in the infected vitreous mass.

2. **Ans. (A) Left medial rectus**
   - **Yoke muscles (contralateral synergists):** It refers to the pair of muscles (one from each eye) which contract simultaneously during version movements.
   - For example, right lateral rectus and left medial rectus act as yoke muscles for dextroversion movements.
   - Other pairs of yoke muscles are: Right MR and left LR, right LR and left MR, right SR and left IO, right IR and left SO, right SO and left IR and right IO and left SR.
3. **Ans. (A) Temporal**
   - **Advanced glaucomatous field defects:** The visual field loss gradually spreads centrally as well as peripherally, and eventually only a small island of central vision *(tubular vision)* and an accompanying temporal island are left. With the continued damage, these islands of vision also progressively diminish in size until the tiny central island is totally extinguished. The *temporal island of the vision* is more resistant and is lost in the end leaving the patient with no light perception.
   - The damage to visual fields in glaucoma occurs in the order of superior-inferior-nasal-temporal-central.
4. **Ans. (A) +2D**

   Treatment of Presbyopia:

   A. Optical treatment: The treatment of presbyopia is the prescription of appropriate convex glasses for near work. A rough guide for providing presbyopic glasses in an emmetrope can be made from the age of the patient. ***Presbyopic spectacles*** may be unifocal, bifocal or varifocal
   - About +1 DS is required at the age of 40-45 years,
   - +1.5 DS at 45-50 years,
   - + 2 DS at 50-55 years, and
   - +2.5 DS at 55-60 years.
   - However, it should be estimated individually in each eye in order to determine how much is necessary to provide a comfortable range.

   Basic principles for presbyopic correction are:
   - Always find out refractive error for distance and first correct it.
   - Find out the presbyopic correction needed in each eye separately and add it to the distant correction.

- Near point should be fixed by taking due consideration for profession of the patient.
- The weakest convex lens with which an individual can see clearly at the near point should be prescribed, since overcorrection will also result in asthenopic symptoms.

B. Surgical Treatment of presbyopia is still in infancy.

5. **Ans. (D) Both are normal**
   - Diabetes mellitus (DM) leads to intrinsic ischemic damage ultimately leading to IIIrd nerve palsy. As the pupillomotor fibers travel outside the sheath of the IIIrd nerve, they avoid damage resulting in normal pupillary reactions.
   - In diabetics, a third nerve palsy is most common followed by sixth nerve, and less frequently, fourth nerve palsies. Diabetic third nerve palsies are characteristically pupil-sparing.
6. **Ans. (A) Central retinal vein occlusion (CRVO)**

   Central retinal vein occlusion (CRVO):
   - **Predisposing factors:**
     - Increasing age–6 to 7th decade
     - Systemic hypertension [most common]
     - Blood dyscrasias–hyperviscosity due to chronic leukemias and polycythemia
     - Raised IOP (POAG)
     - Periphlebitis–sarcoidosis, Behçet's disease
   - **Classification of CRVO:**
     - Nonischemic
     - Ischemic
   - **C/F:**
     - Tortuosity and dilation of retinal veins
     - Flame–shaped hemorrhage–**Splash tomato/Tomato ketchup fundus**
     - Cotton wool spots
     - Optic disc edema and hyperemia
   - **Complications:** Rubeosis iridis and neovascular glaucoma (NVG) occur in more than 50 percent cases within 3 months (so also called as 90 days glaucoma), a few cases develop vitreous hemorrhage and proliferative retinopathy.
   - **Treatment:** Panretinal photocoagulation (PRP) or cryoapplication, if the media is hazy, may be required to prevent neovascular glaucoma in patients with widespread capillary occlusion. Photocoagulation should be carried out when most

of the intraretinal blood is absorbed, which usually takes about 3-4 months.

- 100 day glaucoma or NVG results from conditions which lead to neovascularization in the eye, e.g. PDR, CRVO, retinal malignancies and rarely in CRAO.

7. **Ans. (D)** ***(Ref.Parsons' Diseases of the eye,21st edition)***

Trachoma: Trachoma (previously known as Egyptian ophthalmia) is a chronic keratoconjunctivitis primarily affecting the superficial epithelium of conjunctiva and cornea simultaneously. It is characterized by a mixed follicular and papillary response of conjunctival tissue. It is still one of the leading causes of preventable blindness in the world. The word 'trachoma' comes from the Greek word for 'rough' which describes the surface appearance of the conjunctiva in chronic trachoma.

Prevalence: It is a worldwide disease but it is highly prevalent in North Africa, Middle East and certain regions of South-East Asia. It is believed to affect some 500 million people in the world. There are about 150 million cases with active trachoma and about 30 million having trichiasis needing lid surgery. It is responsible for 15-20 percent of the world's blindness, being second only to cataract.

Sequelae of trachoma:

- Sequelae in the lids may be trichiasis, entropion, tylosis (thickening of lid margin), ptosis, madarosis and ankyloblepharon.
- Conjunctival sequelae include concretions, pseudocyst, xerosis and symblepharon.
- Corneal sequelae may be corneal opacity, ectasia, corneal xerosis and total corneal pannus (blinding sequelae).
- Other sequelae may be chronic dacryocystitis, and chronic dacryoadenitis.

Complications: The only complication of trachoma is corneal ulcer which may occur due to rubbing by concretions, or trichiasis with superimposed bacterial infection.

8. **Ans. (B) Floor**

Bony orbit: The bony orbits are quadrangular truncated pyramids situated between the anterior cranial fossa above and the maxillary sinuses below. Each orbit is about 40 mm in height, width and depth and is formed by portions of seven bones: (1) frontal, (2) maxilla,(3) zygomatic, (4) sphenoid, (5) palatine, (6) ethmoid and (7) lacrimal. It has four walls (medial, lateral, superior and inferior), base and an apex.

- ***The medial walls*** of two orbits are parallel to each other and being thinnest are frequently fractured during injuries as well as during orbitotomy operations, and it also accounts for ethmoiditis being the most common cause of orbital cellulitis.
- ***The inferior orbital wall*** (floor) is triangular in shape and being quite thin is commonly involved in blowout fractures and is easily invaded by tumors of the maxillary antrum.
- ***The lateral wall of the orbit*** is triangular in shape. It covers only posterior half of the eyeball. Therefore, palpation of the retrobulbar tumours is easier from this side. Because of its advantageous anatomical position, a surgical approach to the orbit by lateral orbitotomy is popular.
- ***The roof*** is triangular in shape and is formed mainly by the orbital plate of frontal bone.
- ***Base of the orbit*** is the anterior open end of the orbit. It is bounded by thick orbital margins.
- ***The orbital apex*** is the posterior end of orbit. Here the four orbital walls converge. It has two orifices, the *optic canal* which transmits optic nerve and ophthalmic artery and the *superior orbital fissure* which transmits a number of nerves, arteries and veins.

9. Ans. (B) *Streptococus*

Streptococcus is the most common organism implicated in ocular surface infections as it remains stable at cooler temperatures and is a conjunctival commensal.

10. Ans. (A) Acute leukemia

- *Subacute retinitis of Roth:* It typically occurs in patients suffering from subacute bacterial endocarditis (SABE). It is characterized by multiple superficial retinal hemorrhages involving posterior part of the fundus. Most of the hemorrhages have a white spot in the center (Roth's spot). Vision may be blurred due to involvement of the macular region or due to associated papillitis.
- Roth's spots may be observed in leukemia, diabetes, pernicious anemia, ischemic events, hypertensive retinopathy and rarely in HIV retinopathy.

11. Ans. (B) Treatment will be cylindrical/plano (-) lens

Combination of concave cylinder with plano sphere indicates myopia in one axis and normal neutralisation in other, the indicator of simple myopic astigmatism.

Refractive types of regular astigmatism: Depending upon the position of the two focal lines in relation to retina, the regular astigmatism is further classified into three types:

1. ***Simple astigmatism,*** wherein the rays are focused on the retina in one meridian and either in front (*simple myopic astigmatism*) or behind (*simple hypermetropic astigmatism*) the retina in the other meridian.
2. **Compound astigmatism:** In this type, the rays of light in both the meridian are focused either in front or behind the retina and the condition is labelled as *compound myopic* or *compound hypermetropic astigmatism*, respectively.
3. ***Mixed astigmatism*** refers to a condition wherein the light rays in one meridian are focused in front and in other meridian behind the retina. Thus in one meridian eye is myopic and in another hypermetropic. Such patients have comparatively less symptoms as 'circle of least *diffusion*' is formed on the retina.

Treatment:

1. ***Optical treatment*** of regular astigmatism comprises the prescribing appropriate cylindrical lens, discovered after accurate refraction.
   i. *Spectacles* with full correction of cylindrical power and appropriate axis should be used for distance and near vision.
   ii. *Contact lenses:* Rigid contact lenses may correct upto 2–3 of regular astigmatism, while soft contact lenses can correct only little astigmatism. For higher degrees of astigmatism toric contact lenses are needed. In order to maintain the correct axis of toric lenses, ballasting or truncation is required.
2. ***Surgical correction of astigmatism*** is quite effective.

10

ENT

1. High tracheostomy is done in a patient with consideration of the following in future?

A. Diphtheria infection
B. Ca larynx
C. Papillomatosis
D. Vocal polyps

2. Stimulater of auditory brainstem implant is placed in:

A. Recess of 4th ventricle
B. Scala tympanum
C. Oval window
D. EAC

3. Which of the following is the tensor of vocal cords?

A. Posterior cricoarytenoids
B. Lateral arytenoid
C. Thyroarytenoids
D. Cricothyroid

4. MC fungus causing orbital cellulitis in diabetic patients is?

A. Mucor
B. Rhizopus
C. Aspergillus
D. Candida

5. Water's view is used for:

A. Maxillary sinus
B. Frontal sinus
C. Sphenoid sinus
D. Mastoid air cells

6. Tracheostomy is indicated in all except?

A. Vocal cord replacement
B. Pharynx replacement
C. Tracheomalacia
D. Foreign body obstructing airway

Answers with Explanations

1. **Ans. (B) Ca larynx**

Tracheostomy is making an opening in the anterior wall of trachea and converting it into a stoma on the skin surface. Sometimes, the term tracheotomy has been interchangeably used but the latter actually means opening the trachea, which is a step in the tracheostomy operation.

Types of Tracheostomy

- Emergency tracheostomy
- Elective or tranquil tracheostomy
- Permanent tracheostomy
- Percutaneous dilatational tracheostomy
- Mini tracheostomy (cricothyroidotomy)
  It has also been divided into high, mid or low.
- A **high tracheostomy** is done above the level of thyroid isthmus (isthmus lies against II, III and IV tracheal rings). It violates the first ring of trachea. Tracheostomy at this site can cause perichondritis of the cricoid cartilage and subglottic stenosis and is always avoided. Only indication for high tracheostomy is carcinoma of larynx because in such cases, total larynx anyway would ultimately be removed and a fresh tracheostome made in a clean area lower down.
- A **mid tracheostomy** is the preferred one and is done through the II or III ring and would entail division of the thyroid isthmus or its retraction upwards or downwards to expose this part of trachea.
- A **low tracheostomy** is done below the level of isthmus. Trachea is deep at this level and close to several large vessels; also there are difficulties with tracheostomy tube which impinges on suprasternal notch.

2. **Ans. (A) Recess of 4th ventricle**

Auditory brainstem implant (ABI)

- This implant is designed to stimulate the cochlear nuclear complex in the brainstem directly by placing the implant in the lateral recess of the fourth ventricle. Such an implant is needed when CN VIII has been severed in surgery of vestibular schwannoma. In these cases, cochlear implants are obviously of no use.

- In unilateral acoustic neuroma, ABI is not necessary as hearing is possible from the contralateral side but in bilateral acoustic neuromas as in NF2, rehabilitation is required by ABI.
- Brainstem implant is similar to 'Nucleus' multichannel cochlear implant except that the multielectrode array is attached to a Dacron mesh, which is placed on the brainstem. Receiver/stimulator has a removable magnet so that MRI can be safely performed in such cases if need arises.
- ABIs help in communication, awareness and recognition of environmental sounds; however, they are not as efficient as multichannel cochlear implants. Only limited numbers of such implants have been performed in the world and are under constant technological developments.

3. Ans. (D) Cricothyroid

Muscles of Larynx

They are of two types—intrinsic, which attach laryngeal cartilages to each other and extrinsic, which attach larynx to the surrounding structures.

1. **Intrinsic muscles:** They may act on vocal cords or laryngeal inlet.
   - Acting on vocal cords
     - Abductors: Posterior cricoarytenoid
     - Adductors: Lateral cricoarytenoid, interarytenoid (transverse arytenoid), thyroarytenoid (external part)
     - Tensors: Cricothyroid, vocalis (internal part of thyroarytenoid)
   - Acting on laryngeal inlet
     - **Openers of laryngeal inlet:** Thyroepiglottic (part of thyroarytenoid)
     - **Closers of laryngeal inlet:** Interarytenoid (oblique part), aryepiglottic (posterior oblique part of interarytenoids)
2. **Extrinsic muscles:** They connect the larynx to the neighboring structures and are divided into elevators or depressors of larynx.
   - **Elevators:** Primary elevators act directly as they are attached to the thyroid cartilage and include stylopharyngeus, salpingopharyngeus, palatopharyngeus and thyrohyoid. Secondary elevators act indirectly as they are attached to the hyoid bone and include mylohyoid (main), digastric, stylohyoid and geniohyoid.

- **Depressors:** They include sternohyoid, sternothyroid and omohyoid.

4. **Ans. (A) Mucor**

Mucormycosis: It is a fungal infection of nose and paranasal sinuses which may prove rapidly fatal. It is seen in uncontrolled diabetics or in those taking immunosuppressive drugs.

- From the nose and sinuses, infection can spread to orbit, cribriform plate, meninges and brain. The rapid destruction associated with the disease is due to affinity of the fungus to invade the arteries and cause endothelial damage and thrombosis.
- Typical finding is the presence of a black necrotic mass filling the nasal cavity and eroding the septum and hard palate. Special stains help to identify the fungus in tissue sections.
- Treatment is by amphotericin B and surgical debridement of the affected tissues and control of underlying predisposing cause.
- Mucormycosis must be suspected in all diabetic patients, particularly those in ketoacidosis, and any debilitated or immunocompromised individual with multiple cranial nerve palsies with or without proptosis.
- It requires immediate hospitalization because this is a rapidly progressive and possibly life-threatening disease and the treatment is complex both medical and surgical and must be conducted in a multidisciplinary team.

5. **Ans. (A) Maxillary sinus**

Maxillary sinus (antrum of highmore): It is the largest of paranasal sinuses and occupies the body of maxilla. It is pyramidal in shape with base towards lateral wall of nose and apex directed laterally into the zygomatic process of maxilla and sometimes in the zygomatic bone itself. On an average, maxillary sinus has a capacity of 15 mL in an adult. It is 33 mm high, 35 mm deep and 25 mm wide.

Relations

- Anterior wall is formed by facial surface of maxilla and is related to the soft tissues of cheek.
- Posterior wall is related to infratemporal and pterygopalatine fossa.
- Medial wall is related to the middle and inferior meatuses. At places, this wall is thin and membranous. It is related to uncinate process, anterior and posterior fontanelle and inferior turbinate and meatus.

- Floor is formed by alveolar and palatine processes of the maxilla and is situated about 1 cm below the level of floor of nose. Usually it is related to the roots of second premolar and first molar teeth. Depending on the age of the person and pneumatization of the sinus, the roots of all the molars, sometimes the premolars and canine are in close relation to the floor of maxillary sinus separated from it by a thin lamina of bone or even no bone at all. Oroantral fistula can result from extraction of any of these teeth. Dental infection is also an important cause of maxillary sinusitis. Ostium of the maxillary sinus is situated high up in medial wall and opens in the posteroinferior part of ethmoidal infundibulum into the middle meatus. It is unfavorably situated for natural drainage. An accessory ostium is also present behind the main ostium in 30% of cases.
- Roof of the maxillary sinus is formed by the floor of the orbit. It is traversed by infraorbital nerve and vessels.

Acute Maxillary Sinusitis

Etiology

- Most commonly, it is viral rhinitis which spreads to involve the sinus mucosa. This is followed by bacterial invasion.
- Diving and swimming in contaminated water.
- Dental infections are important source of maxillary sinusitis. Roots of premolar and molar teeth are related to the floor of sinus and may be separated only by a thin layer of mucosal covering. Periapical dental abscess may burst into the sinus; or the root of a tooth, during extraction may be pushed into the sinus. In case of oroantral fistula, following tooth extraction, bacteria from oral cavity enter the maxillary sinus.
- Trauma to the sinus such as compound fractures, penetrating injuries or gunshot wounds may be followed by sinusitis.

Predisposing factors: One or more of the predisposing factors enumerated for sinusitis in general may be responsible for acute or recurrent infection.

Clinical features: Clinical features depend on—(i) severity of inflammatory process and (ii) efficiency of ostium to drain the exudates. Closed ostium sinusitis is of greater severity and leads more often to complications.

- **Constitutional symptoms:** It consist of fever, general malaise and bodyache. They are the result of toxemia.
- **Headache:** Usually, this is confined to forehead and may thus be confused with frontal sinusitis.

- **Pain:** Typically, it is situated over the upper jaw, but may be referred to the gums or teeth. For this reason patient may primarily consult a dentist. Pain is aggravated by stooping, coughing or chewing. Occasionally, pain is referred to the ipsilateral supraorbital region and thus may simulate frontal sinus infection.
- **Tenderness:** Pressure or tapping over the anterior wall of antrum produces pain.
- **Redness and edema of cheek:** Commonly seen in children. The lower eyelid may become puffy.
- **Nasal discharge:** Anterior rhinoscopy/nasal endoscopy shows pus or mucopus in the middle meatus. Mucosa of the middle meatus and turbinate may appear red and swollen. Postural test: If no pus seen in the middle meatus, it is decongested with a pledget of cotton soaked with a vasoconstrictor and the patient is made to sit with the affected sinus turned up. Examination after 10–15 min may show discharge in the middle meatus.
- **Postnasal discharge:** Pus may be seen on the upper soft palate on posterior rhinoscopy or nasal endoscopy.

Diagnosis:

- **Transillumination test:** Affected sinus will be found opaque.
- **X-rays:** Waters' view will show either an opacity or a fluid level in the involved sinus.
- **Computed tomography (CT) scan** is the preferred imaging modality to investigate the sinuses.

Treatment

A. *Medical*

- **Antimicrobial drugs:** Ampicillin and amoxicillin are quite effective and cover a wide range of organisms. Erythromycin or doxycycline or cotrimoxazole are equally effective and can be given to those who are sensitive to penicillin. β-lactamase-producing strains of *H. influenzae* and *M. catarrhalis* may necessitate the use of amoxicillin/clavulanic acid or cefuroxime axetil. Sparfloxacin is also effective and has the advantage of single daily dose.
- **Nasal decongestant drops:** One percent ephedrine or 0.1% xylo- or oxymetazoline are used as nasal drops or sprays to decongest sinus ostium and encourage drainage.
- **Steam inhalation:** Steam alone or medicated with menthol or Tincture Benzoin Compound provides symptomatic relief and

encourages sinus drainage. Inhalation should be given 15–20 min after nasal decongestion for better penetration.

- **Analgesics:** Paracetamol or any other suitable analgesic should be given for relief of pain and headache.
- **Hot fomentation:** Local heat to the affected sinus is often soothing and helps in the resolution of inflammation.

B. *Surgical*

- **Antral lavage:** Most cases of acute maxillary sinusitis respond to medical treatment. Lavage is rarely necessary. It is done only when medical treatment has failed and that too only under cover of antibiotics.

Complications

- Acute maxillary sinusitis may change to subacute or chronic sinusitis.
- Frontal sinusitis: Due to obstruction of frontal sinus drainage pathway because of edema.
- Osteitis or osteomyelitis of the maxilla.
- Orbital cellulitis or abscess: Infection spreads to the orbit because of edema either directly from the roof of maxillary sinus or indirectly after involvement of ethmoid sinuses.

6. Ans. (C) Tracheomalacia

Indications for tracheostomy

- Respiratory obstruction
  - Infections
    - Acute laryngo-tracheo-bronchitis, acute epiglottitis, diphtheria
    - Ludwig's angina, peritonsillar, retropharyngeal or parapharyngeal abscess, tongue abscess
  - Trauma
    - External injury of larynx and trachea
    - Trauma due to endoscopies especially in infants and children
    - Fractures of mandible or maxillofacial injuries
  - **Neoplasms:** Benign and malignant neoplasms of larynx, pharynx, upper trachea, tongue and thyroid
  - Foreign body larynx
  - Edema larynx due to steam, irritant fumes or gases, allergy (angioneurotic or drug sensitivity), radiation
  - Bilateral abductor paralysis
  - Congenital anomalies–laryngeal web, cysts, tracheoesophageal fistula–bilateral choanal atresia

- Retained secretions
  - Inability to cough
    - Coma of any cause, e.g. head injuries, cerebrovascular accidents, narcotic overdose
    - Paralysis of respiratory muscles, e.g. spinal injuries, polio, Guillain–Barre syndrome, myasthenia gravis
    - Spasm of respiratory muscles, tetanus, eclampsia, strychnine poisoning
  - Painful cough chest injuries, multiple rib fractures, pneumonia
  - Aspiration of pharyngeal secretions bulbar polio, polyneuritis, bilateral laryngeal paralysis
- Respiratory insufficiency chronic lung conditions, viz. emphysema, chronic bronchitis, bronchiectasis, atelectasis conditions listed in A and B.

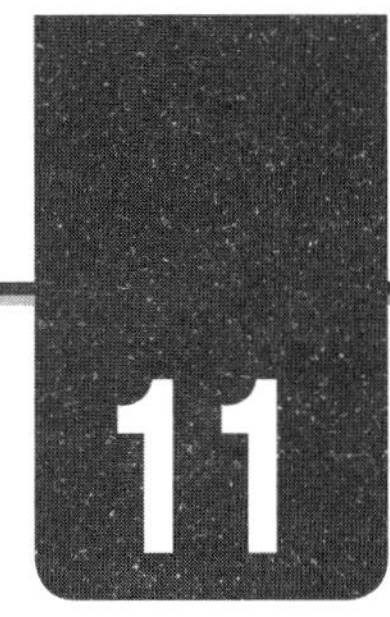

11 Preventive and Social Medicine

1. New RNTCP software online TB monitoring is:

A. Nikshay
B. Nirbhya
C. e-DOT
D. Nischay

2. In a study, the remission rate of the new drug was found to be equal to the remission rate of a drug already in use. P value = 0.4. Which of the following is true?

A. Insufficient data to compare the two drugs
B. Both drugs are ineffective
C. Both drugs are effective
D. Power of study is 60 percent

3. Iodine requirement in pregnant women in micrograms per ml is:

A. 200
B. 150
C. 100
D. 250

4. Most peripheral unit of microscopic center of TB is:

A. District microscopy center
B. TB unit
C. PHC
D. Peripheral microscopy unit

5. Prevalence of Kala-azar is not seen in:

A. UP
B. Bihar
C. West Bengal
D. Assam

6. Screening test was applied on a particular disease, out of 1000 population 90 were tested positive, it was compared with gold standard test which showed 100 were positive. What is the sensitivity of the new screening test?

A. 90/1000
B. 90/100
C. 100/100
D. 90–10/100

7. Which one of the following is not included in the mission Indradhanush scheme of vaccine?

A. TB
B. Diphtheria
C. Polio
D. Japanese encephalitis

8. Hardness of water is not due to:

A. Calcium carbonate
B. Calcium sulphate
C. Calcium bicarbonate
D. Magnesium bicarbonate

9. 10 women got pregnant out of 100 women, mean interval was 2 years. Calculate Pearl index.

A. 5
B. 10
C. 2
D. 4

10. For Net NFR to be 1 couple protection rate should be:

A. 60%
B. 100%
C. 40%
D. 80%

11. Cytotoxic and expired drugs are disposed by:

A. Incineration
B. Deep burial
C. Chemical treatment
D. Autoclaving

12. Chlorine disinfection of water is due to which ions?

A. Hypochlorous acid
B. Hypochlorite ions
C. Hydrogen ions
D. Hydrochloric acid

13. Study unit of ecological study is:

A. Population
B. Individual
C. Society
D. Community

14. Which of the following constitutional article is not related to children rights?

A. 46
B. 39
C. 45
D. 23

15. Which of the following statement regarding Factory Act is correct?

A. Child age less than 14 years cannot be employed in dangerous work
B. Child age less than 18 years cannot be employed
C. Working hours should not be more than 40 hours per week for adults
D. Working hours are 8 hours per day for children

16. Incidence of a disease is 4 per 1000 of population with duration of 2 years. Calculate the prevalence.

A. 8/1000
B. 4/1000
C. 2/1000
D. 6/1000

17. Risk among exposed by risk among non-exposed is defined to be?

A. Relative risk
B. Odds ratio
C. Attributable risk
D. None of the above

18. Pasteurization of milk is done at:

A. 73°C for 20 minutes
B. 63°C for 30 minutes
C. 72°C for 30 seconds
D. 63°C for 30 seconds

19. Susceptible person developed disease within range of IP after coming in contact with primary case is known as:

A. Secondary attack rate
B. Case fatality rate
C. Primary attack rate
D. Tertiary attack rate

20. Which of the following is not an example of direct transmission in communicable diseases?

A. Transplacental
B. Soil
C. Respiratory
D. STDs

Answers with Explanations

1. **Ans. (A) Nikshay**
   - **New initiatives in RNTCP:** The RNTCP has completed the feasibility study of introducing GeneXpert in RNTCP in 18 Tuberculosis Units in 12 states. RNTCP is currently using CB-NAAT for the diagnosis of tuberculosis and MDR-TB in high-risk population like HIV positive and pediatric groups.
   - **Nikshay: TB surveillance using case-based web-based IT system.** Central TB Division in collaboration with National Informatics Center has undertaken the initiative to develop a case-based web-based application named Nikshay. This software was launched in May 2012 and has following functional components:
     - Master management
     - User details
     - TB patient registration and details of diagnosis, DOT provider, HIV status, follow-up, contact tracing, outcomes.
     - Details of solid and liquid culture and DST, LPA, CBNMT details
     - MDR-TB patient registration with details
     - Referral and transfer of patients
     - Private health facility registration and TB notification
     - Mobile application for TB notification
     - SMS alerts to patients on registration
     - SMS alerts to programme officers
     - Automated periodic reports
       - Case finding
       - Sputum conversion
       - Treatment outcome.
   - **TB notification:** In order to ensure proper diagnosis and management of TB cases, and to reduce TB transmission and the emergence and spread of MDR-TB, it is essential to have complete information of all TB cases. According to the Government of India notification dated 7th May 2012, it is now mandatory for all healthcare providers to notify every TB case to local authorities, i.e. District Health Officer/Chief Medical Officer of a district and Municipal Health Officer, every month in a given format. At present, 57,000 health facilities have been registered and 35,000 patients have been notified.

- **Ban on TB serology:** The serological tests are based on antibody response, which is highly variable in TB and may reflect remote infection rather than active disease. Currently available serological tests are having poor specificity and should not be used for the diagnosis of pulmonary or extrapulmonary TB. Their import, manufacturing, sale, distribution and use are banned by the Government of India.

2. **Ans. (C) Both drugs are effective**

   According to convention, if *P* is less than or equal to 0.05, it is regarded as 'statistically significant'. The smaller the *P* value, the greater the statistical significance or probability that the association is not due to chance alone. However, statistical association (*P* value) does not imply causation. Statement of *P* value is thus an inadequate, although common end-point of case-control studies.
   - A small *p*-value (typically ≤ 0.05) indicates strong evidence against the null hypothesis, so you reject the null hypothesis.
   - A large *p*-value (> 0.05) indicates weak evidence against the null hypothesis, so you fail to reject the null hypothesis.
   - *p*-values very close to the cutoff (0.05) are considered to be marginal (could go either way). Always report the *p*-value so that readers can draw their own conclusions.

3. **Ans. (D) 250**

   The daily requirement of iodine for adults is placed at 150 micrograms. The recommendations of WHO of 250 mcg per day for iodine during pregnancy have also been adopted. This amount is normally supplied by the well balanced diet and drinking water except in regions where food and water are deficient in iodine.

4. **Ans. (D) Peripheral microscopy unit**

   Designated microscopy center (DMC): The most peripheral laboratory under the RNTCP network is the DMC which serves a population of around 100,000 (50,000 in tribal and hilly areas).
   - Currently all the districts in the country are implementing EQA. For quality improvement purposes, the NRL on-site evaluation (OSE) recommendations to IRLs and districts are discussed in the RNTCP laboratory committee meetings, quarterly at CTD.
   - Quality improvement workshops for the state level TB officers and laboratory managers are conducted at NRLs based on the observations of the NRL-OSEs. These workshops focus on issues such as human resources,trainings, AMC for binocular microscopes, quality specifications for ZN stains, RBRC blinding and coding issues, bio-medical waste disposal, infection control measures, etc.

- The quality assurance activities include:
  - On-site evaluation
  - Panel testing
  - Random blinded rechecking.

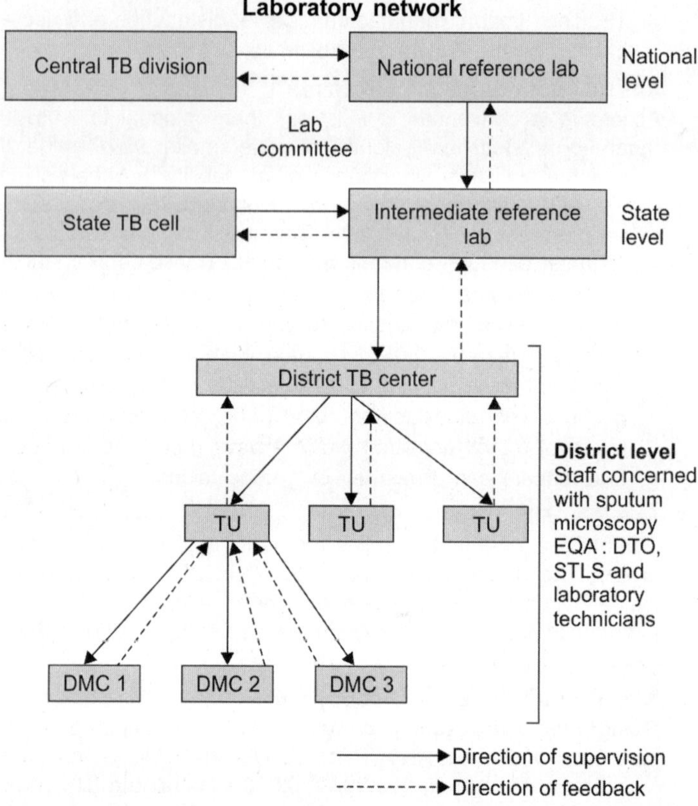

5. Ans. (D) Assam

- Kala-azar has re-emerged from near eradication. The annual estimate for the incidence and prevalence of kala-azar cases worldwide is 0.5 million and 2.5 million, respectively. Of these, 90% of the confirmed cases occur in India, Nepal, Bangladesh and Sudan.
- In India, it is a serious problem in Bihar, West Bengal and eastern Uttar Pradesh where there is underreporting of kala-azar and post kala-azar dermal leishmaniasis in women and children 0–9 years of age.
- Untreated cases of kala-azar are associated with up to 90% mortality, with treatment reduces to 15% and 3.4% even in

specialized hospitals. It is also associated with up to 20% in subclinical infection.

- Spraying of DDT helped control kala-azar; however, there are reports of the vector Phlebotomus argentipes developing resistance. Also lymphadenopathy, a major presenting feature in India raises the possibility of a new vector or a variant of the disease.
- The widespread coexistence of malaria and kala-azar in Bihar may lead to a difficulty in diagnosis and inappropriate treatment. In addition, reports of the organism developing resistance to sodium antimony gluconate—the main drug for the treatment—would make its eradication difficult.
- Clinical trials in India have reported encouraging results with amphotericin B (recommended as a third-line drug by the National Malaria Eradication Programme).
- Phase III Trials with a first-generation vaccine (killed Leishmania organism mixed with a low concentration of BCG as an adjuvant) have also yielded promising results. Preliminary studies using autoclaved Leishmania major mixed with BCG have been successful in preventing infection with *Leishmania donovani*.
- Until a safe and effective vaccine is developed, a combination of sandfly control, detection and treatment of patients and prevention of drug resistance is the best approach for controlling kala-azar.

6. **Ans. (B) 90/100**

Evaluation of a screening test

Screening test result by diagnosis

Screening test results	*Diagnosis*		*Total*
	Diseased	*Not diseased*	
Positive	a (True-positive)	b (False-negative)	a + b
Negative	c (False-negative)	d (True-positive)	c + d
Total	a + c	b + d	a + b + c + d

The following measures are used to evaluate a screening test:

- Sensitivity = a/(a + c) x 100
- Specificity = d/(b + d) x 100
- Predictive value of a positive test = a/(a + b) x 100
- Predictive value of a negative test = d/(c + d) x 100
- Percentage of false-negative = c/(a + c) x 100
- Percentage of true-positive = b/(b + d) x 100s

From the question, a here is 90 and a + c = 100
So, sensitivity of screening test is = 90/100.

7. **Ans. (D) Japanese encephalitis**

Mission Indradhanush: The Government of India has launched Mission Indradhanush on 25th December 2014 to cover children who are either unvaccinated or partially vaccinated against seven vaccine preventable diseases, i.e. diphtheria, whooping cough, tetanus, polio, tuberculosis, measles and hepatitis B. The goal is to vaccinate all under-fives by the year 2020. Under the programme, four special vaccination campaigns will be conducted between January and June 2015. Intensive planning and monitoring experience of pulse polio immunization programme will be used. 201 high focus districts will be covered in the first phase. Of these 82 districts are from Uttar Pradesh, Bihar, Madhya Pradesh and Rajasthan. These 201 districts have nearly 50 percent of all unvaccinated children of the country. The drive will be through a 'catch-up' campaign mode. The mission will be technically supported by WHO, UNICEF, Rotary International and other donor partners.

8. **Ans. (A) Calcium carbonate**

- Hardness may be defined as the soap destroying power of water. The consumer considers water is hard if large amounts of soap are required to produce lather. The hardness in water is caused mainly by four dissolved compounds. These are:
  1. Calcium bicarbonate
  2. Magnesium bicarbonate
  3. Calcium sulphate
  4. Magnesium sulphate

  The presence of any one of these compounds produces hardness. There are others which are of less importance. Chlorides and nitrates of calcium and magnesium can also cause hardness but they occur generally in small amounts. Iron, manganese and aluminium compounds also cause hardness, but as they generally are present in such small amounts, it is customary not to consider them in connection with hardness.
- Hardness is classified as carbonate and non-carbonate. The carbonate hardness which was formerly designated as 'temporary' hardness is due to the presence of calcium and magnesium bicarbonates. The non-carbonate hardness formerly designated as 'permanent' hardness is due to calcium and magnesium sulphates, chlorides and nitrates.

- Hardness in water is expressed in terms of 'milliequivalents per litre (mEq/L)'. One mEq/L of hardness producing ion is equal to 50 mg $CaCO_3$ (50 ppm) in 1 litre of water. The terms soft and hard water are used when the levels of hardness are as given in the table.

- Drinking water should be moderately hard. Softening of water is recommended when the hardness exceeds 3 mEq/L (150 mg per liter).

Classification of hardness in water	
Classification	*Level of hardness (mEg/liter)*
Soft water	Less than 1 (<50 mg/L)
Moderately hard	1–3 (50–150 mg/L)
Hard water	3–6 (150–300 mg/L)
Very hard water	Over 6 (> 300 mg/L)

9. **Ans. (A) 5**

   The Pearl index is defined as the number of 'failures per 100 woman-years of exposure (HWY).' This rate is given by the formula:

   Failure rate per HWY = Total accidental pregnancies/total months of exposure x 1200

   From question, Pearl index = 10/24 x 1200 = 500 or 5%.

10. **Ans. (A) 60%**
    - The acceptance of the primary health care approach to the achievement of HFA/2000 AD led to the formulation of a National Health Policy in 1982. The National Health Policy was approved by the Parliament in 1983.
    - It laid down the long-term demographic goal of NRR = 1 by the year 2000 which implies a 2-child family norm - through the attainment of a birth rate of 21 and a death rate of 9 per thousand population, and a couple protection rate of 60 percent by the year 2000.
    - The Sixth and Seventh Five-Year Plans were accordingly set to achieve these goals. The National Health Policy also called for restructuring the healthcare delivery system to achieve HFA/2000 AD, and family planning has been accorded a central place in the health development.
    - Couple protection rate (CPR) is an indicator of the prevalence of contraceptive practice in the community. It is defined as the percent of eligible couples effectively protected against childbirth by one or the other approved methods of family planning, viz. sterilization, IUD, condom or oral pills. Sterilization accounts for over 60 percent of effectively protected couples. Demographers are of the view that the demographic goal of NRR= 1 can be achieved only if the CPR exceeds 60 percent.

11. Ans. (A) incineration

Schedule I: Categories of biomedical wastes (BMW)		
Waste category no.	*Waste category type*	*Treatment and disposal options*
Category 1	**Human anatomical waste:** Human tissues, organs, body parts	Incineration/deep burial
Category 2	**Animal waste:** Animal tissues, organs, body parts carcasses, bleeding parts, fluid, blood and experimental animals used in research, waste generated by veterinary hospital, animal house	Incineration/deep burial
Category 3	**Microbiology and biotechnology waste:** Wastes from laboratory cultures, stocks or specimens of microorganisms live or attenuated vaccines, human and animal cell culture used/research and infectious agents from research and industrial laboratories, wastes from production of biologicals, toxins, dishes and devices used for transfer of cultures	Local autoclaving/ micro waving/ incineration
Category 4	**Waste sharps:** Needles, syringes, scalpels, blades, glass, etc. that may cause puncture and cuts. This includes both used and unused sharps	Disinfection (chemical treatment/ autoclaving/ microwaving and mutilation/shredding)
Category 5	**Discarded Medicines and cyto-toxic drugs:** Wastes comprising of outdated, contaminated and discarded medicines	Incineration/ autoclaving/micro-waving
Category 6	**Soiled waste:** Items contaminated with blood, and body fluids including cotton, dressings, soiled plaster casts, lines, bedding, other material contaminated with blood	Incineration/ autoclaving/micro waving
Category 7	**Solid waste:** Wastes generated from disposable items other than the waste sharps such as tubing, catheters, intravenous sets, etc.	Disinfection by chemical treatment/ autoclaving/ microwaving and mutilation/shredding

Contd...

Contd...

Waste category no.	*Waste category type*	*Treatment and disposal options*
Category 8	**Liquid waste:** Waste generated from laboratory and washing, cleaning, housekeeping and disinfecting activities	Disinfection by chemical treatment and discharge into drain
Category 9	**Incineration ash:** Ash from incineration of any biomedical waste	Disposal in municipal landfill
Category 10	**Chemical waste:** Chemicals used in the production of biologicals, chemicals used in disinfection, insecticides, etc.	Chemical treatment and discharge into drains for liquids and secured landfill for solids

12. Ans. (A) Hypochlorous acid

- Chlorination is one of the greatest advances in water purification. It is a supplement not a substitute to sand filtration. Chlorine kills pathogenic bacteria, but it has no effect on spores and certain viruses (e.g. polio, viral hepatitis) except in high doses. Apart from its germicidal effect, chlorine has several important secondary properties of value in water treatment: It oxidizes iron, manganese and hydrogen sulphide; it destroys some taste and odor producing constituents; it controls algae and slime organisms; and aids coagulation.
- **Action of chlorine:** When chlorine is added to water, there is a formation of hydrochloric and hypochlorous acids. The hydrochloric acid is neutralized by the alkalinity of the water. The hypochlorous acid ionizes to form hydrogen ions and hypochlorite ions, as follows:

  H2O + Cl2 = HCl + HOCl

  HOCL= H + OCl
- The disinfecting action of chlorine is mainly due to the hypochlorous acid, and to a small extent due to the hypochlorite ions. The hypochlorous acid is the most effective form of chlorine for water disinfection. It is more effective (70-80 times) than the hypochlorite ion. Chlorine acts best as a disinfectant when the pH of water is around 7 because of the predominance of hypochlorous acid. When the pH value exceeds 8.5 it is unreliable as a disinfectant because about 90 percent of the hypochlorous acid gets ionized to hypochlorite ions. It is fortunate that most waters have a pH value between 6-7.5.

- **Principles of chlorination:** The mere addition of chlorine to water is not chlorination. There are certain rules which should be obeyed in order to ensure proper chlorination:
  - First of all, the water to be chlorinated should be clear and free from turbidity. Turbidity impedes efficient chlorination.
  - Secondly, the 'chlorine demand' of the water should be estimated. 'The chlorine demand of water is the difference between the amount of chlorine added to the water and the amount of residual chlorine remaining at the end of a specific period of contact (usually 60 minutes) at a given temperature and pH of the water'. In other words, it is the amount of chlorine that is needed to destroy bacteria and to oxidize all the organic matter and ammoniacal substances present in the water. The point at which the chlorine demand of the water is met is called the 'breakpoint'. If further chlorine is added beyond the breakpoint, free *chlorine* (HOCl and OCl) begins to appear in the water.
  - Thirdly the contact period. The presence of free residual chlorine for a contact period of at least 1 hour is essential to kill bacteria and viruses. It should be noted however, that chlorine has no effect on spores, protozoan cysts and helminthic ova, except in higher doses.
  - The minimum recommended concentration of free chlorine is 0.5 mg/L for one hour. The free residual chlorine provides a margin of safety against subsequent microbial contamination such as may occur during storage and distribution.
  - The sum of the chlorine demand of the specific water plus the free residual chlorine of 0.5 mg/L constitutes the correct dose of chlorine to be applied.

13. Ans. (A) Population

Epidemiological studies can be classified as observational studies and experimental studies with further subdivisions, which are as follows:

Observational studies

- Descriptive studies
- Analytical studies
  - Ecological or correlational with populations as unit of study
  - Cross-sectional or prevalence with individuals as unit of study
  - Case-control or case reference with individuals as unit of study
  - Cohort or follow-up with individuals as unit of study

Experimental studies or intervention studies

- Randomized controlled trails or clinical trials with patients as unit of study

- Field trials with healthy people as unit of study
- Community trials or community intervention studies with communities as unit of study.

14. Ans. (A) 46

Constitution of India

The Indian constitution accords rights to children as citizens of the country, and in keeping with their special status the state has even enacted special laws. The government has the flexibility to undertake appropriate legislative and administrative measures to ensure children's rights; no court can make the government ensure them, as these are essentially directives. These directives have enabled the judiciary to give some landmark judgements promoting children's rights, leading to Constitutional Amendments as is in the case of the 86th Amendment to the Constitution that made Right to Education a fundamental right.

Constitutional guarantees that are meant specifically for children include

- Right to free and compulsory elementary education for all children in the 6–14 year age group (Article 21 A)
- Right to be protected from any hazardous employment till the age of 14 years (Article 24)
- Right to be protected from being abused and forced by economic necessity to enter occupations unsuited to their age or strength (Article 39(e))
- Right to equal opportunities and facilities to develop in a healthy manner and in conditions of freedom and dignity and guaranteed protection of childhood and youth against exploitation and against moral and material abandonment (Article 39 (f))
- Right to early childhood care and education to all children until they complete the age of six years (Article 45).

Besides, children also have rights as equal citizens of India, just as any other adult male or female

- Right to equality (Article 14)
- Right against discrimination (Article 15)
- Right to personal liberty and due process of law (Article 21)
- Right to being protected from being trafficked and forced into bonded labour (Article 23)
- Right of minorities for protection of their interests (Article 29)
- Right of weaker sections of the people to be protected from social injustice and all forms of exploitation (Article 46)
- Right to nutrition and standard of living and improved public health (Article 47)

15. **Ans. (A) Child age less than 14 years cannot be employed in dangerous work**

- **Employment of young persons:** The Factory Act prohibits employment of children below the age of 14 years and declares persons between the ages 15 and 18 to be adolescents. Adolescents should be duly certified by the 'certifying surgeons' regarding their fitness for work. Restrictions have been laid down on employment of women and children in certain dangerous occupations. Child who has not completed his fourteenth year of age has been restricted from employment in any factory. Adolescent employee is allowed to work only between 6 am and 7 pm.
- **Hours of work:** The Act has prescribed a maximum of 48 working hours per week, not exceeding 9 hours per day with rest for at least half hour after 5 hours of continuous work. For adolescents, the hours of work have been reduced from 5 to 4½ per day. The 1976 amendment makes a provision to increase the spread-over period of work (including rest intervals) of an employee in a factory upto 12 hours from the existing 101/2 hours. The total number of hours of work in a week including overtime shall not exceed 60.

16. **Ans. (A) 8/1000**

The term 'disease prevalence' refers specifically to all current cases (old and new) existing at a given point in time, or over a period of time in a given population. A broader definition of prevalence is as follows: 'the total number of all individuals who have an attribute or disease at a particular time (or during a particular period) divided by the population at risk of having the attribute or disease at this point in time or midway through the period'. Although referred to as a rate, prevalence rate is really a ratio.

Prevalence is of two types:

1. Point prevalence
2. Period prevalence

Its calculated as: P = I x D = Incidence x mean duration

So from question, P = 4 x 2 per 1000 = 8/1000.

17. **Ans. (A) Relative risk**

The estimation of disease risk associated with exposure is obtained by an index known as 'Relative Risk' (RR) or 'risk ratio' which is defined as the ratio between the incidence of disease among exposed persons and incidence among non-exposed. It is given by the formula:

Relative risk = Incidence among exposed/incidence among non-exposed

A typical case control study does not provide incidence rates from which relative risk can be calculated directly because there is no appropriate denominator or population at risk to calculate these rates. In general, the relative risk can be exactly determined only from a cohort study.

18. Ans. (B) 63°C for 30 minutes

Pasteurization of milk

- It may be defined as the heating of milk to such temperatures and for such periods of time as are required to destroy any pathogens that may be present while causing minimal changes in the composition, flavor and nutritive value. There are several methods of pasteurization. Three are widely used:
    1. **Holder (Vat) method:** In this process, milk is kept at 63–66°C for at least 30 minutes, and then quickly cooled to 5°C. Vat method is recommended for small and rural communities. In larger cities, it is going out of use.
    2. **HTST method:** Also known as 'high temperature and short time method'. Milk is rapidly heated to a temperature of nearly 72°C is held at that temperature for not less than 15 seconds, and is then rapidly cooled to 4°C. This is now the most widely used method. Very large quantities of milk per hour can be pasteurized by this method.
    3. **UHT method:** Also known as 'ultra-high temperature method.' Milk is rapidly heated usually in 2 stages (the second stage usually being under pressure) to 125°C for a few seconds only. It is then rapidly cooled and bottled as quickly as possible.
- Pasteurization is a preventive measure of public health importance and corresponds in all respects to the modern principles of supplying safe milk. It kills nearly 90 percent of the bacteria in milk including the more heat-resistant tubercle bacillus and the Q fever organisms.
- But it will not kill thermoduric bacteria nor the bacterial spores. Therefore, despite pasteurization, with subsequent rise in temperature, the bacteria are bound to multiply. In order to check the growth of microorganisms, pasteurized milk is rapidly cooled to 4°C. It should be kept cold until it reaches the consumer. Hygienically produced pasteurized milk has a keeping quality of not more than 8 to 12 hours at 18°C.

Tests of pasteurized milk

- **Phosphatase test:** This test is widely used to check the efficiency of pasteurization. The test is based on the fact that raw milk contains an enzyme called phosphatase which is destroyed on heating at a temperature which corresponds closely with the standard time and temperature required for pasteurization. At 60°C for 30 minutes phosphatase is completely destroyed. Consequently, the test is used to detect inadequate pasteurization or the addition of raw milk.

- **Standard plate count:** The bacteriological quality of pasteurized milk is determined by the standard plate count. Most countries in the West enforce a limit of 30,000 bacterial count per ml of pasteurized milk.
- **Coliform count:** Coliform organisms are usually completely destroyed by pasteurization, and therefore, their presence in pasteurized milk is an indication either of improper pasteurization or post-pasteurization contamination. The standard in most countries is that coliforms be absent in 1 mL of milk.

19. Ans. (A) Secondary attack rate

- Secondary attack rate (SAR) is defined as 'the number of exposed persons developing the disease within the range of the incubation period following exposure to the primary case'. It is given by the formula:

  SAR = Number of exposed persons developing the disease within the range of the incubation period/total number of exposed/'susceptible' contacts x 100

- The denominator consists of all persons who are exposed to the case. More specifically, the denominator may be restricted only to 'susceptible' contacts, if means are available to distinguish the susceptible persons from the immune. The primary case is excluded from both the numerator and denominator.
- Supposing there is a family of 6 consisting of 2 parents (already immune) and 4 children who are susceptible to a specific disease, say measles. There is a primary case and within a short time 2 secondary cases among the remaining children. The secondary attack rate is 2/3 or 66.6 percent. The primary case is excluded from both numerator and denominator.
- Secondary attack rate is limited in its application to infectious diseases in which the primary case is infective for only a short period of time measured in days (e.g. measles and chickenpox). When the primary case is infective over a long-period of time (e.g. tuberculosis), duration of exposure is an important factor in determining the extent of spread.
- Another limitation of secondary attack rate is to identify 'susceptibles'. It is feasible only in diseases such as measles and

chickenpox where history can be used as a basis for identification; but in many others, susceptibles cannot be readily identified (e.g. influenza). In such cases, secondary attack rate is based on all exposed family members and still remains a useful tool. Where there are numerous subclinical cases, secondary attack rate has a limited meaning.

- Further spread cannot be measured without laboratory investigations. An additional advantage of the secondary attack rate is that vaccines and non-vaccines from several families can be added to determine the overall attack rates in the vaccinated and unvaccinated populations, provided the same definitions for cases and immunization status are used.
- Secondary attack rate was initially developed to measure the spread of an infection within a family, household or any closed aggregate of persons who have had contact with a case of disease. It is also useful to determine whether a disease of unknown aetiology (e.g. Hodgkin's disease) is communicable or not; and in evaluating the effectiveness of control measures such as isolation and immunization.

20. Ans. (B) Soil

Modes of Transmission

Once an infectious agent leaves a reservoir, it must get transmitted to a new host if it is to multiply and cause disease. The route by which an infectious agent is transmitted from a reservoir to another host is called the mode of transmission. Various direct and indirect modes of transmission are:

- **Direct modes of transmission:** Direct transmission refers to the transfer of an infectious agent from an infected host to a new host without the need for intermediates such as air, food, water or other animals. Direct modes of transmission can occur in two main ways:
  1. **Person to person:** The infectious agent is spread by direct contact between people through touching, biting, kissing, sexual intercourse or direct projection of respiratory droplets into another person's nose or mouth during coughing, sneezing or talking. A familiar example is the transmission of HIV from an infected person to others through sexual intercourse.
  2. **Transplacental transmission:** This refers to the transmission of an infectious agent from a pregnant woman to her fetus through the placenta. An example is mother-to-child transmission (MTCT) of HIV.

- **Indirect modes of transmission:** Indirect transmission is when infectious agents are transmitted to new hosts through intermediates such as air, food, water, objects or substances in the environment, or other animals. Indirect transmission has three subtypes:
  1. **Airborne transmission:** The infectious agent may be transmitted in dried secretions from the respiratory tract, which can remain suspended in the air for sometime. For example, the infectious agent causing tuberculosis can enter a new host through airborne transmission.
  2. **Vehicle-borne transmission:** A vehicle is any non-living substance or object that can be contaminated by an infectious agent which then transmits it to a new host. Contamination refers to the presence of an infectious agent in or on the vehicle.
  3. **Vector-borne transmission:** A vector is an organism, usually an arthropod which transmits an infectious agent to a new host. Arthropods which act as vectors include houseflies, mosquitoes, lice and ticks.

12 Medicine

1. Which condition is caused by congenital adrenal hyperplasia?

A. Male pseudohermaphroditism
B. Female pseudohermaphroditism
C. True hermaphroditism
D. Sequential pseudohermaphroditism

2. High artificial ankle brachial pressure index suggests the diagnosis of:

A. DVT
B. CAD/Arteriosclerosis calcified arteries
C. Varicose veins
D. Ischemic ulcers

3. True regarding upper GI bleeding is:

A. Most common cause is variceal bleeding
B. It is bleeding upto ampulla of vater
C. Most common management is endoscopic banding
D. Rockall scoring is used for risk stratification

4. Most common site of peptic ulcer is:

A. Upper part of lesser curvature
B. Lower part of lesser curvature
C. Pyloric antrum
D. Incisura angularis

5. Most common infection after transplantation is with:

A. Herpes simplex
B. CMV
C. Toxoplamosis
D. HPV

6. Weber's syndrome includes all except:

A. Cranial 3rd nerve palsy
B. Contralateral hemiparesis
C. Dorsal midbrain involvement
D. Anterior cerebellar peduncle

7. Embolism of PICA causes:

A. Horner syndrome
B. Wallenberg syndrome
C. Weber syndrome
D. Medial medullary syndrome

8. A child presents with neurological symptoms and has following feature what test is to be done next?

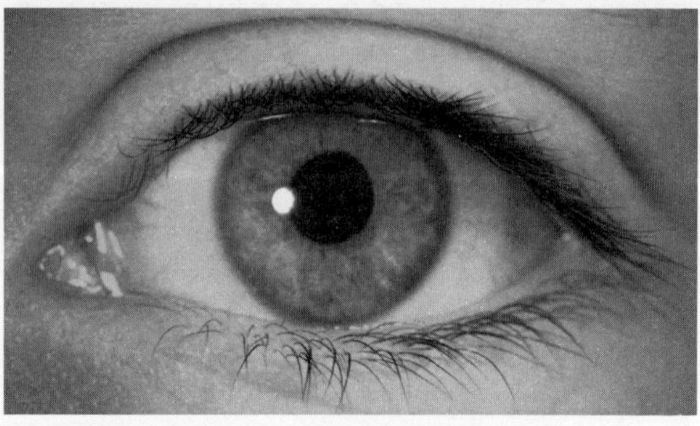

A. Serum ceruloplasmin
B. Karyotyping
C. Serum copper
D. PCR

9. A 55-year-old male having bone pains for the last 2 years with X-ray of skull shown below. Most probable diagnosis is?

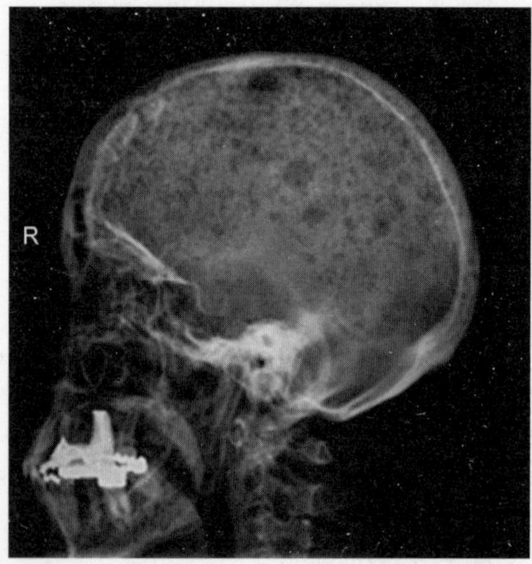

A. Multiple myeloma
B. Paget's disease
C. Hyperparathyroidism
D. Eosinophilic granuloma

10. What is the value of BMI considered fatal to man?

A. 11 B. 13
C. 15 D. 12

11. Child with alkalosis, hypertension and hypokalemia. What can be the cause?

A. Bartter syndrome B. Gitelman syndrome
C. Liddle's syndrome D. Fanconi syndrome

12. Brown-Sequard syndrome is characterized by all except:

A. Contralateral loss of pain
B. Contralateral loss of temperature
C. Contralateral loss of vibration
D. Ipsilateral loss of joint sensation

13. Prosopagnosia is seen due to defect in:

A. Frontal lobe B. Temporal lobe
C. Parietal lobe D. Occipital lobe

14. Postpartum cardiomyopathy can occur till how many weeks of delivery:

A. 6 weeks B. 6 months
C. 6 days D. 3 months

15. Which thyroid test is altered in pregnancy?

A. Free T3 B. Total T3
C. Free T4 D. TSH

16. For prophylaxis of meningococcal meningitis, drug used is?

A. Rifampicin B. Tetracycline
C. Ceftriaxone D. Azithromycin

17. Pseduo 'P' pulmonale is seen in:

A. Hypercalcemia B. Hypernatremia
C. Hypokalemia D. Hypocalcemia

18. Patient presents with pancreatitis and shock what to be done?

A. Access CVL and give hypertonic crystalloids
B. Access IV line and give hypertonic crystalloids
C. Access IV line and give hypotonic saline
D. Access IV line and give isotonic saline

19. Basiliximab mechanism of action is:

A. IL 2 inhibitor B. CD20 inhibitor
C. Antithrombin D. IL 17 inhibitor

20. Which of the following causes AV block?

A. Hypothyroidism
B. Hyperthyroidism
C. Pheochromocytoma
D. Carcinoid

21. Antiviral drug used in both HIV and HBV infection is:

A. Abacavir
B. Emtricitabine
C. Stavudine
D. Enfuvirtide

22. Ischemic dactylitis is seen in:

A. Hemophilia
B. Thalassemia
C. Sickle cell anemia
D. Hereditary spherocytosis

23. Cystinuria have malabsorption of all the amino acids except:

A. Cystine
B. Cysteine
C. Arginine
D. Lysine

24. Hyperprolactinemia is diagnostic when serum prolactin is more than?

A. 50 microgram per ml
B. 100 microgram per ml
C. 150 microgram per ml
D. 200 microgram per ml

25. All are seen in ARDS except:

A. PCWP more than 18 mm of Hg
B. Severe hypoxemia
C. Decreased pulmonary compliance
D. Pulmonary edema

26. Which of the following is not seen in ABPA?

A. Wheeze, cough, fever
B. Peripheral eosinophilia
C. Skin rash
D. Recurrent pneumonia

27. Criteria of NF1 include all except?

A. Lisch nodule
B. Optic gliomas
C. Bilateral schwannomas
D. Café au lait spots

28. Earliest feature of Crohn's disease is?

A. Aphthous ulcers
B. Fissures
C. Perforation
D. Granuloma

29. True about ataxia telangiectasia are all except:

A. Autosomal dominant
B. Occurs in adults
C. Poor coordination and telangiectasia present
D. Oculomotor apraxia

30. Which of these is associated with recurrent bouts of acute gout?

A. Beryllium
B. Cadmium
C. Antimetabolites
D. Lead

31. Saturnine gout is seen with:

A. Lead
B. Arsenic
C. Mercury
D. Cadmium

32. A 50-year-old male patient presenting with cutaneous vasculitis, proteinuria and cryoglobulinemia and glomerulonephritis. What test should be most appropriate for diagnosis?

A. ANCA
B. HBsAg
C. Anti-HCV antibody
D. MIF

33. Characteristic features of hemophilia:

A. Hematemesis
B. Hemarthrosis
C. Hemoptysis
D. Bleeding varices

34. 5-HIAA is increased in which of the following condition?

A. Carcinoid syndrome
B. Cushing syndrome
C. Addison disease
D. GIST

35. Drug of choice for treatment of rheumatic chorea:

A. Sodium valproate
B. Haloperidol
C. Risperidone
D. Diazepam

36. Severe pulmonary failure is when:

A. FEV1/FVC <0.7 and FEV1 <50%
B. FEV1/FVC <0.7 and FEV1 <30%
C. FEV1/FVC <0.7 and FEV1 >80%
D. FEV1/FVC <0.7 and FEV1 <80%

37. Vitamin K is reduced in gut by:

A. Bacterial overgrowth
B. Antibiotic use
C. Low dietary intake
D. Liver disease

38. What is seen in relation to LDH levels in MI?

A. LDH2 <LDH1
B. LDH2 >LDH1
C. LDH1 = LDH2
D. LDH3 >LDH2

39. Implantable cardioverter defibrillator (ICD) would benefit which of the following?

A. A postcardiac arrest case of Brugada syndrome
B. CAD associated with post MI cardiac arrest
C. Post cardiac arrest patient of idiopathic VF
D. All of these

40. Feline esophagus is seen in:

A. Eosinophilic esophagitis
B. Herpetic esophagitis
C. Reflux esophagitis
D. Radiation induced esophagitis

41. Mean time interval from HIV to AIDS manifestation is?

A. 7.5 years
B. 10 years
C. 15 years
D. 12 years

42. Oxygen therapy may not be useful in:

A. Asthma
B. Pneumonia
C. Subglottic stenosis
D. Pulmonary fibrosis

43. About myasthenia gravis pathogenesis, true is?

A. Antibody against ach receptor
B. Antibody against Ca receptor
C. Ach is not secreted
D. Blockage of nerve conduction through myoneural junction

44. Chromosome involved in myotonic dystrophy is:

A. Chromosome 19
B. Chromosome 20
C. Chromosome 21
D. Chromosome 22

45. Urea breath test is used for diagnosis of:

A. *H. pylori*
B. *Campylobacter jejuni*
C. *E. coli*
D. *Lactobacillus*

46. Myocardial stunning pattern is not matching the ECG findings, what is the diagnosis?

A. Takotsubo cardiomyopathy
B. Restrictive cardiomyopathy
C. Brigade's cardiomyopathy
D. Pericardial calcification

Answers with Explanations

1. **Ans. (B) Female pseudohermaphroditism**
   - **21-Hydroxylase deficiency (congenital adrenal hyperplasia):** The *classic form* of 21-hydroxylase deficiency (21-OHD) is the most common cause of CAH. It has an incidence between 1 in 10,000 and 1 in 15,000 and is the most common cause of androgenization in chromosomal 46,XX females.
   - Affected individuals are homozygous or compound heterozygous for severe mutations in the enzyme 21-hydroxylase (*CYP21A2*). This mutation causes a block in adrenal glucocorticoid and mineralocorticoid synthesis, increasing 17-hydroxyprogesterone and shunting steroid precursors into the androgen synthesis pathway.
   - Glucocorticoid insufficiency causes a compensatory elevation of adrenocorticotropin (ACTH), resulting in adrenal hyperplasia and additional synthesis of steroid precursors proximal to the enzymatic block.
   - Increased androgen synthesis in utero causes androgenization of the 46,XX fetus in the first trimester.
   - Ambiguous genitalia are seen at birth with varying degrees of clitoral enlargement and labial fusion. Excess androgen production causes gonadotropin-independent precocious puberty in males with 21-OHD.
2. **Ans. (B) CAD/Arteriosclerosis calcified arteries**
   - **Noninvasive Testing in PAD:** The history and physical examination are often sufficient to establish the diagnosis of PAD. An objective assessment of the presence and severity of disease is obtained by noninvasive techniques.
   - Arterial pressure can be recorded noninvasively in the legs by placement of sphygmomanometric cuffs at the ankles and the use of a Doppler device to auscultate or record blood flow from the dorsalis pedis and posterior tibial arteries. Normally, systolic blood pressure in the legs and arms is similar.
   - Indeed, ankle pressure may be slightly higher than arm pressure due to pulse-wave amplification. In the presence of hemodynamically significant stenoses, the systolic blood pressure in the leg is decreased. Thus, the ratio of the ankle and brachial artery pressures (termed the *ankle:brachial index* or ABI) is 1.00–1.40 in normal individuals.

- ABI values of 0.91–0.99 are considered 'borderline,' and those <0.90 are abnormal and diagnostic of PAD.
- ABIs >1.40 indicate noncompressible arteries secondary to vascular calcification.

3. **Ans. (D) Rockall scoring is used for risk stratification**
   - **Bleeding peptic ulcer:**
     - It is **bleeding either from duodenal ulcer, or gastric ulcer or stomal ulcer**.
     - In bleeding from stomal ulcer, partial gastrectomy is required.
     - Mortality in bleeding peptic ulcer is high (20–30%). Elderly age, associated systemic diseases increase the mortality.
     - NSAIDs and *H. pylori* infection, coagulopathy and anticoagulant drugs are common precipitating factors. Concomitant use of NSAID and steroids increase risk by 10-fold.
     - Need of more than 5 units of blood transfusion during hospital stay is called as *massive hemorrhage*.
   - **Bleeding duodenal ulcer:**
     - 10% common.
     - Risk of bleeding in chronic duodenal ulcer increases to 35% if patient has not taken specific anti-*Helicobacter pylori* therapy and PPI.
     - Bleeding from DU is either from the *small vessels in the wall of ulcer* crater or due to erosion into the *gastroduodenal artery*.
     - Usually *posterior* duodenal ulcer bleeds.
     - Bleeding from small vessels in the wall of ulcer is due to sloughing of the ulcer. It is less severe, gradual and most often well-controlled by conservative treatment.
     - Bleeding from erosion of gastroduodenal artery is severe, torrential and almost always needs early surgical intervention.
   - **Clinical features:**
     - *Hematemesis and melena.*
     - **Features of shock:** Pallor, tachycardia, sweating, hypotension, tachypnea, dry tongue, cold periphery.
     - Past history of chronic DU may be present.
     - History of pain and tenderness in epigastric region which has increased in intensity recently.

- **Investigations:**
  - To look for in endoscopy, in bleeding ulcer
    - Spurter
    - Clot
    - Visible vessel
    - Aneurysmal dilatation of the arteriole in the wall of ulcer
    - Ooze
  - **Gastroscopy is confirmative:** It is a must. It identifies ulcer bleed in 90% of cases clearly. Possibility of rebleed is also assessed by endoscopy. A flat clear based ulcer is less likely to rebleed. Active ulcer/fresh clot/visible vessel/pseudoaneurysm/large ulcer are more likely to rebleed.
  - *Rockall scoring system* is used to predict rebleed.
  - *Celiac angiogram* to identify the bleeder may be helpful.
  - Hb% and PCV—should be repeated at regular intervals (once in 2–3 hours).
  - Blood group and cross-matching.
  - Estimation of serum electrolytes, blood urea, serum creatinine, platelet count.
- **Treatment:**
  - Seventy percent of bleeding duodenal ulcers are treated conservatively.
  - The shock is corrected initially by: Foot end elevation, IV fluids, plasma expanders (haemaccel, dextran, crystalloids).
  - Catheterization—to assess urine output.
  - Blood transfusion to replace the lost blood.
  - Stomach wash is given—1:2,00,000 adrenaline in saline wash is given to the stomach through Ryle's tube.
  - IV ranitidine 50 mg 6th or 8th hourly.
  - IV pantoprazole 80 mg in 100 ml dextrose saline is given slow IV as starting dose and later 40 mg in dextrose saline IV OD/BD. Slow continuous infusion of pantoprazole 40 mg in dextrose saline, 500 ml IV can also be given.
  - *Endoscopic cauterization* of small vessel with either gastroscopic bipolar cautery or through laser or through heater probe or through hemoclips can be tried to stop the bleeding.
  - *Sclerotherapy*—ethanolamine oleate, distilled water.
  - *Epinephrine injection* is also used *commonly.* Other agents used are absolute alcohol, polidocanol.
  - Observation is done for patients with bleeding from small vessels in the wall of DU will commonly respond to conservative treatment.
  - Angiographic embolization of gastroduodenal artery.

- **Surgery:**
  - After laparotomy, pyloric channel and first part of the duodenum (gastroduodenum) is opened longitudinally, bleeder is identified.
  - *Underruning of* the bleeding area with vicryl is done.
  - If the bleed is from gastroduodenal artery, then it has to be *ligated* to stop the bleeding. Opened gastroduodenum is closed by ***Finney's pyloroplasty.***
  - Truncal vagotomy may be done together, if the general condition of the patient is good.

4. Ans. (C) Pyloric antrum

Types of gastric ulcer (Daintree Johnson)			
Types	*Location*	*Incidence*	*Acid level*
I	In the antrum, near the lesser curve	55%	Normal
II	Combined gastric ulcer (in the body) with duodenal ulcer	25%	High
III	Prepyloric ulcer	15%	High
IV	Gastric ulcer in the proximal stomach or cardia	5%	Normal

5. Ans. (B) CMV

Infections after transplantation:

- Wound infection is the most common complication after renal transplantation.
- Infections are the most common complications after transplantation.
- They may be common (e.g. pneumococcal pneumonia) or unusual (e.g. necrotizing fasciitis from a rare fungus).
- Organisms that cause clinical infection in the immunosuppressed host include cytomegalovirus (CMV), common bacteria, fungi, and protozoa such as *Pneumocystis (carinii) jirovecii.*
- For this reason, all patients receive antifungals and trimethoprim/sulfamethoxazole (for *Pneumocystis* prophylaxis).
- CMV infection is one of the most common infections in post-transplant. It is manifested by fever, malaise, weakness, gastrointestinal bleeding and esophagitis.
- The disease results from the infection of a seronegative recipient by a positive donor or from reactivation of the recipient endogenous viral load by excessive immunosuppression, especially in the context of biologic agents.
- Prophylactic therapy with Valganciclovir is commonly used.

6. **Ans. (D) Anterior cerebellar peduncle**

   Two clinical syndromes are commonly observed with occlusion of the PCA:

   1. **P1 syndrome:** Midbrain, subthalamic, and thalamic signs, which are due to disease of the proximal P1 segment of the PCA or its penetrating branches (thalamogeniculate, Percheron, and posterior choroidal arteries); and
   2. **P2 syndrome:** Cortical temporal and occipital lobe signs due to occlusion of the P2 segment distal to the junction of the PCA with the posterior communicating artery.

   1. **P1 syndromes:** Infarction usually occurs in the ipsilateral subthalamus and medial thalamus and in the ipsilateral cerebral peduncle and midbrain.
      - A third nerve palsy with contralateral ataxia (Claude's syndrome) or with contralateral hemiplegia (Weber's syndrome) may result. The ataxia indicates involvement of the red nucleus or dentatorubrothalamic tract; the hemiplegia is localized to the cerebral peduncle.
      - If the subthalamic nucleus is involved, contralateral hemiballismus may occur. Occlusion of the artery of Percheron produces paresis of upward gaze and drowsiness and often abulia.
      - Extensive infarction in the midbrain and subthalamus occurring with bilateral proximal PCA occlusion presents as coma, unreactive pupils, bilateral pyramidal signs, and decerebrate rigidity.
      - Occlusion of the penetrating branches of thalamic and thalamogeniculate arteries produces less extensive thalamic and thalamocapsular lacunar syndromes.
      - The *thalamic or Dejerine-Roussy syndrome* consists of contralateral hemisensory loss followed later by an agonizing, searing or burning pain in the affected areas. It is persistent and responds poorly to analgesics.
      - Anticonvulsants (carbamazepine or gabapentin) or tricyclic antidepressants may be beneficial.
   2. **P2 syndromes:** Occlusion of the distal PCA causes infarction of the medial temporal and occipital lobes. Contralateral homonymous hemianopia with macula sparing is the usual manifestation.
      - Medial temporal lobe and hippocampal involvement may cause an acute disturbance in memory, particularly if it occurs in the dominant hemisphere. The defect usually clears because memory has bilateral representation.

- If the dominant hemisphere is affected and the infarct extends to involve the splenium of the corpus callosum, the patient may demonstrate alexia without agraphia. Visual agnosia for faces, objects, mathematical symbols, and colors and anomia with paraphasic errors (amnestic aphasia) may also occur even without callosal involvement.
- Occlusion of the posterior cerebral artery can produce *peduncular hallucinosis* (visual hallucinations of brightly colored scenes and objects).
- Bilateral infarction in the distal PCAs produces cortical blindness (blindness with preserved pupillary light reaction). The patient is often unaware of the blindness or may even deny it (*Anton's syndrome*). Tiny islands of vision may persist, and the patient may report that vision fluctuates as images are captured in the preserved portions. Rarely, only peripheral vision is lost and central vision is spared resulting in 'gun-barrel' vision.
- Bilateral visual association area lesions may result in *Balint's syndrome*, a disorder of the orderly visual scanning of the environment usually resulting from infarctions secondary to low flow in the 'watershed' between the distal PCA and MCA territories as occurs after cardiac arrest.
- Patients may experience persistence of a visual image for several minutes despite gazing at another scene (*palinopsia*) or an inability to synthesize the whole of an image (*simultanagnosia*). Embolic occlusion of the top of the basilar artery can produce any or all of the central or peripheral territory symptoms. The hallmark is the sudden onset of bilateral signs including ptosis.

7. Ans. (B) Wallenberg syndrome

Lateral medullary syndrome (occlusion of any of five vessels may be responsible—vertebral, posterior inferior cerebellar, superior, middle or inferior lateral medullary arteries).

- **On side of lesion:**
  - **Pain, numbness, impaired sensation over one-half the face:** *Descending tract and nucleus fifth nerve*
  - **Ataxia of limbs, falling to side of lesion:** *Uncertain—restiform body, cerebellar hemisphere, cerebellar fibers, spinocerebellar tract*
  - **Nystagmus, diplopia, oscillopsia, vertigo, nausea, vomiting:** *Vestibular nucleus*

  - **Horner's syndrome (miosis, ptosis, decreased sweating):** *Descending sympathetic tract*
  - **Dysphagia, hoarseness, paralysis of palate, paralysis of vocal cord, diminished gag reflex:** *Issuing fibers ninth and tenth nerves*
  - **Loss of taste:** *Nucleus and tractus solitarius*
  - **Numbness of ipsilateral arm, trunk, or leg:** *Cuneate and gracile nuclei*
  - **Weakness of lower face:** *Genuflected upper motor neuron fibers to ipsilateral facial nucleus*
- **On side opposite lesion:** Impaired pain and thermal sense over half the body, sometimes face: *Spinothalamic tract.*

8. **Ans. (A) Serum ceruloplasmin**

Image showing KF ring, seen in Wilson's disease and among all the options,option (a) is the answer here.

Diagnosis of Wilson's disease:

- Serum ceruloplasmin levels should not be used for definitive diagnosis because they are normal in up to 10% of affected patients and are reduced in 20% of carriers.
- Kayser-Fleischer rings can be definitively diagnosed only by an ophthalmologist using a slit-lamp. They are present in >99% of patients with neurologic/psychiatric forms of the disease and have been described very rarely in the absence of Wilson's disease. They are present in only ~30–50% of patients diagnosed in the hepatic or presymptomatic state; thus, the absence of rings does not exclude the diagnosis.
- Urine copper measurement is an important diagnostic tool, but urine must be collected carefully to avoid contamination. Symptomatic patients invariably have urine copper levels >1.6 μmol (>100 μg) per 24 h. Heterozygotes have values <1.3 μmol (<80 μg) per 24 h. About half of presymptomatic patients who are ultimately affected have diagnostically elevated urine copper values, but the other half have levels that are in an intermediate range between 0.9 and 1.6 μmol (60–100 μg) per 24 h. Because heterozygotes may have values up to 1.3 μmol (80 μg) per 24 h, patients in this range may require a liver biopsy for definitive diagnosis.
- The gold standard for diagnosis remains liver biopsy with quantitative copper assays. Affected patients have values >3.1 μmol/g [>200 μg/g (dry weight) of liver].
- Copper stains are not reliable. False positive results can occur with longstanding obstructive liver disease which can elevate

hepatic and urine copper concentrations and rarely causes Kayser-Fleischer rings.

9. **Ans. (A) Multiple myeloma**
   - The skull demonstrates the typical 'punched out' lesions characteristic of multiple myeloma.
   - The lesion represents a purely osteolytic lesion with little or no osteoblastic activity.

10. **Ans. (B) 13**
   - A recent study has examined the literature on starvation using body mass index (BMI) to define the limits of human survival to starvation. Data included is based on normal weight subjects who died from starvation, famine or anorexia nervosa.
   - Despite the diversity of sources, the data shows a remarkable consistency. In particular, the review illustrates a sex difference in the limits of survival when based on BMI classification.
   - In males, a BMI of around 13 appears to be fatal. The coefficient of variation (CV) of the BMI is 8.7%. In contrast, females survive to a lower BMI of around 11, although with greater index variability (CV 14%). Several females had BMI's as low as 9 and 10.
   - Based on these figures a mean BMI of 12 as the lower limit for human survival emerges.
   - The ability of females to withstand a greater degree of food deprivation may be due to the following reasons:
     - Females have greater body stores of fat than males, and this can be used as a source of energy for a much longer period (fat is more energy dense than protein)
     - The contribution of fat energy to total energy expenditure is greater in the female resulting in a greater conservation of protein
     - Females appear better able to mobilize adipose tissue from most sites in the body.

11. **Ans. (C) Liddle's syndrome**
   - Liddle's syndrome is caused by autosomal dominant gain-in-function mutations of ENaC subunits. Disease associated mutations either activate the channel directly or abrogate aldosterone-inhibited retrieval of ENaC subunits from the plasma membrane; the end result is increased expression of activated ENaC channels at the plasma membrane of principal cells.

- Patients with Liddle's syndrome classically manifest severe hypertension with hypokalemia, unresponsive to spironolactone yet sensitive to amiloride.
- Hypertension and hypokalemia are, however, variable aspects of the Liddle's phenotype; more consistent features include a blunted aldosterone response to ACTH and reduced urinary aldosterone excretion.

12. **Ans. (C) Contralateral loss of vibration**

    Brown-Sequard syndrome: This consists of ipsilateral weakness (corticospinal tract) and loss of joint position and vibratory sense (posterior column) with contralateral loss of pain and temperature sense (spinothalamic tract) one or two levels below the lesion. Segmental signs such as radicular pain, muscle atrophy, or loss of a deep tendon reflex are unilateral. Partial forms are more common than the fully developed syndrome.

13. **Ans. (D) Occipital lobe**
    - A patient with *prosopagnosia* cannot recognize familiar faces, including, sometimes, the reflection of his or her own face in the mirror. This is not a perceptual deficit because prosopagnosic patients easily can tell whether two faces are identical.
    - Furthermore, a prosopagnosic patient who cannot recognize a familiar face by visual inspection alone can use auditory cues to reach appropriate recognition if allowed to listen to the person's voice.
    - Prosopagnosic patients characteristically have no difficulty with the generic identification of a face as a face or a car as a car, but may not recognize the identity of an individual face or the make of an individual car. This reflects a visual recognition deficit for proprietary features that characterize individual members of an object class. When recognition problems become more generalized and extend to the generic identification of common objects, the condition is known as *visual object agnosia*.
    - A patient with anomia cannot name the object but can describe its use. In contrast, a patient with visual agnosia is unable either to name a visually presented object or to describe its use.
    - Face and object recognition disorders can also result from the simultanagnosia of Balint's syndrome, in which case they are known as *apperceptive* agnosias as opposed to the *associative* agnosias that result from inferior temporal lobe lesions.
    - **Causes of prosopagnosia are:** The occipitotemporal network for face and object recognition.

- The characteristic lesions in prosopagnosia and visual object agnosia of acute onset consist of bilateral infarctions in the territory of the posterior cerebral arteries.
- Associated deficits can include visual field defects (especially superior quadrantanopias) and a centrally based color blindness known as achromatopsia.
- Rarely, the responsible lesion is unilateral. In such cases, prosopagnosia is associated with lesions in the right hemisphere, and object agnosia with lesions in the left.
- Degenerative diseases of anterior and inferior temporal cortex can cause progressive associative prosopagnosia and object agnosia. The combination of progressive associative agnosia and a fluent aphasia is known as *semantic dementia*. Patients with semantic dementia fail to recognize faces and objects and cannot understand the meaning of words denoting objects.

14. Ans. (B) 6 months

- Peripartum cardiomyopathy (PPCM), also known as postpartum cardiomyopathy is an uncommon form of heart failure that happens during the last month of pregnancy or up to five months after giving birth.
- PPCM is a dilated form of the condition which means the heart chambers enlarge and the muscle weakens. This causes a decrease in the percentage of blood ejected from the left ventricle of the heart with each contraction.
- PPCM is rare in the United States, Canada, and Europe. About 1,000 to 1,300 women develop the condition in the US each year. In some countries, PPCM is much more common and may be related to differences in diet, lifestyle, other medical conditions or genetics.
- PPCM may be difficult to detect because symptoms of heart failure can mimic those of third trimester pregnancy, such as swelling in the feet and legs, and some shortness of breath.
- PPCM is diagnosed when the following three criteria are met:
  1. Heart failure develops in the last month of pregnancy or within 5 months of delivery.
  2. Heart pumping function is reduced with an ejection fraction (EF) less than 45% (typically measured by an echocardiogram).
  3. No other cause for heart failure with reduced EF can be found.

- **Symptoms of the condition include:**
  - Fatigue
  - Feeling of heart racing or skipping beats (palpitations)
  - Increased night time urination (nocturia)
  - Shortness of breath with activity and when lying flat
  - Swelling of the ankles
  - Swollen neck veins
  - Low blood pressure, or it may drop when standing up.
- The underlying cause is unclear. Heart biopsies in some cases show women have inflammation in the heart muscle. This may be because of prior viral illness or abnormal immune response. Other potential causes include poor nutrition, coronary artery spasm, small-vessel disease, and defective antioxidant defenses. Genetics may also play a role.
- Initially thought to be more common in women older than 30, PPCM has since been reported across a wide range of age groups. Risk factors include:
  - Obesity
  - History of cardiac disorders, such as myocarditis (inflammation of the heart muscle)
  - Use of certain medications
  - Smoking
  - Alcoholism
  - Multiple pregnancies
  - African-American descent
  - Poor nourishment
- The objective of peripartum cardiomyopathy treatment is to keep extra fluid from collecting in the lungs and to help the heart recover as fully as possible.
  - **Angiotensin-converting enzyme (ACE) inhibitor:** Help the heart work more efficiently
  - **Beta blockers:** Cause the heart to beat more slowly so it has recovery time
  - **Diuretics:** Reduce fluid retention
  - **Digitalis:** It strengthens the pumping ability of the heart
  - **Anticoagulants:** To help thin the blood. Patients with PPCM are at increased risk of developing blood clots, especially if the EF is very low.
  - A low-salt diet, fluid restrictions, or daily weighing.
  - Women who smoke and drink alcohol will be advised to stop.

15. **Ans. (B) Total T3**
    - **Thyroid function in pregnancy:** Five factors alter thyroid function in pregnancy:
        1. The transient increase in hCG during the first trimester, which stimulates the TSHR;
        2. The estrogen-induced rise in TBG during the first trimester, which is sustained during pregnancy;
        3. Alterations in the immune system leading to the onset, exacerbation or amelioration of an underlying autoimmune thyroid disease;
        4. Increased thyroid hormone metabolism by the placenta; and
        5. Increased urinary iodine excretion which can cause impaired thyroid hormone production in the areas of marginal iodine sufficiency.
    - Women with a precarious iodine intake (<50 μg/d) are most at risk of developing a goiter during pregnancy or giving birth to an infant with a goiter and hypothyroidism.
    - The World Health Organization recommends a daily iodine intake of 250 μg during pregnancy and prenatal vitamins should contain 150 μg per tablet.
    - In pregnancy, the estrogen-induced increase in thyroxine-binding globulin increases circulating levels of total T3 and total T4.
    - The normal range of circulating levels of free T4, free T3, and TSH remain unaltered by pregnancy.
    - The thyroid gland normally enlarges during pregnancy. Many physiologic adaptations to pregnancy may mimic subtle signs of *hyperthyroidism*. Maternal hyperthyroidism occurs at a rate of ~2 per 1000 pregnancies and is generally well tolerated by pregnant women.
    - Hyperthyroidism in pregnancy is most commonly caused by Graves' disease, but autonomously functioning nodules and gestational trophoblastic disease should also be considered.
    - Testing for *hypothyroidism* using TSH measurements before or early in pregnancy may be warranted in symptomatic women and in women with a personal or family history of thyroid disease.

16. **Ans. (A) Rifampicin**
    - **Meningococcal Meningitis:** Although ceftriaxone and cefotaxime provide adequate empirical coverage for *N. meningitidis*, penicillin G remains the antibiotic of choice for meningococcal meningitis caused by susceptible strains. Isolates of

N. meningitides with moderate resistance to penicillin have been identified and are increasing in incidence worldwide.

- CSF isolates of *N. meningitides* should be tested for penicillin and ampicillin susceptibility, and if resistance is found, cefotaxime or ceftriaxone should be substituted for penicillin. A 7-day course of intravenous antibiotic therapy is adequate for uncomplicated meningococcal meningitis.
- The index case and all close contacts should receive chemoprophylaxis with a 2-day regimen of rifampicin (600 mg every 12 h for 2 days in adults and 10 mg/kg every 12 h for 2 days in children >1 year). Rifampicin is not recommended in pregnant women.
- Alternatively, adults can be treated with one dose of azithromycin (500 mg) or one intramuscular dose of ceftriaxone (250 mg). Close contacts are defined as those individuals who have had contact with oropharyngeal secretions, either through kissing or by sharing toys, beverages, or cigarettes.

17. Ans. (C) Hypokalemia

Assess p-wave morphology:

- In some cases there can be a notched (or bifid) p-wave known as 'p mitrale', indicative of left atrial hypertrophy which may be caused by mitral stenosis. There may be tall peaked p-waves. This is called 'p-pulmonale' and is indicative of right atrial hypertrophy often secondary to tricuspid stenosis or pulmonary hypertension.
- A similar picture can be seen in hypokalemia (known as 'pseudo p-pulmonale').

18. Ans. (B) Access IV line and give hypertonic crystalloids

- **Fluid Resuscitation and Monitoring in Pancreatitis:** The most important treatment intervention for acute pancreatitis is safe, aggressive intravenous fluid resuscitation.
- The patient is made NPO to rest the pancreas and is given intravenous narcotic analgesics to control abdominal pain and supplemental oxygen (2 L) via nasal cannula.
- Intravenous fluids of lactated Ringer's or normal saline are initially bolused at 15–20 cc/kg (1050–1400 mL), followed by 3 mg/kg per hour (200–250 mL/h), to maintain urine output >0.5 cc/kg per hour.
- Serial bedside evaluations are required every 6–8 h to assess vital signs, oxygen saturation, and change in physical examination.

- Lactated Ringer's solution has been shown to decrease systemic inflammation and may be a better crystalloid than normal saline.
- A *targeted resuscitation strategy* with measurement of hematocrit and BUN every 8–12 h is recommended to ensure adequacy of fluid resuscitation and monitor response to therapy, noting less aggressive resuscitation strategy may be needed in milder forms of pancreatitis.
- A rising BUN during hospitalization is not only associated with inadequate hydration but also higher in-hospital mortality. A decrease in hematocrit and BUN during the first 12–24 h is strong evidence that sufficient fluids are being administered.
- Serial measurements and bedside assessment for fluid overload are continued,and fluid rates are maintained at the current rate. Adjustments in fluid resuscitation may be required in patients with cardiac, pulmonary, or renal disease.
- A rise in hematocrit or BUN during serial measurement should be treated with a repeat volume challenge with a 2-L crystalloid bolus followed by increasing the fluid rate by 1.5 mg/kg per hour.
- If the BUN or hematocrit fails to respond (i.e. remains elevated or does not decrease) to this bolus challenge and increase in fluid rate, consideration of transfer to an intensive care unit is strongly recommended for hemodynamic monitoring.

19. Ans. (A) IL 2 inhibitor

- Monoclonal antibodies to the CD25 (IL-2a) receptor (basiliximab) are being used for treatment of graft-versus-host disease in bone marrow transplantation.
- Anti-CD20 MAb (rituximab) is used to treat hematologic neoplasms, autoimmune diseases, kidney transplant rejection, and rheumatoid arthritis.
- The anti-IgE monoclonal antibody (omalizumab) is used for blocking antigen-specific IgE that causes *hay fever* and *allergic rhinitis*; however, side effects of anti-IgE include increased risk of anaphylaxis. Studies have shown that TH17 cells, in addition to TH1, are mediators of inflammation in Crohn's disease, and anti–IL-12/IL-23p40 antibody therapy has been studied as a treatment.
- Natalizumab is a humanized monoclonal IgG antibody against an alpha 4 integrin that inhibits leukocyte migration into tissues and has been approved for the treatment of multiple sclerosis in the United States.

- Both it and anti-CD20 (rituximab) have been associated with the onset of progressive multifocal leukoencephalopathy (PML)—a serious and usually fatal CNS infection caused by JC polyomavirus.
- Efalizumab, a humanized IgG monoclonal antibody previously approved for treatment of plaque psoriasis, has now been taken off the market due to reactivation of JC virus leading to fatal PML.

20. Ans. (A) Hypothyroidism

- Hypothyroidism can cause a variety of manifestations including cardiovascular dysfunction. The more common presenting signs are sinus bradycardia and pericardial effusion. The affected patient usually has severe symptoms.
- It rarely causes complete atrioventricular (AV) block. The cardiac electrical activity changes that can be observed in hypothyroid patients are sinus bradycardia, QT interval prolongation, T wave inversion and AV block.
- Other cardiovascular effects include increased peripheral vasoconstriction; decreased cardiac contractility; and prolonged diastolic relaxation. Subsequently, cardiac output decreases due to a reduction in stroke volume and heart rate. Changes ensue as a result of the decrease in inotropy and chronotropy, such as narrowing of pulse pressure, prolongation of circulatory time and decrease in peripheral blood flow.

21. Ans. (B) Emtricitabine

- Lamivudine, emtricitabine, adefovir/tenofovir/entecavir, and telbivudine alone or in combination are useful in the treatment of hepatitis B in patients with HIV infection. It is important to remember that all the above mentioned drugs also have activity against HIV and should not be used alone in patients with HIV infection, in order to avoid the emergence of HIV resistant to these drugs. For this reason, the need to treat hepatitis B infection in a patient with HIV infection is an indication to treat HIV infection in that same patient, regardless of $CD4^+$ T cell count.
- In addition to the seven approved antiviral drugs for hepatitis B, emtricitabine, a fluorinated cytosine analogue very similar to lamivudine in structure, efficacy, and resistance profile, offers no advantage over lamivudine. A combination of emtricitabine and tenofovir is approved for the treatment of HIV infection and is an appealing combination therapy for hepatitis B, especially for lamivudine-resistant disease.

22. Ans. (C) Sickle cell anemia

- **Sickle cell disease:** It is associated with several musculoskeletal abnormalities. Children under the age of 5 years may develop diffuse swelling, tenderness, and warmth of the hands and feet lasting 1–3 weeks. This condition, referred to as *sickle cell dactylitis* or *hand-foot syndrome*, has also been observed in sickle cell thalassemia.
- Dactylitis is believed to result from infarction of the bone marrow and cortical bone leading to periostitis and soft tissue swelling. Radiographs show periosteal elevation, subperiosteal new-bone formation, and areas of radiolucency and increased density involving the metacarpals, metatarsals, and proximal phalanges.
- These bone changes disappear after several months. The syndrome leaves little or no residual damage. Because hematopoiesis ceases in the small bones of the hands and feet with age, the syndrome is rarely seen after age 5.
- Sickle cell crisis is associated with periarticular pain and occasionally with joint effusions. The joint and periarticular area are warm and tender. Knees and elbows are most often affected, but other joints can be involved. Joint effusions are usually noninflammatory.
- Acute synovial infarction can cause a sterile effusion with high neutrophil counts in synovial fluid. Synovial biopsies have shown mild lining-cell proliferation and microvascular thrombosis with infarctions.
- Scintigraphic studies have shown decreased marrow uptake adjacent to the involved joint. Patients with sickle cell disease seem predisposed to osteomyelitis, which commonly involves the long tubular bones.
- *Salmonella* is a particularly common cause. Radiographs of the involved site initially show periosteal elevation, with subsequent disruption of the cortex.
- Treatment of the infection results in healing of the bone lesion. In addition, sickle cell disease is associated with bone infarction resulting from vaso-occlusion secondary to the sickling of red cells. Bone infarction also occurs in hemoglobin sickle cell disease and sickle cell thalassemia. The bone pain in sickle cell crisis is due to infarction of bone and bone marrow. In children, infarction of the epiphyseal growth plate interferes with normal growth of the affected extremity.

- Radiographically, infarction of the bone cortex results in periosteal elevation and irregular thickening of the bone cortex. Infarction in the bone marrow leads to lysis, fibrosis, and new bone formation.

23. Ans. (B) Cysteine

- Cystinuria is an autosomal-recessive defect in reabsorptive transport of cystine and the dibasic amino acids ornithine, arginine, and lysine from the luminal fluid of the renal proximal tubule and small intestine.
- The only phenotypic manifestation of cystinuria is cystine urolithiasis, which often recurs throughout an affected individual's lifetime. Surgical intervention is necessary, but the cornerstones of treatment are dietary and medical prevention of recurrent stone formation.
  - **Type I cystinuria:** The pure autosomal recessive form: mutations in the SLC3A1 gene on chromosome 2p16.
  - **Non-type 1 cystinuria:** Inherited in a dominant mode with incomplete penetrance: mutations in the SLC7A9 gene on chromosome 19q13.11

24. Ans. (D) 200 microgram per ml

- Hyperprolactinemia is the most common pituitary hormone hypersecretion syndrome in both men and women. PRL-secreting pituitary adenomas (prolactinomas) are the most common cause of PRL levels >200 μg/L. Less pronounced PRL elevation can also be seen with microprolactinomas but is more commonly caused by drugs, pituitary stalk compression, hypothyroidism, or renal failure.
- **Presentation and diagnosis:** Women usually present with amenorrhea, infertility, and galactorrhea. If the tumor extends outside the sella, visual field defects or other mass effects may be seen. Men often present with impotence, loss of libido, infertility, or signs of central nervous system (CNS) compression including headaches and visual defects.
- Assuming that physiologic and medication-induced causes of hyperprolactinemia are excluded, the diagnosis of prolactinoma is likely with a PRL level >200 μg/L. PRL levels <100 μg/L may be caused by microadenomas, other sellar lesions that decrease dopamine inhibition,or nonneoplastic causes of hyperprolactinemia. For this reason, an MRI should be performed in all patients with hyperprolactinemia.
- It is important to remember that hyperprolactinemia caused secondarily by the mass effects of nonlactotrope lesions is also

corrected by treatment with dopamine agonists despite failure to shrink the underlying mass. Consequently, PRL suppression by dopamine agonists does not necessarily indicate that the underlying lesion is a prolactinoma.

25. Ans. (A) PCWP more than 18 mm of Hg

Diagnostic criteria for ARDS			
Severity: Oxygenation	*Onset*	*Chest radiograph*	*Absence of left atrial hypertension*
Mild: 200 mm Hg $< Pao_2/Fio_2 \leq 300$ mm Hg Moderate: 100 mm Hg $< Pao_2/Fio_2 \leq 200$ mm Hg Severe: $Pao_2/Fio_2 \leq 100$ mm Hg	Acute	Bilateal alveolar or interstitial infiltrates	PCWP <18 mm Hg or no clinical evidence of increased left atrial pressure

26. Ans. (C) Skin rash

- **Allergic bronchopulmonary aspergillosis:** It is an eosinophilic pulmonary disorder that occurs in response to allergic sensitization to antigens from *Aspergillus* species fungi. The predominant clinical presentation of ABPA is an asthmatic phenotype, often accompanied by cough with production of brownish plugs of mucus. It has also been well described as a complication of cystic fibrosis.
- A workup for ABPA may be beneficial in patients who carry a diagnosis of asthma but have proven refractory to usual therapy. It is a distinct diagnosis from simple asthma, characterized by prominent peripheral eosinophilia and elevated circulating levels of IgE (>417 IU/mL).
- Establishing a diagnosis of ABPA also requires establishing sensitivity to *Aspergillus* antigens by skin test reactivity, positive serum precipitins for *Aspergillus*, and/or direct measurement of circulating specific IgG and IgE to *Aspergillus*. Central bronchiectasis is described as a classic finding on chest imaging in ABPA but is not necessary for making a diagnosis. Other possible findings on chest imaging include patchy infiltrates and evidence of mucus impaction.
- Systemic glucocorticoids may be used in the treatment of ABPA that is persistently symptomatic despite the use of inhaled therapies for asthma. Courses of glucocorticoids should be tapered over 3–6 months, and their use must be balanced against the risks of prolonged steroid therapy.

- Antifungal agents such as fluconazole and voriconazole given over a 4-month course reduce the antigenic stimulus in ABPA and may therefore modulate disease activity in selected patients. The use of monoclonal antibody against IgE (omalizumab) has been described in treating severe ABPA particularly in individuals with ABPA as a complication of cystic fibrosis.
- ABPA-like syndromes have been reported as a result to sensitization to several non-*Aspergillus* species fungi. However, these conditions are substantially rarer than ABPA, which may be present in a significant proportion of patients with refractory asthma.

27. Ans. (C) Bilateral schwannomas
Neurofibromatosis:

- Neurofibromatosis type 1 (NF1) which is also referred to as von Recklinghausen's disease is an autosomal dominant disorder characterized by the following manifestations: neurologic (e.g. peripheral and spinal neurofibromas); ophthalmologic (e.g. optic gliomas and iris hamartomas such as Lisch nodules); dermatologic (e.g. café au lait macules); skeletal (e.g. scoliosis, macrocephaly, short stature and pseudoarthrosis); vascular (e.g. stenoses of renal and intracranial arteries); and endocrine (e.g. pheochromocytoma, carcinoid tumors, and precocious puberty).
- Neurofibromatosis type 2 (NF2) is also an autosomal dominant disorder but is characterized by the development of bilateral vestibular schwannomas (acoustic neuromas) that lead to deafness, tinnitus, or vertigo. Some patients with NF2 also develop meningiomas, spinal schwannomas, peripheral nerve neurofibromas, and cafe au lait macules.
- Endocrine abnormalities are not found in NF2 and are associated solely with NF1. Pheochromocytomas, carcinoid tumors, and precocious puberty occur in about 1% of patients with NF1, and growth hormone deficiency has been also reported. The features of pheochromocytomas in NF1 are similar to those in non-NF1 patients with 90% of tumors being located within the adrenal medulla and the remaining 10% at an extra-adrenal location which often involves the para-aortic region. Primary carcinoid tumors are often periampullary and may also occur in the ileum but rarely in the pancreas, thyroid or lungs.
- The *NF1* gene which is located on chromosome 17q11.2 and acts as a tumor suppressor consists of 60 exons that span

more than 350 kb of genomic DNA. Mutations in *NF1* are of diverse types and are scattered throughout the exons. The NF1 gene product is the protein neurofibromin, which has homologies to the p120GAP (GTPase activating protein) and acts on p21ras by converting the active GTP bound form to its inactive GDP form. Mutations of *NF1* impair this downregulation of the p21ras signalling pathways, which in turn results in abnormal cell proliferation.

28. Ans. (A) Aphthous ulcers

Crohn's disease: Microscopic features:

- The earliest lesions are aphthoid ulcerations and focal crypt abscesses with loose aggregations of macrophages, which form non-caseating granulomas in all layers of the bowel wall.
- Granulomas can be seen in lymph nodes, mesentery, peritoneum, liver, and pancreas. Although granulomas are a pathognomonic feature of CD,they are rarely found on mucosal biopsies. Surgical resection reveals granulomas in about one-half of cases.
- Other histologic features of CD include submucosal or subserosal lymphoid aggregates, particularly away from the areas of ulceration, gross and microscopic skip areas, and transmural inflammation that is accompanied by fissures that penetrate deeply into the bowel wall and sometimes form fistulous tracts or local abscesses.

29. Ans. (A) Autosomal dominant

- **Ataxia-telangiectasia** (**AT** or **A-T**), also referred to as **ataxia-telangiectasia syndrome** or **Louis–Bar syndrome**, is a rare, neurodegenerative, autosomal recessive disease causing severe disability. A-T is caused by a defect in the ATM gene, which is responsible for managing the cell's response to multiple forms of stress including double-strand breaks in DNA. The protein produced by the ATM gene recognizes that there is a break in DNA, recruits other proteins to fix the break, and stops the cell from making new DNA until the repair is complete. The condition occurs in about 1 in 70,000 people.
- **Symptoms:**
  - Ataxia (difficulty with control of movement) that is apparent early but worsens in school to preteen years.
  - Oculomotor apraxia (difficulty with coordination of head and eye movement when shifting gaze from one place to the next).
  - Involuntary movements.

- Telangiectasia (dilated blood vessels) over the white (sclera) of the eyes, making them appear bloodshot. These are not apparent in infancy and may first appear at age 5–8 years. Telangiectasia may also appear on sun-exposed areas of skin.
- Problems with infections, especially of the ears, sinuses and lungs
- Increased incidence of cancer (primarily, but not exclusively, lymphomas and leukemias).
- Delayed onset or incomplete pubertal development, and very early menopause.
- Slowed rate of growth (weight and/or height).
- Drooling particularly in young children when they are tired or concentrating on activities.
- Dysarthria (slurred, slow, or distorted speech sounds).
- Diabetes in adolescence or later.
- Premature changes in hair and skin.

30. Ans. (D) Lead

Causes of hyperuricemia and gout	
Diminished renal excretion	
• Increased renal tubular reabsorption • Renal failure • Lead toxicity • Lactic acidosis • Alcohol	• Drugs Thiazide and loop diuretics Low-dose aspirin Ciclosporin Pyrazinamide
Increased intake	
• Red meat • Seafood	• Offal
Over-production of uric acid	
• Myeloproliferative and lymphoproliferative disease • Psoriasis • High fructose intake • Glycogen storage disease	• Inherited disorders Lesh-Nyhan syndrome (HPRT mutations) Phosphoribosyl pyrophosphate synthetase 1 mutations

31. Ans. (A) Lead

- **Heavy metal (lead) nephropathy:** Heavy metals, such as lead or cadmium can lead to a chronic tubulointerstitial process after prolonged exposure. The disease entity is no longer commonly diagnosed because such heavy metal exposure has been greatly reduced due to the known health risks from lead and the consequent removal of lead from most commercial products and fuels.

- Nonetheless, occupational exposure is possible in workers involved in the manufacture or destruction of batteries, removal of lead paint, or manufacture of alloys and electrical equipment (cadmium) in countries where industrial regulation is less stringent.
- In addition, ingestion of moonshine whiskey distilled in lead-tainted containers has been one of the more frequent sources of lead exposure. Early signs of chronic lead intoxication are attributable to proximal tubule dysfunction, particularly hyperuricemia as a result of diminished urate secretion. The triad of "saturnine gout," hypertension, and renal insufficiency should prompt a practitioner to ask specifically about lead exposure.
- Unfortunately, evaluating lead burden is not as straightforward as ordering a blood test; the preferred methods involve measuring urinary lead after infusion of a chelating agent or by radiographic fluoroscopy of bone.
- Several recent studies have shown an association between chronic low-level lead exposure and decreased renal function, although either of these two factors may have been the primary event. In those patients who have CIN of unclear origin and an elevated total body lead burden, repeated treatments of lead chelation therapy have been shown to slow the decline in renal function.

32. Ans. (C) Anti-HCV antibody

Cryoglobulinemic vasculitis:

- The most common clinical manifestations of cryoglobulinemic vasculitis are cutaneous vasculitis, arthritis, peripheral neuropathy, and glomerulonephritis. Renal disease develops in 10–30% of patients. Life-threatening rapidly progressive glomerulonephritis or vasculitis of the CNS, gastrointestinal tract, or heart occurs infrequently.
- The presence of circulating cryoprecipitates is the fundamental finding in cryoglobulinemic vasculitis. Rheumatoid factor is almost always found and may be a useful clue to the disease when cryoglobulins are not detected.
- Hypocomplementemia occurs in 90% of patients. An elevated ESR and anemia occur frequently. Evidence for hepatitis C infection must be sought in all patients by testing for hepatitis C antibodies and hepatitis C RNA.

33. Ans. (B) Hemarthrosis

- Hemarthroses and spontaneous muscle hematomas are characteristic of moderate or severe congenital factor VIII or IX deficiency. They can also be seen in moderate and severe deficiencies of fibrinogen, prothrombin, and factors V, VII, and

X. Spontaneous hemarthroses occur rarely in other bleeding disorders except for severe VWD with associated factor VIII levels <5%.

- Muscle and soft tissue bleeds are also common in acquired factor VIII deficiency. Bleeding into a joint results in severe pain and swelling, as well as loss of function, but is rarely associated with discoloration from bruising around the joint.
- Life-threatening sites of bleeding include bleeding into the oropharynx, where bleeding can obstruct the airway into the central nervous system, and into the retroperitoneum.
- Central nervous system bleeding is the major cause of bleeding related deaths in patients with severe congenital factor deficiencies.

34. Ans. (A) Carcinoid syndrome

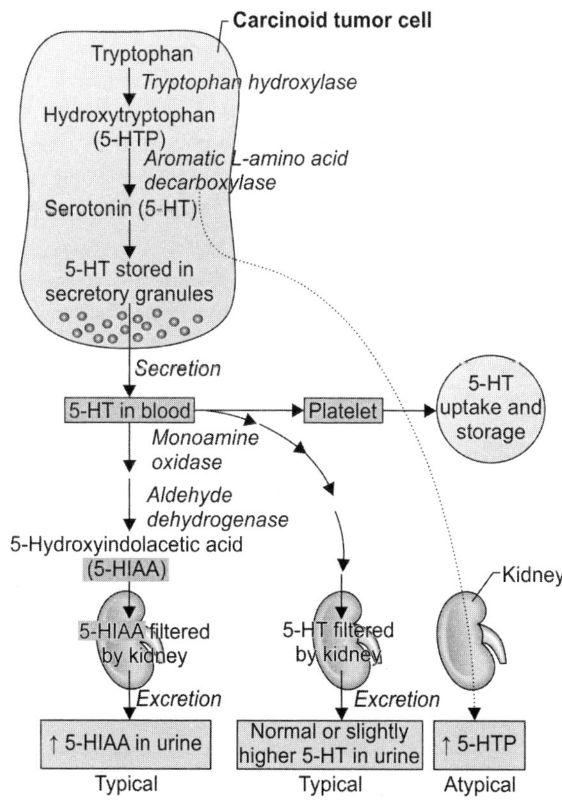

Synthesis, secretion, and metabolism of serotonin (5-HT) in patients typical and atypical syndromes. 5-HIAA, 5-hydroxyindolacetic acid. 5-HT, 5-hydroxytryptamine

35. Ans. (A) sodium valproate

Chorea:

- Medications to control the abnormal movements do not alter the duration or outcome of chorea. Milder cases can usually be managed by providing a calm environment. In patients with severe chorea, carbamazepine or sodium valproate is preferred to haloperidol. A response may not be seen for 1–2 weeks, and medication should be continued for 1–2 weeks after symptoms subside.
- There is recent evidence that corticosteroids are effective and lead to more rapid symptom reduction in chorea. They should be considered in severe or refractory cases. Prednisone or prednisolone may be commenced at 0.5 mg/kg daily with weaning as early as possible, preferably after 1 week if symptoms are reduced, although slower weaning or temporary dose escalation may be required if symptoms worsen.
- Small studies have suggested that IVIg may lead to more rapid resolution of chorea but have shown no benefit on the short- or long-term outcome of carditis in ARF without chorea. In the absence of better data, IVIg is *not* recommended except in cases of severe chorea refractory to other treatments.

36. Ans. (A) FEV1/FVC <0.7 and FEV1 <50%

Gold criteria for COPD severity *(Ref: Harrison 19th ed. p. 1704)*

Gold stage	*Severity*	*Symptoms*	*Spirometry*
0	At risk	Chronic cough, sputum production	FEV1/FVC >0.7 (Normal) FEV1 ≥80% (Normal)
I	Mild	With or without chronic cough or sputum production	FEV1/FVC >0.7 and FEV1 ≥80% predicted
II	Moderate	With or without chronic cough or sputum production	FEV1/FVC >0.7 and FEV1 50 to 80% predicted
III	Severe	With or without chronic cough or sputum production	FEV1/FVC >0.7 and FEV1 30 to 50% predicted
IV	Very severe	With or without chronic cough or sputum production	FEV1/FVC >0.7 and FEV1 <30% predicted or FEV1 <50% predicted with respiratory failure or signs of right heart failure

37. Ans. (C) Low dietary intake

Vitamin K:

- There are two natural forms of vitamin K: vitamin K1 also known as *phylloquinone*, from vegetable and animal sources, and vitamin K2, or *menaquinone*, which is synthesized by bacterial flora and found in hepatic tissue. Phylloquinone can be converted to menaquinone in some organs.
- Vitamin K is required for the post-translational carboxylation of glutamic acid, which is necessary for calcium binding to γ-carboxylated proteins such as prothrombin (factor II); factors VII, IX, and X; protein C; protein S; and proteins found in bone (osteocalcin) and vascular smooth muscle (e.g. matrix Gla protein).
- **Dietary sources:** It is found in green leafy vegetables such as kale and spinach, and appreciable amounts are also present in margarine and liver. It is present in vegetable oils; olive, canola, and soybean oils are particularly rich sources.
- **Deficiency:** The symptoms of vitamin K deficiency are due to hemorrhage; newborns are particularly susceptible because of low fat stores, low breast milk levels of vitamin K, relative sterility of the infantile intestinal tract, liver immaturity, and poor placental transport. Intracranial bleeding as well as gastrointestinal and skin bleeding can occur in vitamin K–deficient infants 1–7 days after birth.
- Thus, vitamin K (0.5–1 mg IM) is given prophylactically at delivery. Vitamin K deficiency in adults may be seen in patients with chronic small-intestinal disease (e.g. celiac disease, Crohn's disease), in those with obstructed biliary tracts, or after small-bowel resection.
- Broadspectrum antibiotic treatment can precipitate vitamin K deficiency by reducing numbers of gut bacteria which synthesize menaquinones, and by inhibiting the metabolism of vitamin K.
- In patients with warfarin therapy, the anti-obesity drug orlistat can lead to international normalized ratio changes due to vitamin K malabsorption.
- Vitamin K deficiency is usually diagnosed on the basis of an elevated prothrombin time or reduced clotting factors,although vitamin K may also be measured directly by high-pressure liquid chromatography.
- Vitamin K deficiency is treated with a parenteral dose of 10 mg. For patients with chronic malabsorption, 1–2 mg/d should be given orally or 1–2 mg per week can be taken parenterally.

- Patients with liver disease may have an elevated prothrombin time because of liver cell destruction as well as vitamin K deficiency. If an elevated prothrombin time does not improve during vitamin K therapy, it can be deduced that this abnormality is not the result of vitamin K deficiency.
- Inherited deficiency of the functional activity of the enzymes involved in vitamin K metabolism, notably the GGCX or VKORC1 results in bleeding disorders. The amount of vitamin K in the diet is often limiting for the carboxylation reaction; thus recycling of the vitamin K is essential to maintain normal levels of vitamin K–dependent proteins.
- In adults, low dietary intake alone is seldom reason for severe vitamin K deficiency but may become common in association with the use of broad-spectrum antibiotics. Disease or surgical interventions that affect the ability of the intestinal tract to absorb vitamin K, either through anatomic alterations or by changing the fat content of bile salts and pancreatic juices in the proximal small bowel can result in significant reduction of vitamin K levels.
- Prolongation of PT values is the most common and earliest finding in vitamin K–deficient patients due to reduction in prothrombin, FVII, FIX, and FX levels. FVII has the shortest half-life among these factors that can prolong the PT before changes in the aPTT.
- Parenteral administration of vitamin K at a total dose of 10 mg is sufficient to restore normal levels of clotting factor within 8–10 h. In the presence of ongoing bleeding or a need for immediate correction before an invasive procedure, replacement with FFP or PCC is required.

38. Ans. (A) LDH2 <LDH1

- **Lactate dehydrogenase** (**LDH**) is an enzyme found in nearly all living cells catalyzes the conversion of lactate to pyruvic acid and converts NAD^+ to NADH and back.
- **Isozymes:** Lactate dehydrogenase is composed of four subunits (tetramer). The two most common subunits are the LDH-M and LDH-H protein, encoded by the *LDHA* and *LDHB* genes, respectively. These two subunits can form five possible tetramers (isoenzymes): 4H, 4M, and the three mixed tetramers (3H1M, 2H2M, 1H3M).
- These five isoforms are enzymatically similar but show different tissue distribution: The major isoenzymes of skeletal muscle and liver, M_4 has four muscle (M) subunits, while H_4 is the

main isoenzymes for heart muscle in most species containing four heart (H) subunits.

- LDH-1 (4H)—in the heart and in red blood cells (RBC), as well as the brain.
- LDH-2 (3H1M)—in the reticuloendothelial system
- LDH-3 (2H2M)—in the lungs
- LDH-4 (1H3M)—in the kidneys, placenta, and pancreas
- LDH-5 (4M)—in the liver and striated muscle.

- Usually LDH-2 is the predominant form in the serum. A LDH-1 level higher than the LDH-2 level (a 'flipped pattern') suggests myocardial infarction (damage to heart tissues releases heart LDH which is rich in LDH-1 into the bloodstream). The use of this phenomenon to diagnose infarction has been largely superseded by the use of Troponin I or T measurement.

39. Ans. (D) All of these

Implantable cardioverter-defibrillators (ICDs)

- ICDs are highly effective for termination of VT and VF and also provide bradycardia pacing. ICDs decrease mortality in patients at risk for sudden death due to structural heart diseases. In all cases, ICDs are recommended only if there is also expectation for survival of at least a year with acceptable functional capacity. The exception is in cases of patients with end-stage heart disease who are awaiting cardiac transplantation outside the hospital, or who have left bundle branch block. QRS prolongation such that they are likely to have improvement in ventricular function with cardiac resynchronization therapy from a biventricular ICD.
- ICDs can often terminate monomorphic VT by a burst of rapid pacing faster than the VT known as antitachycardia pacing (ATP). If ATP fails or is not a programed treatment, as is often the case for rapid VT or VF, a shock is delivered. Shocks are painful if the patient is conscious.
- The most common ICD complication is the delivery of unnecessary therapy (either ATP or shocks) in response to a rapid supraventricular tachycardia or electrical noise as a result of an ICD lead fracture.
- Despite prompt termination of VT or VF by an ICD, the occurrence of these arrhythmias predicts subsequent increased mortality and risk of heart failure. Occurrence of VT or VF should therefore prompt assessment for potential causes including worsening heart failure, electrolyte abnormalities, and ischemia.

- Patients who survive an episode of SCD are considered to be at very high-risk and qualify for placement of an implantable cardioverter-defibrillator.

Long-term management after survival of out-of-hospital cardiac arrest:

- Patients who survive cardiac arrest without irreversible damage to the central nervous system and who achieve hemodynamic stability should have diagnostic testing to define appropriate therapeutic interventions for their long-term management. This approach is driven by the fact that survival after out-of-hospital cardiac arrest is followed by a 10–25% mortality rate during the first 2 years after the event, and there are data suggesting that significant survival benefits can be achieved by prescription of an ICD.
- Among patients in whom an acute ST elevation MI or transient and reversible myocardial ischemia is identified as the specific mechanism triggering an out-of-hospital cardiac arrest, the management is dictated in part by the transient nature of life-threatening arrhythmia risk during the acute coronary syndrome (ACS) and in part by the extent of permanent myocardial damage that results.
- Cardiac arrest during the acute ischemic phase is not an ICD indication, but survivors of cardiac arrest not associated with an ACS do benefit.
- In addition, patients who survive MI with an EF less than 30–35% appear to benefit from ICDs.
- For patients with cardiac arrest determined to be due to a treatable transient ischemic mechanism, particularly with higher EFs, catheter interventional, surgical, and/or pharmacologic anti-ischemic therapy is generally accepted for long-term management.
- Survivors of cardiac arrest due to other categories of disease, such as the hypertrophic or dilated cardiomyopathies and the various rare inherited disorders (e.g. right ventricular dysplasia, long QT syndrome, Brugada syndrome, catecholaminergic polymorphic VT, and so-called idiopathic VF), are all considered ICD candidates.

40. Ans. (A) Eosinophilic esophagitis

- Eosinophilic esophagitis with multiple circular rings of the esophagus creating a corrugated appearance, and an impacted grape at the narrowed esophagogastric junction. The diagnosis requires biopsy with histologic finding of >15–20 eosinophils per high-power field.

- The presence of linear furrows and multiple corrugated rings throughout a narrowed esophagus (*feline esophagus*) should raise suspicion for eosinophilic esophagitis, an increasingly recognized cause for recurrent dysphagia and food impaction.

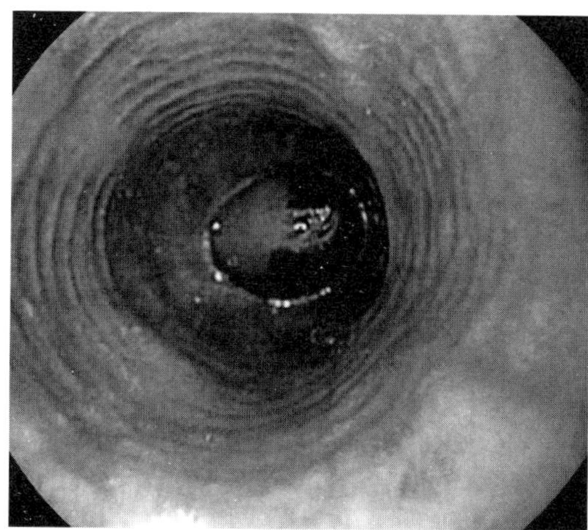

Feline esophagus

41. **Ans. (B) 10 years**

HIV:

- The original infection may be asymptomatic, or followed by a glandular fever-like illness at the time of seroconversion. After a variable latent phase which may last several years a persistent generalized lymphadenopathy develops.
- The term AIDS-related complex refers to the next stage in which many of the symptoms of AIDS (e.g. fever, weight-loss, fatigue or diarrhea) may be present without the opportunistic infections or tumors characteristic of full-blown AIDS.
- Not all of those infected with HIV will develop AIDS but, for those who do, the average time from infection to the onset of AIDS is about 10 years without treatment.
- Once AIDS develops, if untreated, about half will die within 1 year and three quarters within 4 years.
- The use of HAART has led to marked reductions in the rates of illness and death in HIV infected individuals, and a life expectancy following diagnosis now measured in decades.

42. **Ans. (C) Subglottic stenosis**

Oxygen therapy is useful in all the options given in the question,but if one has to choose one out of the four given options, subglottic stenosis is the answer here.

43. Ans. (A) Antibody against ach receptor

- Myasthenia gravis (MG) is a neuromuscular disorder characterized by weakness and fatigability of skeletal muscles.
- The underlying defect is a decrease in the number of available acetylcholine receptors (AChRs) at neuromuscular junctions due to an antibody-mediated autoimmune attack.
- **Pathophysiology:** In MG, the fundamental defect is a decrease in the number of available AChRs at the postsynaptic muscle membrane. In addition, the postsynaptic folds are flattened, or 'simplified'. These changes result in decreased efficiency of neuromuscular transmission. Therefore, although ACh is released normally, it produces small endplate potentials that may fail to trigger muscle action potentials. Failure of transmission at many neuromuscular junctions results in weakness of muscle contraction. The amount of ACh released per impulse normally declines on repeated activity (termed *presynaptic rundown*). In the myasthenic patient, the decreased efficiency of neuromuscular transmission combined with the normal rundown results in the activation of fewer and fewer muscle fibers by successive nerve impulses and hence increasing weakness, or *myasthenic fatigue*. This mechanism also accounts for the decremental response to repetitive nerve stimulation seen on electrodiagnostic testing.
- The neuromuscular abnormalities in MG are caused by an autoimmune response mediated by specific anti-AChR antibodies. The anti-AChR antibodies reduce the number of available AChRs at neuromuscular junctions by three distinct mechanisms:
    1. Accelerated turnover of AChRs by a mechanism involving cross-linking and rapid endocytosis of the receptors;
    2. Damage to the postsynaptic muscle membrane by the antibody in collaboration with complement; and
    3. Blockade of the active site of the AChR, i.e. the site that normally binds ACh. An immune response to muscle-specific kinase (MuSK), a protein involved in AChR clustering at neuromuscular junctions can also result in MG with reduction of AChRs demonstrated experimentally.
- Anti-MuSK antibody occurs in about 40% of patients without AChR antibody. A small proportion of patients whose sera are negative for both AChR and MuSK antibodies have antibodies to another protein at the neuromuscular junction—low-density lipoprotein receptor related protein 4 (lrp4)—that is important for clustering of AChRs.

- The pathogenic antibodies are IgG and are T cell dependent. Thus, immunotherapeutic strategies directed against either the antibody-producing B cells or helper T cells are effective in this antibody-mediated disease.
- How the autoimmune response is initiated and maintained in MG is not completely understood, but the thymus appears to play a role in this process. The thymus is abnormal in ~75% of patients with AChR antibody–positive MG; in ~65% the thymus is "hyperplastic," with the presence of active germinal centers detected histologically, although the hyperplastic thymus is not necessarily enlarged.
- An additional 10% of patients have thymic tumors (thymomas). Muscle-like cells within the thymus (myoid cells) which express AChRs on their surface may serve as a source of autoantigen and trigger the autoimmune reaction within the thymus gland.

44. Ans. (A) Chromosome 19

Myotonic dystrophy:

- It is also known as *dystrophia myotonica* (DM). The condition is composed of at least two clinical disorders with overlapping phenotypes and distinct molecular genetic defects: Myotonic dystrophy type 1 (DM1), the classic disease and myotonic dystrophy type 2 (DM2) also called *proximal myotonic myopathy* (PROMM).
- Type 1 DM (DM1) occurs when a gene on chromosome 19 called DMPK contains an abnormally expanded section.
- Type 2 DM (DM2) is caused by an abnormally expanded section in a gene on chromosome 3 called ZNF9.

45. Ans. (A) *H. pylori*

Tests commonly used to detect *H. Pylori*		
Test	*Advantages*	*Disadvantages*
Test based on endoscopic biopsy		
Rapid urease test	Quick, simple	Some commercial tests not fully sensitive before 24 hour
Histology	May give additional histologic information	Sensitivity dependent on experience and use of special stains
Culture	Permits determination of antibiotic susceptibility	Sensitivity dependent on experience

Contd...

Contd...

Test	*Advantages*	*Disadvantages*
Noninvasive tests		
Serology	Inexpensive and convenient; not affected by recent antibiotics or proton pump inhibitors to the same extent as breath and stool tests	Cannot be used for early follow-up after treatment; some commercial kits inaccurate, and most less accurate than urea breath test
13C urea breath	Inexpensive and simpler than endoscopy; useful for follow-up after treatment	Requires fasting; not as convenient as blood or stool tests
Stool antigen test	Inexpensive and convenient; useful for follow-up after treatment; may be useful in children	Stool-based tests are disliked by people from some cultures

46. Ans. (A) Takotsubo cardiomyopathy

Takotsubo cardiomyopathy:

- The apical ballooning syndrome, or stress-induced cardiomyopathy occurs typically in older women after sudden intense emotional or physical stress. The ventricle shows global ventricular dilation with basal contraction, forming the shape of the narrow-necked jar (*takotsubo*) used in Japan to trap octopi. Originally described in Japan, it is increasingly recognized elsewhere during emergency cardiac catheterization and intensive care unit admissions for noncardiac conditions.
- **Transient vasospasm:** Some of the original researchers of takotsubo suggested that multiple simultaneous spasms of coronary arteries could cause enough loss of blood flow to cause transient stunning of the myocardium. Other researchers have shown that vasospasm is much less common than initially thought. It has been noted that when there are vasospasms, even in multiple arteries, that they do not correlate with the areas of myocardium that are not contracting.
- Presentations include pulmonary edema, hypotension, and chest pain with ECG changes mimicking an acute infarction. The left ventricular dysfunction extends beyond a specific coronary artery distribution and generally resolves within days to weeks. Animal models and ventricular biopsies suggest that this acute cardiomyopathy may result from intense sympathetic activation with heterogeneity of myocardial autonomic

innervation, diffuse microvascular spasm, and/or direct catecholamine toxicity. Coronary angiography may be required to rule out acute coronary occlusion.

- No therapies have been proven beneficial, but reasonable strategies include nitrates for pulmonary edema, intra-aortic balloon pump if needed for low output, combined alpha and beta blockers rather than selective beta blockade if hemodynamically stable, and magnesium for arrhythmias related to QT prolongation.
- Anticoagulation is generally withheld due to the occasional occurrence of ventricular rupture. While the prognosis is generally good, recurrences have been described in up to 10% of patients.

13

Surgery

1. A 50 kg man having 40% second degree burns. So how much fluid will be needed in first 8 hours:

A. 8 liters
B. 4 liters
C. 2 liters
D. 6 liters

2. Plan KUB showing what procedure done?

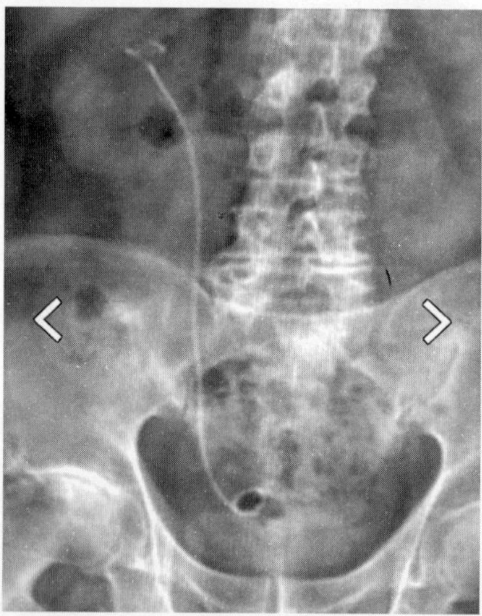

A. ESWL for renal stone
B. ESWL for bladder stones
C. ESWL for renal TB
D. Stent for benign prostatic hyperplasia

3. A 50-year-old male with symptoms of obstructive uropathy. A retrograde urethrogram was done which shows?

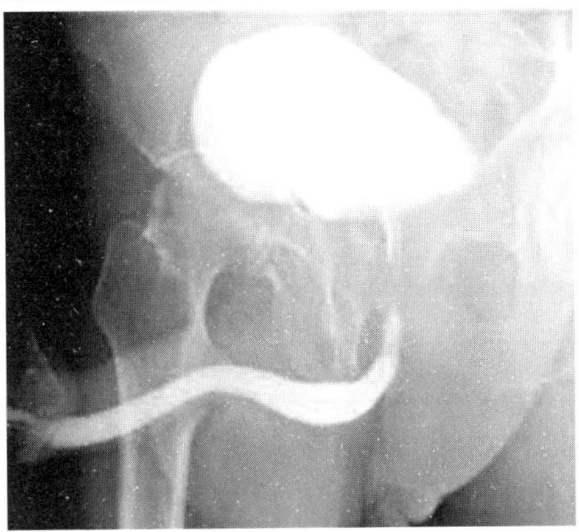

A. Urethral stone
B. Bladder stone
C. Benign prostatic hyperplasia
D. Hydronephrosis

4. Heller's operation is done for?

A. Achalasia cardia
B. Zenker's diverticulum
C. Esophageal spasm
D. Esophageal perforation

5. Van Nuy's classification of DCIS include all except:

A. Grade
B. Size
C. Microinvasion
D. Receptors

6. Best investigation for carcinoma head of pancreas?

A. FNAC by endoscopic ultrasound
B. CT guided biopsy
C. ERCP
D. USG

7. Asymtomatic aortic aneurysm is to be operated when more than:

A. 55 mm
B. 75 mm
C. 50 mm
D. 60 mm

8. Paget's disease seen in site other than breast is?

A. Cevix
B. Vagina
C. Uterus
D. Vulva

9. Identify the retractor?

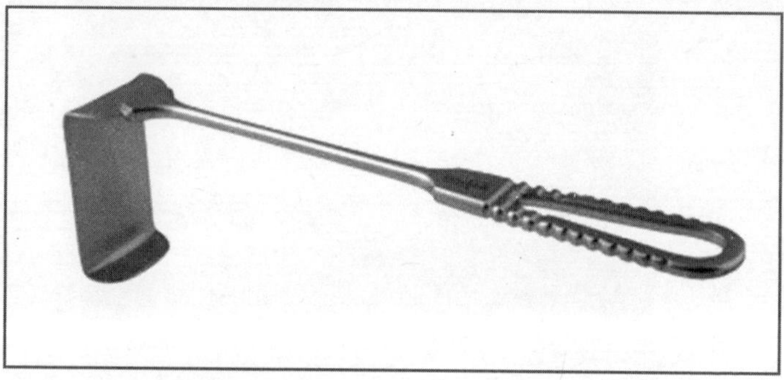

A. Morris retractor
B. Langenbeck retractor
C. Richardson retractor
D. Deaver retractor

10. Most common stones formed due to excess laxative use:

A. Urate
B. Struvite
C. Oxalate
D. Cystine

11. What is the Glasgow Coma Scale of a patient presenting after injury, confused, eye opening on painful stimulus, flexion withdrawal on left side and localising to pain on right side?

A. 8
B. 9
C. 10
D. 11

12. Most common cause of chronic pancreatitis:

A. Alcoholism
B. Pancreatic stones
C. Pancreas divisum
D. Gallstones

13. True about Crohn's disease on endoscopy are all except:

A. Whole length shows involvement
B. Skip lesions are seen
C. Non caseating granulomas are seen
D. Biopsy can be taken

14. Which organism causing acute bacterial prostatitis?

A. *Enterococcus*
B. *Streptococcus viridans*
C. *Peptostreptococcus*
D. *E. coli*

15. Which of the following statement is true about suture material in the image?

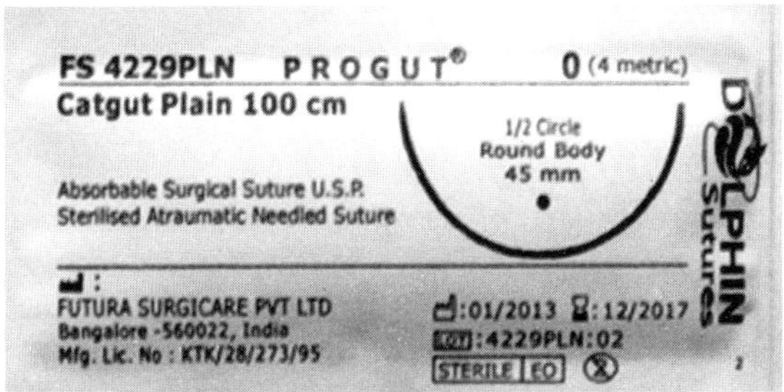

A. Made of rabbit submucosa
B. Made of cat submucosa
C. Not degraded
D. Degraded by enzymatic degradation

16. The following statement about Keloid is true?

A. It contains growth factors
B. Extended excision is the treatment of choice
C. Do not extend beyond the wound
D. None of the above

17. Which of the following is best stent for femoropopliteal bypass graft?

A. Dacron
B. Reversed saphenous vein
C. Polytetrafluoroethyline
D. None

Answers with Explanations

1. **Ans. (B) 4 liters**

   Resuscitation in a burn patient: Two large-bore (18 gauge or larger) IV lines should be placed into the bilateral antecubital fossae; lactated Ringer is the classical fluid of choice.
   - **Adults:** Parkland formula for second and third degree burns.
   - **Fluid resuscitation:** Should be tailored to urine output; calculated requirement of fluid is from the time of burn.
     - **Timing:** First 50% of fuid is given in the initial 8 hours, with the rest in the remaining 16 hours.
     - **Urinary catheter:** Placed to monitor urine output.

   Parkland formula or burn resuscitation:
   - 4 mL X total body surface area burned (TBSA) X weight (kg) = estimated fluid requirements in the first 24 hours.
   - So from question fluid required = 4 X 40 X 50 = 8000 mL
   - So for 1st hour, 4 liters is given.

2. **Ans. (A) ESWL for renal stone, Treatment of renal calculi:**
   - ***PCNL (Percutaneous Nephrolithotomy):***

     Indications
     - Stones more than 2.5 cm in size
     - Multiple stones
     - Stones not responding for ESWL

     Procedure: Initially cystoscopy is done and ureteric stent/catheter is placed and renal pelvicalyceal system is identified under C-Arm guidance. Under the guidance of C-Arm or US, needle puncture is made in the loin percutaneously. Through kidney, calyx and pelvis are approached. Guidewire is passed. Graduated dilators are passed and so track is widened. Then through that, a nephroscope is passed. After fragmentation, stone is removed using different methods [Laser (Holmium), pneumatic, ultrasonic or electrohydraulic].

     Complications of PCNL
     - Hemorrhage
     - Perforation of collecting duct causing extravasation of irrigation fluid
     - Injury to colon or pleura while creating initial track for nephroscope
   - ***ESWL (Extracorporeal Shock Wave Lithotripsy):***
     - *Piezoceramic* or *electromagnetic* shock waves are passed to the stone through water bath or water cushion which

acts as a media. Shocks are produced at 2/sec. 1000-4000 shocks are required for each stone.

- *Dornier Lithotripter* is used for fragmenting stones.
- Stone is located and observed through fluoroscope (C-Arm) or ultrasound. Shock waves are triggered to create *compressive waves* over the stone, to *fragment* it. These fragments are flushed out later.

Advantages

- No anesthesia is required
- Can be done as an OP procedure
- Less than 2.5 cm sized stones are well fragmented
- Hard stones, oxalate stones are better eliminated by ESWL
- ESWL can be done repeatedly in different sittings
- If it is not successful one can switch over to PCNL

Complications

- Renal hematoma
- Severe hematuria
- Injury to adjacent structures
- Fragmented stone retains in the ureter

Contraindications

- Pregnancy
- Bleeding disorders
- Patients with abdominal aneurysms
- Sepsis and renal failure (serum creatinine more than 3 mg%)

- ***Conservative treatment:***
  - Flush therapy—mainly *used for lower ureteric stones.*
  - IV fluids.
  - Inj frusemide 60-80 mg IV.
  - Anti-inflammatory and antispasmodic agents are given to relieve the pain.
- ***Surgery for renal stones:*** Presently most of the renal stones can be removed without open surgery (PCNL, ESWL, URS). But limiting factors are cost and availability.

3. **Ans. (C) BPH**

Retrograde urethrogram is showing filling defect at the level of the bladder neck which can be due to any of the causes of the bladder neck obstruction.

Bladder outlet obstruction (BOO): It is low urinary flow rate with the presence of high voiding pressure. It is an urodynamically confirmed entity.

- It is diagnosed by urodynamic pressure flow study.
- Flow rate will be less than 10 ml/second with voiding pressure more than 80 cm of water.

- Eventually detrusor inefficiency occurs causing significant residual urine.
- *Causes of BOO*—BPH; bladder neck hypertrophy or stenosis; carcinoma of prostate; urethral stricture; functional bladder neck obstruction.
- *Effects of BOO*—acute retention of urine; chronic retention of urine; impaired bladder emptying; uremia; infection; stone formation, hematuria.
- US; renal function tests; IVU; PSA are the investigations.
- *Management* is by treating the cause by cystoscopic bladder neck incision, urethrotomy, TURP, etc.

4. **Ans. (A) Achalasia cardia**

Achalasia cardia (cardiospasm): It is failure of relaxation of cardia (esophagogastric junction) due to disorganized esophageal peristalsis, as a result of failure of integration of parasympathetic impulses causing *functional obstruction.*

- **Etiology:**
  - There is absence or less numbered ganglions in myenteric plexus.
    - Stress.
    - Vit B_1 deficiency.
    - Chaga's disease. It is caused by *Trypanosoma cruzi,* which is common in South America called as sleeping sickness.
    - Diffuse esophageal spasm *(Corkscrew esophagus).*
    - Most commonly it is *idiopathic*. There is *degeneration of Auerbach's myenteric plexus* along the entire length of esophagus more so in LOS.
  - There is pencil shaped narrowing of cardia (O-G junction) with enormous dilatation of proximal esophagus, which contains foul smelling fluid and is more prone for aspiration pneumonia.
  - Achalasia cardia *is a precancerous* condition—seven times chances of getting *squamous cell carcinoma* (8%, after 15 years).
- **Pathology:**
  - Thickening of circular muscle fibers in distal esophagus.
  - Myenteric inflammation; depletion of ganglion cells; neural fibrosis, reduced nitric oxide and Vasoactiveintestinal peptide [mediators of lower esophageal sphincter (LES) relaxation].

  - Absence of peristalsis; raised LES pressure; failure of relaxation with functional obstruction of esophagogastric junction.
  - Dilatation of proximal esophagus with atony.
- **Clinical Features:**
  - Common in females between 20 and 40 years age group.
  - Incidence is 6 per 1,00,000 population.
  - Chest pain occurs in early stage.
  - Achalasia with diffuse esophageal spasm is called as '*vigorous achalasia*'.
  - Presents with progressive dysphagia, which is more for liquid than to solid food.
  - Regurgitation and recurrent pneumonia are common (10%).
  - Walking while eating, chin thrusting, neck and shoulder extension, Valsalva maneuver facilitates emptying of food from the esophagus.
  - Heartburn (50%) is common.
  - Malnutrition and general ill health.
  - Lung abscess formation.
  - Odynophagia and weight loss.
- **Investigations:**
  - *Barium swallow is diagnostic*—shows.
    - Pencil like smooth narrowing of lower esophagus—*Bird beak appearance*
    - Dilatation of proximal esophagus
    - Absence of fundic gas bubble
    - Sigmoid esophagus or megaesophagus
  - Chest X-ray shows patches of pneumonia. *Double mediastinal strip* of dilated esophagus is typical with air fluid level in posterior mediastinum on lateral view.
  - Esophageal manometry shows unrelaxed lower esophageal sphincter with high resting pressure—very useful and gold standard. It shows failure of LES to relax completely during swallowing and complete absence of peristalsis. LES pressure is > 35 mm Hg. Baseline esophageal pressure will be high without progressive esophageal peristalsis with low amplitude muscular tone. Intraesophageal pressure in relation to intragastric pressure is elevated.
  - Esophagoscopy is done to confirm the diagnosis and to rule out carcinoma esophagus. It shows totally closed LES with atonic, dilated proximal esophagus. Biopsy of mucosa at LES should be done.

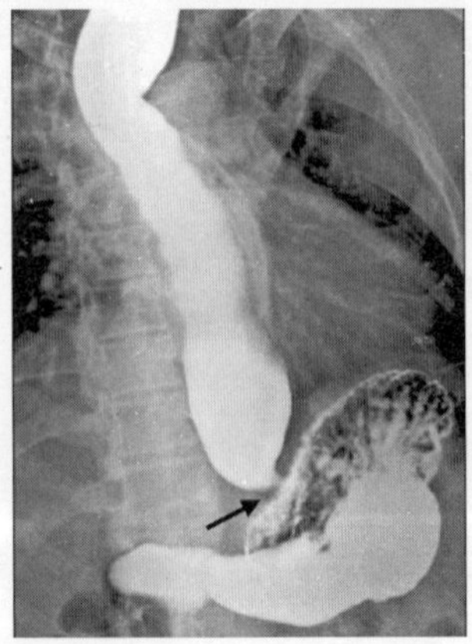

Barium swallow X-ray showing features of achalasia cardia

- **Differential Diagnosis:**
  - Carcinoma esophagus.
  - Stricture esophagus.
  - Scleroderma.
- **Treatment for achalasia:**
  - *Forcible dilatation*:
    - Plummer's pneumatic dilatation
    - Negus hydrostatic balloon dilatation
  - Modified *Heller's* cardiomyotomy
  - *Drugs*
    - Botulinum toxin A
    - Nitroglycernie, nifedipine

5. Ans. (D) Receptors

Van Nuy's prognostic index for DCIS			
Score	*1*	*2*	*3*
Size in mm	< 15 mm	15–40 mm	> 40 mm
Clearance in mm	> 10 mm	1–10 mm	< 1 mm
Grade and necrosis	not high grade	not high grade	high grade
	No necrosis	Necrosis present	Necrosis present
Total score is 9			
Score 3–4 conservative breast surgery (wide local excision)			
Score 5–7 conservative surgery + Radiotherapy			
Score 8–9 total mastectomy			

6. **Ans. (A) FNAC by EUS**

Clinical Presentation and Evaluation of pancreatic carcinoma: The signs and symptoms of pancreatic carcinoma relate to the location of the tumor and the tumors effects on local structures.

- Periampullary tumors often present early with painless jaundice. Most patients have a combination of weight loss, jaundice, and pain as a result of infiltration of the tumor into the peripancreatic region including retroperitoneal nerves carried through the celiac plexus. Invasion of these nerves by tumor often results in pain that is constant, posterior and epigastric in distribution with radiation to the back as opposed to the intermittent colicky pain that is usually associated with biliary tract disease.
- A palpable nontender gallbladder associated with painless jaundice is more commonly associated with malignancy **(Courvoisier's sign)**, while cholecystitis or obstructive jaundice due to choledocholithiasis is typically painful and associated with tenderness on examination. The evaluation of jaundiced patients includes serum chemistries.
- Markedly elevated transaminases (AST, ALT near 1000) are suggestive of hepatitis. Elevation of the total and direct bilirubin, alkaline phosphatase and γ-GGT are suggestive of obstructive jaundice. Transaminases may be mildly elevated into the low hundreds. Liver function studies suggesting obstructive jaundice demand further imaging studies that should begin with ultrasonography.
- Ultrasound is useful in diagnosing a dilated or obstructed biliary ductal system, liver lesions, cholelithiasis, choledocholithiasis, cholecystitis, and in some cases pancreatic neoplasms.
- In patients with a history and physical findings suggestive of a pancreatic neoplasm, CT may be a more informative initial diagnostic test. CT provides information about the level of the biliary tract obstruction, delineates the mass and its relation to vital structures, and identifies liver metastases. A high-quality, contrast-enhanced CT scan is required to preoperatively stage the lesion and to determine tumor resectability as defined by the absence of distant spread of disease, ascites and lack of involvement of the SMV, portal vein (PV), SMA, hepatic artery, vena cava or aorta.
- Endoscopic ultrasound (EUS) is the newest modality for evaluating pancreatic lesions. Its sensitivity and specificity are similar to that of CT in evaluating the mass and adjacent vasculature.

It is not useful for evaluating liver metastases. EUS, unlike CT, however, is invasive and highly operator dependent. MRCP, ERCP and percutaneous transhepatic cholangiography (PTC) can also delineate biliary and pancreatic ductal anatomy. Palliative drainage of the biliary tract to address symptoms due to hyperbilirubinemia can also be achieved endoscopically or transhepatically in unresectable cases, but preoperative drainage of the biliary system is not routinely indicated when imaging studies suggest a resectable pancreatic tumor. Likewise, biopsy of a pancreatic mass in resectable cases is not indicated due to a high false negative rate and difficulty in establishing the diagnosis.

- Biopsy and tissue diagnosis are important if neoadjuvant or palliative chemotherapy or radiation therapy is to be undertaken and may be obtained by percutaneous CT or EUS-guided methods.

7. **Ans. (A) 55 mm**

Abdominal Aneurysm:

- Abdominal aortic aneurysm is the *most common* aortic aneurysm.
- Splenic artery aneurysm is the *second most common* type.
- Incidence is 2%. It is more common in males.
- Transverse diameter of aorta in an aneurysm should be 3 cm or more.
- Common in elderly; common in males (4:1); chance of getting aneurysm in genetically related first degree relatives is 10 times more.
- Common in smokers (8:1 with nonsmokers); in 55% of patients *Chlamydia pneumoniae* is identified.

Causes:

- *Atherosclerosis* (as degenerative process) is the *most common facilitating* cause (95%)—aortic wall contains smooth muscle cell matrix, elastin, collagen; *elastin* (in tunica media) is the main load bearing part with *collagen* (in adventitia) as safe net in the wall to provide tensile strength preventing aneurysm formation. *Elastin in medial layer* of aorta is *degraded* and reduced significantly in infrarenal aorta in relation to collagen, absence or less vasa vasorum in infrarenal aorta and atherosclerotic unstability of the medial wall of aorta cause infrarenal aorta more prone to develop aneurysm. Increased proteolytic activity of aortic medial wall due to increased *matrix metalloproteinases* (MMP) (derived from aortic smooth muscle cells and macrophages) cause elastin and collagen degradation and increase in diameter of aneurysm. *Collagen degradation in adventitia* causes rupture.

- *Familial* aortic aneurysm (associated with 25% of AAA) is more prevalent in females to reduce male to female ratio to 2:1. It is related to decrease in type III collagen, α1 antitrypsin and lysyl oxidase. Marfan's, Ehler-Danlos syndromes are related genetically.
- *Others:* Syphilis, dissection, trauma, collagen diseases, infection, arteritis, cystic medial necrosis, association with *Chlamydia pneumoniae* (55%).

Classification I:

- Infrarenal—most common 95%.
- Suprarenal—5%. Isolated suprarenal type is rare; it is usually associated with thoracic and or infrarenal types.

Classification II:

- Asymptomatic.
- Symptomatic.
- Symptomatic ruptured.

Asymptomatic type is found incidentally either on clinical examination or on angiography or on ultrasound. Repair is required if diameter is over 5.5 cm on ultrasound. It is identified during routine abdominal palpation or while assessing or operating for some other abdominal conditions.

Investigations:

- Blood urea, serum creatinine.
- U/S (*most widely used* noninvasive test; but neck of the aneurysm, dimensions and relation to renal arteries are difficult to assess), aortogram, DSA, CT scan (*most precise*). *U/S is an effective screening tool.* Screening is done in cardiovascular patients in men (60-85 years), in women (60-85 years); men and women above 50 years with family history; annually in asymptomatic AAA with 4.0-4.5 cm size, with size > 4.5 cm once in every 6 months.
- CT angiogram, MR angiogram.
- Blood sugar, lipid profile.
- Other relevant investigations like echocardiography, cardiac and pulmonary assessment.
- X-ray will show *eggshell* calcification. CT scan is *more reliable and precise* investigation of choice gives better information regarding extent on sides/neck, size, dimensions, size and site

of the thrombus, calcification, relation of renal arteries, inflammation and fibrosis and adjacent tissues. MRI may be better only in renal failure patients.

Complications of abdominal aortic aneurysm:

- Rupture, infection
- Thrombosis, embolism
- Distal ischemia/gangrene
- Aortocaval fistula formation
- Aortoenteric fistula
- Erosion of vertebra
- Spinal cord ischemia when thrombosis develops

Differential Diagnosis:

- Retroperitoneal mass, pseudocyst of pancreas, retroperitoneal cyst mimic abdominal aortic aneurysm especially when it is thrombosed.
- Mesenteric ischemia, acute pancreatitis, perforated duodenal ulcer may mimic ruptured aneurysm.
- Other conditions causing back pain like disc prolapse, sciatica.

Treatment:

- **Conservative/Medical Treatment**
  - It is done in *low-risk* abdominal aortic aneurysm (age below 70 years; active physically without cardiac, respiratory, renal impairment and noninflammatory aneurysm); if aneurysm size is < 5 cm; if growth rate is < 0.5 cm/year.
  - It includes risk factor modifications; stopping smoking; control of blood pressure (propranolol), cholesterol; usage of drugs—alpha blockers, elastase inhibitors (NSAID—indomethacin), matrix metalloproteinases (MMP) inhibitor (doxycycline).
  - Periodic size measurement of an aneurysm using ultrasound once in 6 months to find out growth rate is essential during conservative treatment.
- **Surgical Treatment:** *Indications for surgery are:*
  - Asymptomatic aneurysm more than 5.5 cm.
  - Growth rate more than 0.5 cm/year.
  - Painful, tender aneurysm.
  - Thrombosed aneurysm, aneurysm with distal emboli.

8. **Ans. (D) Vulva**

Adenocarcinoma arising from the apocrine glands of skin is called as *extramammary Paget's* disease of skin (intraepidermal adenocarcinoma) commonly observed in perianal region. It can occur in genitalia or in axilla (more apocrine glands). In 25%

of cases, the condition is associated with an *underlying in situ* or invasive carcinoma. *Presentation* is like red plaque/white/depigmented areas/crusts/scales mimicking dermatitis, eczema, fungal infections. Condition is often associated with GI or urinary malignancies (40%). Biopsy of lesion, CT evaluation for other malignancies, wide local excision and radiotherapy—are the management principles.

It is a rare extramammary disease, is comparable to intraductal carcinoma of the breasts, because the apocrine sweat glands are involved. It occurs in a postmenopausal woman as a sharply demarcated and slightly elevated white indurated or eczematous lesion and causes pruritus. The biopsy reveals the characteristic large pale vacuolated cells in the epidermis (See Figure below).

Perianal and perineal areas are rarely involved. The Paget's cells are adenocarcinomatous mucus-secreting cells, round cells with pale cytoplasm and vesicular nuclei. Mitosis is rare. Unlike Paget's disease of the breast, the underlying carcinoma is reported in only 20% due to adenocarcinoma of the Bartholin's gland. In the perianal region, it is associated with adenocarcinoma of the anus. It is important to search for the underlying malignancy which may be involved in 30% cases.

The treatment is local excision or vulvectomy if no underlying lesion is detected. With underlying lesion, treatment is as of invasive cancer. Radiotherapy is employed for women unfit for surgery but prolonged follow-up for recurrence is obligatory. Local and systemic 5 FU and bleomycin is also tried. The tumor recurs in 20%.

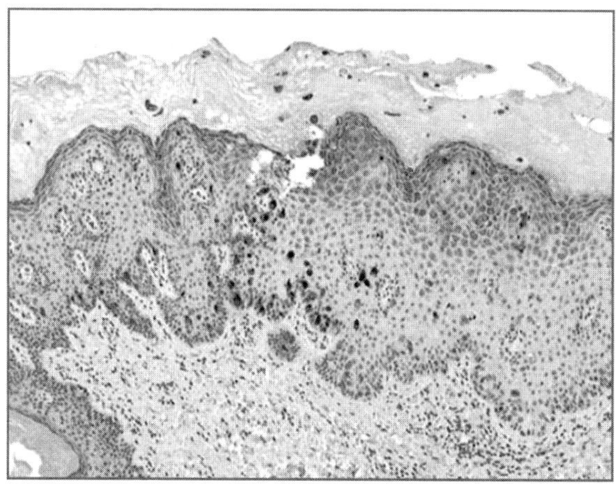

Paget's disease of the vulva

9. **Ans. (A) Morris retractor**

Morris Retractor:

- It may be single blade type or double blade type.
- It is used to retract abdominal wall.
- It helps in keeping the incision open and to keep the skin and tissue away from the bones and the organs while surgery is being performed, allowing the surgeon to go deeper into the surgical site without having to constantly face tissue and skin.
- A retractor such as the Morris retractor is usually curved. The handle of the retractor is made in a manner to provide the surgeon with the utmost grip and for the instrument to be comfortable while being used. There are some Morris retractors which are double ended as well and hence can be used from either side. A retractor may have to be held in place by the surgeon or his assistant or it could even be placed onto the surgical field.

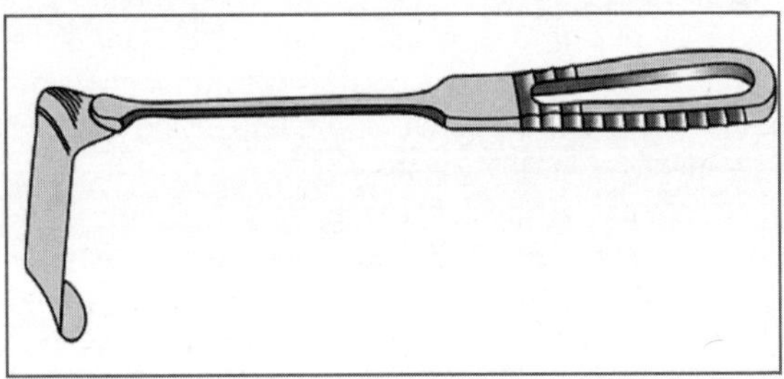

10. **Ans. A. Urate**

- Uric acid stones are one of four major types of kidney stones, which include calcium stones (calcium oxalate and calcium phosphate), struvite stones and cystine stones.
- Among men, the lifetime risk is about 19%; in women, it is 9%. Usually, the first incidence of kidney stones occurs after age 30. However, there are many cases that occur sooner, some in children as young as five years of age.
- Uric acid stones form when the levels of uric acid in the urine is too high, and/or the urine is too acidic (pH level below 5.5) on a regular basis. High acidity in urine is linked to the following causes:
  - Inherited problems in how the body processes uric acid or protein in the diet can increase the acid in urine. This can be seen in conditions such as gout, which is known for its high levels of uric acid in the blood and painful deposits of crystals in the joints.

- Uric acid can result from a diet high in purines, which are found especially in animal proteins such as beef, poultry, pork, eggs and fish. The highest levels of purines are found in organ meats, such as liver and fish. Eating large amounts of animal proteins can cause uric acid to build up in the urine. The uric acid can settle and form a stone by itself or in combination with calcium. It is important to note that a person's diet alone is not the cause of uric acid stones. Other people might eat the same diet and not have any problems because they are not prone to developing uric acid stones.
- There is an increased risk of uric acid stones in those who are obese or diabetic.
- Patients on chemotherapy are prone to developing uric acid stones.
- Laxative abuse should be suspected whenever a woman has an ammonium urate renal calculus in sterile urine.

- All types of kidney stones produce similar symptoms, including one or more of the following:
  i. Pain in the lower back, sides, abdomen or groin; the pain is the result of irritation or blockage inside the kidneys or urinary system
  ii. Blood in the urine
  iii. Nausea or vomiting
  iv. Fever and chills
  v. Urine that smells bad or is cloudy during a urinary tract infection.

11. Ans. D. 11

Glasgow Coma Scale

Behavior	*Response*	*Score*
Eye opening response	Spontaneously To speech To pain No response	4 3 2 1
Best verbal response	Oriented to time, place and person Confused Inappropriate words Incomprehensible sounds No response	5 4 3 2 1

Contd...

Contd...

Behavior	*Response*	*Score*
Best motor response	Obeys commands Moves to localized pain Flexion withdrawal from pain Abnormal flexion (decorticate) Abnormal extension (decerebrate) No response	6 5 4 3 2 1
Total score	Best response Comatose client Totally unresponsive	15 8 or less 3

From this table we can calculate GCS as E=2, V=4, Best motor response=5, so answer is 11.

12. Ans. (A) Alcoholism

Chronic pancreatitis: It is persistent progressive irreversible damage of the pancreas due to chronic inflammation.

- It can be chronic relapsing pancreatitis or chronic pancreatitis (persistent) (which can be chronic noncalcifying or calcifying pancreatitis pancreatitis).
- Chronic pancreatitis is more common in males, common in Kerala (induced by diet, rich in Tapioca).

Etiology:

- Alcohol—80% main cause
- Stones in biliary tree—rare cause
- Malnutrition, diet
- Hyperparathyroidism
- Hereditary (familial hereditary pancreatitis)
- Idiopathic—20%—as mutation
- Trauma
- Congenital anomaly (Pancreatic divisum)
- Cystic fibrosis
- Autoimmune pancreatitis
- Hyperlipidemia

TIGAR-O Risk Factor Classification 2001

T – Toxic - alcohol/tobacco/dietary/drug. Metabolic-hypercalcemia/lipidemia/lipoprotein lipase deficiency.

I – Idiopathic—early/late onset/tropical.

G – Genetic mutations—CFTR/SPINK 1.

A – Autoimmune primary/with Sjogren/Crohn's disease.

R – Recurrent and severe acute/ischemic.

O – Obstructive—pancreas divisum/annular pancreas/stenotic papilla/duodenal obstruction/trauma/pancreatic ductal stones/ choledochocele.

13. **Ans. (A) Whole length shows involvement**

Regional enteritis (Crohn's Disease):

- It is a granulomatous, noncaseating inflammatory condition of the ileum commonly and of the colon often.
- It is independent of age, sex, socioeconomic status and geographic areas.

Causes for Crohn's disease:

- *Infectious—Mycobacterium paratuberculosis* and atypical mycobacteria
- *Immunologic*
- *Genetic*—chromosome 16q—IBDI with CARD15/NOD2 gene (40-fold risk)
- *Environmental*
- *Jews* are more prone
- Smoking, diet, OCPs (controversial), psychosocial factors

Main features of Crohn's disease:

- Ileum—most common site of occurrence—60%
- Rectal sparing is usual and common
- Skip lesion
- Hose-pipe pattern
- Linear ulcers and cobble stone appearance of mucosa
- Transmural

Extraintestinal manifestations of Crohn's disease:

- Skin: Erythema nodosum, pyoderma gangrenosum—most common
- Eyes: Iritis, uveitis
- Joints: Arthritis, ankylosing spondylitis
- Sclerosing cholangitis
- Nephrotic syndrome
- Pancreatitis
- Amyloidosis
- *Blood:* Anemia, thrombocytosis, DVT, arterial thrombosis

Investigations:

- Plain X-ray abdomen, ultrasound abdomen.
- *Barium meal follow through or small bowel enema shows—*
  - Straightening of valvulae conniventes.
  - Multiple defects (*cobblestone* appearance).
  - Cicatrisation of ileum (*string sign of Kantor*).

    - *Rose thorn appearance of the bowel wall.*
    - Radiologically Crohn's disease is classified as nonstenosing type or stenosing type.
- CT scan and CT fistulogram is useful method.
- Colonoscopy usually shows normal rectum; with colon showing aphthoid like ulcers and reddened mucosal margin. Deep ulcers, stricture and fistula will be evident in late cases. Colonoscopy also shows segmental, deep, cobblestone look.
- Blood tests for anemia, protein loss, mineral and trace element loss like magnesium, zinc, and selenium. There will be raised *C reactive protein and orosomucoid* in active disease.
- Capsule endoscopy is useful investigation.
- MRI to diagnose anal disease.
- *Serum markers*: 90% of patients with Crohn's disease show ASCA (anti-Saccharomyces cerevisiae antibodies) positive and pANCA (perineural antineutrophil cytoplasmic antibodies) negative, whereas in 98% of patients with ulcerative colitis, ASCA is negative but pANCA positive.

Complications of Crohn's disease:

- Intestinal obstruction
- Stricture
- Bleeding
- Fistula formation
- Carcinoma small and large bowel
- Perianal abscess
- Peritonitis
- Pericolic abscess

Medical therapy:

- To induce remission—steroids
- For maintenance—immunomodulating drugs like azathioprine
- Antibiotics, metronidazole (as immunomodulator)
- Monoclonal antibody—infliximab
- Nutritional support
- Patients with Crohn's disease should avoid NSAIDs

14. Ans. (D) *E. coli*

Prostatitis

Types: Acute or chronic.

- Acute Prostatitis:

  Causes:
    - Due to instrumentation.
    - Ascending infection from below.
    - Hematogenous.
    - Descending infection from above.

Bacteria involved:
- *E. coli, Klebsiella, Proteus.*
- *Staphylococcus.*
- *Streptococcus faecalis.*
- *Gonococcus.*

Clinical features:
- Pain, frequency, fever with chills and rigors.
- Retention of urine.
- Perineal heaviness, pain on defaecation.
- Tender prostate on per rectal examination.
- Initial fraction of urine is turbid which is sent for culture and sensitivity.

Investigations:
- Urine culture and sensitivity.
- Ultrasound abdomen.

Treatment:
- Prolonged rigorous antibiotics for 2 months.
- Avoidance of alcohol and sexual intercourse for 6 weeks.

Complications:
- Formation of single or multiple abscess. It is common in diabetics
- Chronic prostatitis
- Retention of urine

Chronic prostatitis: Caused by *E. coli, Staphylococcus, Streptococcus, Trichomonas, Chlamydia.*
- There is always associated posterior urethritis.
- Epididymitis.
- Pain in the perineum, rectum, low back pain, leg pain.
- Fever.
- Sexual dysfunction.
- Per rectal examination shows tender prostate.
- Prostatic fluid obtained by prostatic massage shows 15 or more pus cells/HPF.
- In three glass urine test—first glass contains prostatic threads.

Treatment: Antibiotics—Co-trimethoxazole, trimethoprim, doxycycline.

15. Ans. (D) Degraded by enzymatic degradation

Absorbable suture materials should not be used for suturing tendon, nerves, vessels (vascular anastomosis).

- **Plain catgut** is derived from submucosa of jejunum of sheep.
  - It is yellowish white in color.
  - It is absorbed by inflammatory reaction and phagocytosis absorption time is 7 days.
  - It is used for subcutaneous tissue, muscle, circumcision in children.

- **Chronic catgut** is catgut with chronic acid salt.
  - It is brown in color.
  - Its absorption time is 21 days.
  - It is used for suturing muscle, fascia, external oblique aponeurosis, ligating pedicles, etc.
- **Vicryl (polyglactic acid):**
  - It is synthetic absorbable suture material.
  - It gets absorbed in 90 days.
  - Absorption is by hydrolysis.
  - It is violet in color (braided).
  - It is multifilament and braided.
  - It is very good suture material for bowel anastomosis, suturing muscles, closure of peritoneum.
- **Dexon (polyglycolic acid)** is synthetic absorbable suture material like vicryl. It is creamy yellow in color (braided).
- **Maxon (polyglyconate)** monofilament.
- PDS (Polydioxanone Suture material) is absorbable suture material. It is creamy in color with properties like vicryl. It is costly but better suture material than vicryl.
- Monocryl (Polyglecaprone) monofilament.
- Biosyn (Glycomer) monofilament.

Nonabsorbable Suture Materials:

- ***Silk*** is natural, multifilament, braided, nonabsorbable suture material derived from cocoon of silkworm larva. It is black in color. It is coated suture material to reduce capillary action.
- ***Polypropylene*** (Prolene) is synthetic, monofilament suture material. It is blue in color. It has got high memory. (*Memory of suture material* is recoiling tendency after removal from the packet. Ideally suture material should have low memory.) (Prolene mesh used for hernioplasty is white in color).
- ***Polyethylene*** (Ethylene) is synthetic monofilament nonabsorbable suture material. It is black in color.
- ***Cotton*** is twisted multifilament natural nonabsorbable suture material. It is white in color.
- ***Linen*** is derived from bark of cotton tree.
- ***Steel, polyester, polyamide, nylon*** are other nonabsorbable suture materials.

16. **Ans. (A) It contains growth factors**

KELOID: 'Like a claw'

- It is common in blacks. Common in females.
- Genetically predisposed. Often familial. Very rare in Caucasians.
- There is defect in maturation and stabilization of collagen fibrils. Normal collagen bundles are absent.

- It continues to grow even after 6 months, may be for many years. It extends into adjacent normal skin. It is brownish black/ pinkish black (due to vascularity) in color, painful, tender and sometimes hyperaesthetic; spreads and causes itching.
- It may be associated with Ehlers-Danlos syndrome or scleroderma.
- When keloid occurs following an unnoticed trauma without scar formation is called as *spontaneous keloid*, commonly seen in Negroes.
- Some keloids occasionally become nonprogressive after initial growth.
- Pathologically keloid contains proliferating immature fibroblasts, proliferating immature blood vessels and type III thick collagen stroma.
  - Site: Common over the sternum. Other sites are upper arm, chest wall, lower neck in front.
  - Differential diagnosis: Hypertrophic scar.
  - Treatment: Controversial.
    - Steroid injection—***intrakeloidal triamcinolone***, is injected at regular intervals, may be once in 7-10 days, of 6-8 injections.
    - Steroid injection—excision—steroid injection.
    - Methotrexate and vitamin A therapy into the keloid.
    - Silicone gel sheeting; topical retinoids.
    - Laser therapy.
    - Vitamin E/palm oil massage.
    - *Intralesional excision* retaining the scar margin may prevent recurrence. *It is ideal and better than just excision.*
    - Excision and irradiation or irradiation alone.
    - Excision and skin grafting may be done.

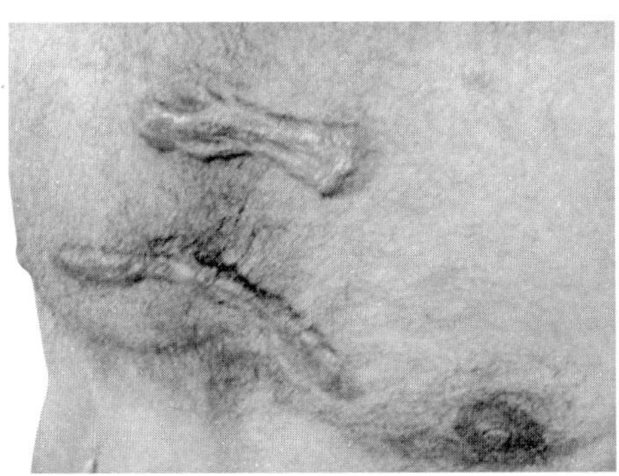

Keloid over sternum (butterfly shaped). Note the typical common site

17. Ans. (B) Reversed saphenous vein

Arterial/venous grafts:

- *Synthetic:*
  - Dacron woven graft
  - Dacron knitted graft
  - PTFE—polytetrafluoroethylene graft
- *Natural:*
  - Internal mammary artery (ideal one)
  - Long saphenous vein either reverse or *in situ*
  - Umbilical vein graft (cryopreserved)—3 mm vein is the minimum diameter required

Reverse saphenous vein graft: In case of femoropopliteal block, saphenous vein is dissected out, reversed and sutured above to the femoral artery and below to popliteal segment so as to bypass the blood through reverse saphenous vein graft. Saphenous vein is reversed to nullify the action of valves so as to allow easy flow of blood.

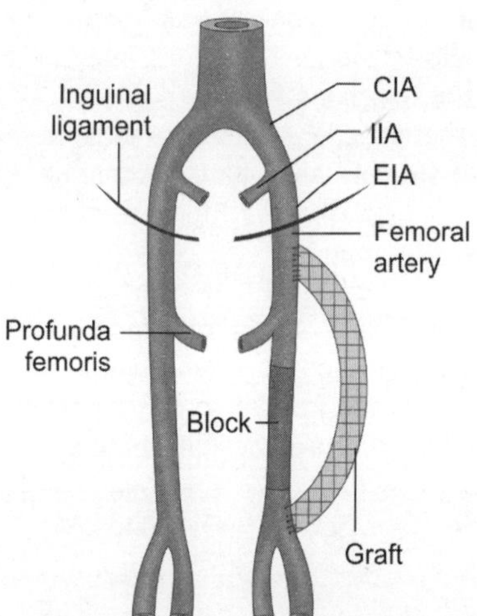

Femoropopliteal bypass graft

14 Pediatrics

1. The abdominal mass swelling of pyloric stenosis can be best felt by?

A. Above umbilicus
B. When baby is being fed milk
C. From right to left upper quadrant
D. When baby is sleeping

2. Time gap between 2 live vaccines is:

A. 2 weeks
B. 4 weeks
C. 8 weeks
D. 6 weeks

3. Which of the following fontanelle is the last to close?

A. Anterolateral
B. Anterior
C. Lateral
D. Occipital

4. True hermaphroditism karyotype is?

A. 45 XO, STREAKED GONADS
B. 46 XX, OVOTESTIS
C. 47 XY+9
D. 47 XX

5. Establishment of fetoplacental circulation seen at?

A. 11 to 13 days
B. 20 to 22 days
C. 7 days
D. 25 to 26 days

6. 1 year child weighing 6 kg is suffering from acute gastroenteritis along with signs of sunken eyes and skin pinch goes back within 2 seconds. What will be your management?

A. RL infusion 120 ml in the first hour followed by 360 ml in the next 5 hours
B. RL infusion 180 ml in the first hour followed by 420 ml in the next 5 hours
C. RL infusion 180 ml in the first hour followed by 480 ml in the next 2 hours
D. RL infusion 240 ml in the first hour followed by 360 ml in the next 5 hours

Answers with Explanations

1. **Ans. (B) When baby is being fed milk**

Idiopathic hypertrophic pyloric stenosis

- Hypertrophic pyloric stenosis is the most common surgical disorder of the gastrointestinal tract in infants.
- The pylorus is thickened and elongated with narrowing of its lumen due to hypertrophy of the circular muscle fibers of pylorus.

Clinical presentation

- The classical presentation is with nonbilious vomiting that gradually increases in frequency and severity to become projectile in nature.
- The disorder is 4–6 times more common in boys than girls.
- Most patients present with vomiting starting beyond 3 weeks of age; however, about 20% are symptomatic since birth and presentation is delayed until 5 months of age in others.
- Constipation is common.
- Recurrent and persistent vomiting causes dehydration, malnutrition and hypochloremic alkalosis.
- As the stomach muscles contract forcibly to overcome the obstruction, a vigorous peristaltic wave can be seen to move from left hypochondrium to umbilicus, particularly on examination after feeding.
- A firm olive-shaped mass is palpable in the mid epigastrium in 75–80% infants, especially after feeds.

Evaluation

Ultrasound abdomen is the diagnostic investigation and shows muscle thickness of > 4 mm and pylorus length of > 16 mm. The ultrasound is 100% sensitive and nearly 90% specific in diagnosis of hypertrophic pyloric stenosis. However, in case of doubt, an upper GI barium study can show a consistent elongation of the pyloric channel or an upper GI endoscopy is performed.

Differential diagnosis

- Gastroesophageal reflux disease
- Cow's milk protein allergy
- Antral or pyloric web are considered in patients without a palpable pyloric mass and normal ultrasound.

Management

- The treatment includes rapid correction of dehydration and electrolyte abnormalities.

- The treatment of choice is surgical; a pyloromyotomy (Ramstedt operation) is performed.

2. Ans. (B) 4 weeks

Principles of Immunization

While immunizing children, certain guidelines are useful in order to maximize the benefit from vaccination. Important considerations during immunization are as follows:

- Compliance with the recommended dose and route of vaccination limits adverse events and loss of efficacy.
- A minimum interval of 4 weeks is recommended between the administrations of two live vaccines, if not administered simultaneously. Exceptions are—OPV and MMR and OPV and oral typhoid (Ty21a), where administration of one before or after another is permitted if necessary.
- Killed antigens may be administered simultaneously or at any interval between the doses. However, a minimum interval of 4 weeks between doses of DPT enhances immune responses. A gap of 3-4 weeks is recommended between two doses of cholera or yellow fever vaccine.
- There is no minimum recommended time interval between two types of vaccines. A live and an inactivated viral vaccine can be administered simultaneously at two different sites.
- A delay or lapse in the administration of a vaccine does not require the whole schedule to be repeated; the missed dose can be administered to resume the course at the point it was interrupted.
- Mixing of vaccines in the same syringe is not recommended, unless approved by the manufacturer.
- The following are not contraindications to immunization: Minor illnesses (e.g. upper respiratory tract infection and diarrhea, mild fever), prematurity, history of allergies, malnutrition, recent exposure to infection and current therapy with antibiotics.
- Live vaccines are contraindicated in children with inherited or acquired immunodeficiency and during therapy with immunosuppressive drugs. Live viral vaccines may be given after short courses (less than 2 weeks) of low dose steroids.
- Immunoglobulins interfere with the immune response to certain live vaccines like measles or MMR. If immunoglobulins are administered within 14 days of the vaccine, vaccination should be repeated after 3–6 months. Immunoglobulins do not interfere with the immune response to OPV, yellow fever or oral typhoid vaccines. Hepatitis B, tetanus and rabies vaccine or toxoid

may be administered concurrently with their corresponding immunoglobulin.
- Active immunization is recommended following exposure to rabies, measles, varicella, tetanus and hepatitis B.

3. Ans. (B) Anterior

In humans, the sequence of fontanelle closure is as follows:
- Posterior fontanelle generally closes 2–3 months after birth.
- Sphenoidal fontanelle is the next to close around 6 months after birth.
- Mastoid fontanelle closes next from 6–18 months after birth.
- The anterior fontanelle is generally the last to close between 1–3 years of age.
- If the sagittal fontanelle is present, it is usually located near the parietal notch and is present at birth in 50–80% of perinatal skulls. It is defined by the sixth prenatal month and is usually obliterated at birth or within a few months after birth.
- The sagittal fontanelle has been clinically associated with Down's syndrome and other abnormalities.
- If the metopic fontanelle is present, it will obliterate between 2 to 4 years of age.
- In humans, all fontanelles are generally fused by the fifth year of life with 38% of fontanelles closed by the end of the first year and 96% of the fontanelles closed by the second year.
- In contrast, apes fuse the fontanelles soon after birth—in chimpanzees the anterior fontanelle is fully closed by 3 months of age.

4. Ans. (B) 46 XX, OVOTESTIS

Disorders of gonadal differentiation

These disorders are associated with abnormal gonadal development.
- The gonad is usually streak (no functional gonadal tissue).
- Combinations of partially functional testis or ovary or ovotestis may be observed.
- SRY gene deletion results in normal female phenotype with 46, XY karyotype. Mutations in genes involved in the testicular differentiation (WTI, SOX9, steroidogenic factor 1 and DAXI) are other causes of 46, XY gonadal dysgenesis. These disorders are associated with renal (WTI mutation), skeletal (SOX9) and adrenal abnormalities (DAXI). 46, XY gonadal dysgenesis is associated with risk of development of gonadoblastoma.
- Asymmetric gonadal location may result in asymmetric genital appearance.

- 46, XX gonadal dysgenesis is usually caused by SRY translocation and presents as normal appearing male. Ovotesticular DSD, new term for true hermaphroditism is characterized by the presence of both ovarian and testicular tissue in the same individual.

Karyotype based classification of disorders of sexual differentiation (DSD)

Karyotype	*Normal genital*	*Genital ambiguity appearance*
46 XX	SRY insertion Severe 21-hydroxylase deficiency	Congenital adrenal hyperplasia Aromatase deficiency Maternal virilization Maternal drug intake
46 XY	SRY deletion SF1 defect Gonadal dysgenesis Severe StAR defect Complete androgen Insensitivity syndrome	Testicular dysgenesis Steroidogenic defects Partial androgen insensitivity syndrome Aromatase dysgenesis
46 XY/ 45 X		Gonadal dysgenesis Ovotesticular DSD

5. **Ans. (B) 20 to 22 days**

Fetoplacental circulation

- Fetal circulation is established by 21st day after fertilization. The heart assumes its normal four-chambered shape by the end of six weeks of intrauterine life. From then on only minor changes occur and consist mainly in the growth of the heart as a whole with increasing age of the fetus. For the exchange of gases the fetus is dependent on placental circulation, whereas the neonate is dependent on the lungs.
- Immediately following birth, with the first inspiration, the lungs expand with air and the gas exchange function is transferred from the placenta to the lungs. This necessitates circulatory adjustments following birth to transform the fetal circulation to the postnatal circulation. Blood oxygenated in the placenta is returned by way of umbilical veins, which enter the fetus at the umbilicus and join the portal vein. The ductus venosus provides a low resistance bypass between the portal vein and the inferior vena cava.
- Most of the umbilical venous blood shunts through the ductus venosus to the inferior vena cava. Only a small proportion mixes with the portal venous blood and passes through the liver. Blood from inferior vena cava comprising that from hepatic veins, umbilical veins and that from lower extremities and

kidneys enters the right atrium. On reaching the right atrium the bloodstream is divided into two by the inferior margin of septum secundum-the crista dividens.

- About one-third of the inferior vena cava blood enters the left atrium, through the foramen ovale, the rest two-third mixes with the venous return from the superior vena cava to enter the right ventricle.
- The blood reaching the left atrium from the right atrium mixes with small amount of blood reaching the left atrium through the pulmonary veins and passes to the left ventricle. The left ventricle pumps out the blood into the ascending aorta for distribution to the coronaries, head and upper extremities.
- The superior vena cava stream, comprising blood returning from the head and arms, passes almost directly to the right ventricle. Only minor quantities (1 to 3%) reaches the left atrium.
- The right ventricle pumps out blood into the pulmonary trunk. A small amount of this blood enters the pulmonary circulation, the rest passes through the ductus arteriosus into the descending aorta to mix with the small amount of blood reaching the descending aorta from the aortic arch (derived from the left ventricle).
- The main differences between the fetal and postnatal circulation are:
  - Presence of placental circulation which provides gas exchange for the fetus
  - Absence of gas exchange in the collapsed lungs; this results in very little flow of blood to the lungs and thus little pulmonary venous return to left atrium
  - Presence of ductus venosus, joining the portal vein with the inferior vena cava, providing a low resistance bypass for umbilical venous blood to reach the inferior vena cava
  - Widely open foramen ovale to enable oxygenated blood (through umbilical veins) to reach the left atrium and ventricle for distribution to the coronaries and the brain and lastly
  - Wide open ductus arteriosus to allow right ventricular blood to reach the descending aorta, since lungs are non-functioning.

6. Ans. (B) RL infusion 180 ml in the first hour followed by 420 ml in the next 5 hours

This child is having symptoms of dehydration that is sunken eyes and skin pinch goes back slowly, so he should be treated according to the treatment plans of dehydration (i.e. Plan C).

Assessment of dehydration in patients with diarrhea			
Look at			
Condition	Well alert	Restless, irritable	Lethargic or unconscious; floppy
Eyes	Normal	Sunken	Very sunken and dry
Tears	Present	Absent	Absent
Mouth and tongue	Moist	Dry	Very dry
Thirst	Drinks normally, not thirsty	Thirsty, drinks eagerly	'Drinks poorly' or is not able to drink
Feel			
Skin pinch	Goes back quickly	Goes back slowly	Goes back very slowly
Decide	The patient has no signs of dehydration	If the patient has two or more signs, there is some dehydration	If the patient has two or more signs, there is severe dehydration
Treat	Use treatment **Plan A**	Weigh the patient, if possible, and use treatment **Plan B**	Weigh the patient and use treatment **Plan C** urgently

Treatment plan A: Treatment of 'No Dehydration'

Such children may be treated at home after explanation of feeding and the danger signs to the mother/caregiver. The mother may be given WHO ORS for use at home. Danger signs requiring medical attention are those of continuing diarrhea beyond 3 days, increased volume/ frequency of stools, repeated vomiting, increasing thirst, refusal to feed, fever or blood in stools.

Oral redehydration therapy to prevent dehydration (Plan A)		
Age	*Amount of ORS or other culturally appropriate ORT fluids to give after each loose stool*	*Amount of ORS to provide for use at home*
< 24 months	50–100 ml	500 ml/day
2–10 year	100–200 ml	1000 ml/day
> 10 year	Ad lib	2000 ml/day

Treatment Plan B: Treatment of 'Some Dehydration'

All cases with obvious signs of dehydration need to be treated in a health center or hospital. However, oral fluid therapy must be commenced promptly and continued during transport. Fluid requirement is calculated under the following three headings:

1. Provision of normal daily fluid requirements
2. Rehydration to correct the existing water or electrolyte deficits
3. Maintenance to replace ongoing losses to prevent recurrence of dehydration.

- The daily fluid requirements in children are calculated as follows:
  Up to 10 kg = 100 ml/kg
  10–20 kg = 50 ml/kg
  > 20 kg = 20 ml/kg
  As an example, the daily fluid requirement in a child weighing 15 kg will be 1250 ml (first 10 kg, 10 x 100 =1000 ml; another 5 kg, 5 x 50 = 250 ml, total 1000 + 250 = 1250 ml).
- Deficit replacement or rehydration therapy is calculated as 75 ml/kg of ORS, to be given over 4 hr. If ORS cannot be taken orally then nasogastric tube can be used. If child's weight cannot be taken then only age may be used to calculate fluid requirement as shown in table.

Guidelines for treating patients with some dehydration (Plan B)

Age	*<4 mo*	*4–11 mo*	*12–23 mo*	*2–4 year*	*5–14 years*	*≥ 15 years*
Weight	<5 kg	5–8 kg	8–11 kg	11–16 kg	16–20 kg	>30 kg
ORS, ml	200–400	400–600	600–800	800–1200	1200–2200	> 2200
No. of glasses	1–2	2–3	3–4	4–6	6–11	12–20

If after 4 hr, the child still has some dehydration then another treatment with ORS (as in rehydration therapy) is to be given. This therapy is effective in 95% cases.

Oral rehydration therapy may be ineffective in children with a high stool purge rate of >5 ml/kg body weight/hr, persistent vomiting >3 per hr, paralytic ileus and incorrect preparation of ORS (very dilute solution).

- Maintenance fluid therapy to replace losses. This phase should begin when signs of dehydration disappear, usually within 4 hr. ORS should be administered in volumes equal to diarrheal losses, usually to a maximum of 10 ml/kg per stool. Breastfeeding and semisolid food are continued after replacement of deficit. Plain water can be offered in between.

Treatment Plan C: Children with 'Severe Dehydration'

Intravenous fluids should be started immediately using Ringer lactate with 5% dextrose. Normal saline or plain Ringer solution may be used as an alternative, but 5% dextrose alone is not effective. A total of 100 ml/kg of fluid is given, over 6 hr in children <12 months and over 3 hr in children >12 months as shown below. ORS solution should be started simultaneously if the child can take orally. If IV fluids cannot be given (for reasons of access, logistic availability or during transport), nasogastric feeding is given at 20 ml/kg/hr for 6 hr (total 120 ml/kg). The child should be reassessed every 1–2 hr; if there is repeated vomiting or abdominal distension, the oral or nasogastric fluids are given more slowly. If there is no improvement in hydration after 3 hr, IV fluids should be started as early as possible. The child should be reassessed every 15–30 min for pulses and hydration status after the first bolus of 100 ml/kg of IV fluid. Management following intravenous hydration end is to be done as follows:

Age	*30 ml/kg*	*70 ml/kg*
< 12 mo	1 hr	5 hr
> 12 mo	30 min	2 ½ hr

- Persistence of severe dehydration. Intravenous infusion is repeated.
- Hydration is improved but some dehydration is present. IV fluids are discontinued; ORS is administered over 4 hr according to Plan B
- There is no dehydration. IV fluids are discontinued; treatment Plan A is followed.

The child should be observed for at least 6 hr before discharge, to confirm that the mother is able to maintain the child's hydration by giving ORS solution.

Unique problems in infants below 2 months of age.

Breastfeeding must continue during the rehydration process, whenever the infant is able to suck. Complications like septicemia, paralytic ileus and severe electrolyte disturbance are more likely in young infants with diarrhea than at later ages. Diarrhea in these infants should be ideally treated as inpatient by experienced physicians at treatment centers with appropriate facilities. This allows for careful assessment of need of systemic antibiotics and monitoring.

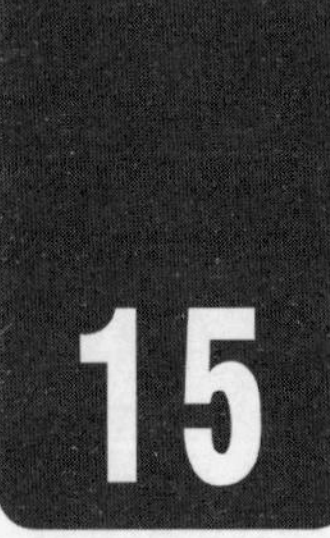

15 Gynecology and Obstetrics

1. Obstetric nerve palsy associated in puerperium causes:

A. Median nerve
B. Facial nerve
C. Wrist drop
D. Foot drop

2. Female with complaints of infertility, HSG showing what?

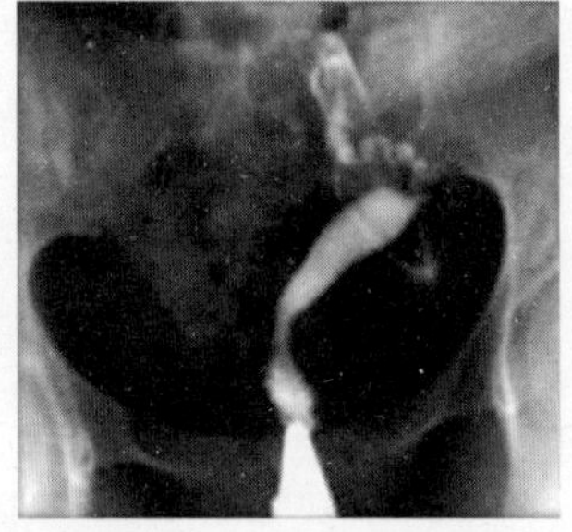

A. Unicornuate uterus
B. Septate uterus
C. Bicornuate uterus
D. Uterus didelphys

3. Section of uterus showing what?

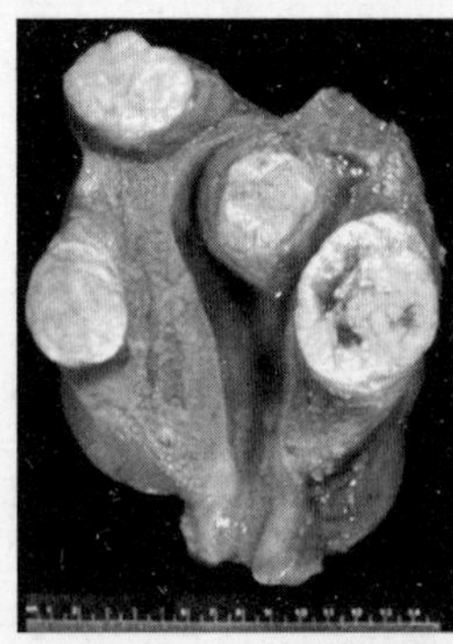

A. Leiomyoma
B. Endometrial polyp
C. Endometriosis
D. Leiomyosarcoma

4. Which is an epithelial cancer?

A. Endometrioid
B. Dysgerminoma
C. Granulose cell tumor
D. Leydig cell tumor

5. In shoulder dystocia, next step in management is:

A. Immediate C-section
B. Flex hips on abdomen
C. O_2 ventilation is least effective
D. Rotate the shoulders 90° manually

6. Anesthesia of choice for pre-eclampsia patients during delivery is:

A. Epidural + Spinal
B. GA
C. Epidural
D. Spinal

7. Sacrospinous fixation is for strengthening:

A. Apical defect
B. Posterior defect
C. Lateral defect
D. Anterior defect

8. How to see if pessary is adequately inserted or not?

A. Patient feels discomfort
B. Do not comes out during voiding
C. After Valsalva pessary do not come out
D. Onc finger gap between vagina and ring

9. A female is found to be positive for HIV in pregnancy. How will you manage this case?

A. Start ART in second trimester and give till pregnancy
B. Start ART immediately and give till pregnancy
C. Start ART in second trimester and continue lifelong
D. Start ART immediately and continue lifelong

10. Fimbriectomy is also known as:

A. Uchida's procedure
B. Kroener procedure
C. Irvings procedure
D. Pomeroy procedure

11. Regarding Progestine only pill incorrect is:

A. Ovulation is stopped completely
B. Ovulation can occur some time
C. Make cervical mucosa thick
D. Interfere with implantation

12. What is meant by Superfecundation?

A. Fertilization of two or more ova in one intercourse
B. Fertilization of two or more ova in different intercourses in same menstrual cycle
C. Fertilization of ova and then it is division
D. Fertilization of second ovum first being implanted

13. Fetal heart starts beating at:

A. 10–12 days
B. 10–12 weeks
C. 3–5 weeks
D. 3–5 month

14. Which of the following is not a high risk pregnancy?

A. Previous history of manual removal of placenta
B. Anemia
C. Infertility history
D. Obesity

15. Dilatation and curettage (D and C) is contraindicated in:

A. Pelvic inflammatory disease (PID)
B. Endometriosis
C. Ectopic pregnancy
D. None

16. Which of the following is correct regarding placenta?

A. Placental artery provides nutrients through umbilical cord to fetus
B. Placenta has Wharton's jelly
C. Placenta has 2 veins and 1 artery
D. Estrogen is secreted by placenta

17. Acute fatty liver commonly seen in pregnancy at:

A. 3rd trimester
B. 1st trimester
C. Immediate postpartum
D. Intrapartum

18. Which one of the following is not a cause of secondary postpartum hemorrhage?

A. Placenta previa
B. Retained bits of placenta
C. Endometritis
D. Polyp

19. Best time to do quadruple test is:

A. 8–12 weeks
B. 11–15 weeks
C. 15–20 weeks
D. 18–22 weeks

20. Drug that is used for fetal lung maturity is:

A. Dexamethasone B. Folic acid
C. Beclomethasone D. None

21. Hormonal replacement therapy is indicated in menopausal women for:

A. Hot flushes B. Ca breast
C. Endometriosis D. Uterine bleeding

22. Anteversion of uterus is maintained by which ligament?

A. Cardinal B. Uterosacral
C. Pubocervical D. Round

Answers with Explanations

1. **Ans. (D) Foot drop**
   - Neurologic injury during childbirth has long been recognized as a potential complication, with the lateral femoral cutaneous nerve as the most common obstetric-related nerve injury.
   - Peroneal nerve injury is less commonly encountered and typically unilateral; the incidence of bilateral peroneal neuropathy following childbirth is extremely rare.
   - According to a large review by Wong et al. evaluating the incidence of lower extremity neuropathies after childbirth, the incidence was found to be 0.92%. Factors associated with lower extremity nerve injury in this study were nulliparous women and a prolonged second stage of labor.
   - Most cases of bilateral peroneal neuropathy associated with childbirth occur in developed countries from prolonged mechanical external knee compression and forceful knee flexion.
   - Additionally, nerve injury can result from an extended period of low pressure as well as a short interval of high pressure.
   - Although the vast majority of neurologic injuries associated with childbirth are intrinsic obstetric palsies, neuraxial anesthesia is a risk factor for an obstetric-related neurologic injury.
   - Regional anesthesia, in particular, increases the risk for developing a peroneal neuropathy as it blocks sensation to the lower extremities and, therefore, recognition of an impending nerve injury such as pain or altered sensation.

2. **Ans. (A) Unicornuate uterus**

   Congenital Müllerian malformations (American Fertility Society Classification System):
   - **Class I (agenesis, hypoplasia):** Uterus is absent in total agenesis. Partial agenesis is identified as unicornuate uterus. In hypoplasia, the endometrial cavity is small with reduced intercornual distance of less than 2 cm.
   - **Class II (unicornuate uterus):** Appears banana-shaped without the rounded fundus and triangular-shaped uterine cavity. If present, rudimentary horn presents as a soft tissue mass with similar myometrial echogenicity. Obstruction in the rudimentary horn is recognized as hematometra on one side.

- **Class III (uterus didelphys):** The two horns are widely separated, but vaginal septum is difficult to identify.
- **Class IV (bicornuate uterus):** Shows two uterine cavities, with concave fundus, with fundal cleft greater than 1 cm, and this differentiates between the bicornuate and the septate uterus. The intercornual distance is more than 4 cm.
- **Class V (septate uterus):** Shows a convex or flattened fundus. The intercornual distance is normal (4 cm) and each cavity is small.
- **Class VI (arcuate uterus):** With no fundus is of no clinical importance.

Congenital müllerian anomalies

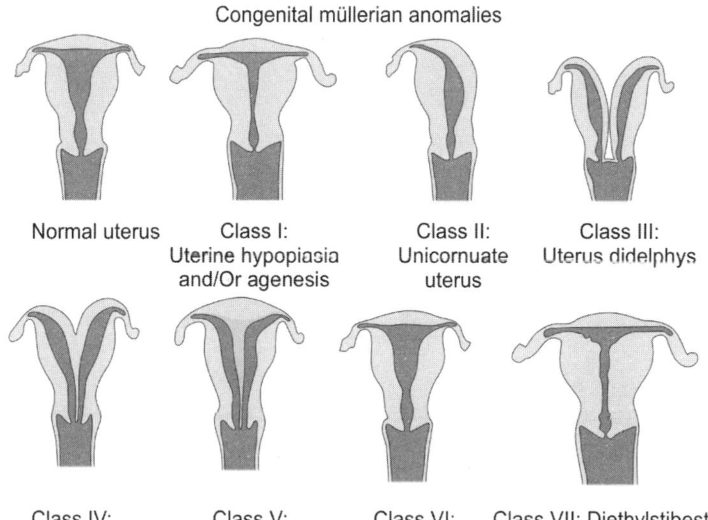

3. **Ans. (A) Leiomyoma**
   - Fibromyomas (leiomyomas, fibroids or simply myomas) are generally benign uterine neoplasms, commonly encountered in gynecological practice (5–20% of women in the reproductive age group). They are slow growing tumors and take 3–5 years to be clinically palpable, unlike ovarian tumors. The presence of myoma causes hyperplasia of the myometrial wall.
   - The cavity of the uterus is often distorted and enlarged. The endometrium tends to be thicker due to endometrial hyperplasia. The ovaries at times are enlarged, cystic and hyperemic with evidence of salpingo-oophoritis in about 15% cases.

Cervical, submucous and broad ligament fibroids are usually single. Interstitial and subserous fibroids may be single or multiple, varying in size from a seedling fibroid to a huge neoplasm.

- **Etiology:** Each myoma is derived from smooth muscle cell rests, either from vessel walls or uterine musculature. Although estrogen, progesterone growth hormone and possibly human placental lactogen have been implicated in the growth of myomas. The fibroids are often associated with adenomyosis, pelvic endometriosis and pelvic inflammatory disease. The distribution of myoma in the body of the uterus is broadly classified as follows:
  - Intramural (interstitial): 75%
  - Submucous: 15%
  - Subserous: 10%

4. **Ans. (A) Endometrioid**

   WHO classification of ovarian tumors (major groups):
   - **Common epithelial tumors:**
     - Serous tumors
     - Mucinous tumors
     - Endometrioid tumors
     - Clear cell (mesonephroid tumors)
     - Brenner tumors
     - Mixed epithelial tumors
     - Undifferentiated carcinoma
     - Unclassified epithelial tumors
   - **Sex cord (gonadal stromal) tumors:**
     - Granulosa stromal cell tumors, theca cell tumors
     - Androblastomas: Sertoli-Leydig cell tumors
     - Gynandroblastomas
     - Unclassified
   - **Lipid (lipoid) cell tumors**
   - **Germ cell tumors:**
     - Dysgerminoma
     - Endodermal sinus tumor
     - Embryonal carcinoma
     - Polyembryoma
     - Choriocarcinoma
     - Teratoma
     - Mixed forms

- **Gonadoblastoma:**
  - Pure
  - Mixed with dysgerminoma or other germ cell tumors
- Soft tissue tumors not specific to ovary
- Unclassified tumors
- Secondary (metastatic) tumors
- Tumor-like conditions

5. **Ans. (B) Flex hips on abdomen**

The term shoulder dystocia is defined to describe a wide range of additional obstetric maneuvers to deliver the fetus after the head has been born and gentle traction has failed to deliver the shoulder. **Shoulder dystocia** occurs when either the anterior or the posterior (rare) fetal shoulder impacts on the maternal symphysis or on the sacral promontory respectively. Overall incidence varies between 0.2% and 1%. All maternity staff should have shoulder dystocia training.

Risk factors: (1) Previous shoulder dystocia, (2) Macrosomia (>4.5 kg), (3) Diabetes, (4) Obesity (BMI >30 kg/m^2), (5) Induced labor, (6) Prolonged first stage or second stage of labor, (7) Secondary arrest of labor,(8) Postmaturity, (9) Multiparity, (10) Anencephaly, (11) Mid-pelvic instrumental delivery (more following ventouse than forceps), (12) Fetal ascites.

Management: The following maneuvers are commonly employed. There is no evidence that any method is superior to another in releasing the impacted shoulder or reducing the chance.

Injury:

- Head and neck should be grasped and taken posteriorly while suprapubic pressure is applied by an assistant slightly toward the side of fetal chest. This will reduce the bisacromial diameter and rotate the anterior shoulder toward the oblique diameter. **This maneuver is simple as well as effective. It needs only one assistant.**
- **McRoberts maneuver:** Abduct the maternal thighs and sharply hyperflex them onto her abdomen. There is rotation of symphysis pubis upward and decrease in angle of pelvic inclination. This straightens the lumbosacral angle, rotates the maternal pelvis upward and increases the anterior-posterior diameter of the pelvis. This maneuver is effective and is successful in about 90% of cases. Suprapubic pressure may be used together.

- **Wood's maneuver:** General anesthesia is administered. The posterior shoulder is rotated to anterior position (180°) by a corkscrew movement. This is done by inserting two fingers in the posterior vagina. Simultaneous suprapubic pressure is applied. This pushes the bisacromial diameter from the anteroposterior diameter to an oblique diameter. This helps easy entry of the bisacromial diameter into the pelvic inlet.
- **Extraction of the posterior arm:** The operator's hand is introduced into the vagina along the fetal posterior humerus in the sacral hollow. The arm is then swept across the chest and thereafter delivered by gentle traction. This procedure may cause either fracture clavicle or humerus or both.
- **"All Fours" Position:** Changing the mother on to all fours may increase the pelvic dimensions and allow the fetal position to shift. Downward traction on the posterior shoulder helps to free the impacted shoulder. This may be done for a mobile and slim woman in a community setting.
- Other techniques may be used when all the above maneuvers have failed:
  - Deliberate fracture of the clavicle by finger pressure (fracture heals rapidly) or **cleidotomy:** One or both clavicles may be cut with scissors to reduce the shoulder girth. This is applicable to a living anencephalic baby as a first choice or in a dead fetus.
  - **Zavanelli maneuver** (pushing the fetus back to the uterus and delivering by cesarean section) or **symphysiotomy** is done rarely.

6. Ans. (C) Epidural

Management of pre-eclampsia: Principles of management are same as that of pre-eclampsia and eclampsia. Antiseizure prophylaxis with magnesium sulphate is started. Careful assessment of maternal and fetal status followed by delivery is done. Administration of corticosteroids improves perinatal (↑ pulmonary maturity, ↓ IVH and ↓ necrotizing enterocolitis) and maternal (↑ thrombocyte count, ↑ urinary output) outcome. Cesarean section is the common mode of delivery. Epidural anesthesia can be used safely if the platelet count is >1,00,000/mm^3).Platelet transfusion should be given if the count is <50,000/mm^3. Patient should be managed in an ICU until there is improvement in platelet count, urine output, BP and liver enzymes. Recurrence risk of HELLP syndrome is 3–19%.

Cesarean section: The operation should be done by an experienced surgeon with the help of an expert anesthetist. **Epidural anesthesia is preferred,** unless there is coagulopathy.

Indications: (1) **When an urgent termination is indicated and the cervix is unfavorable** (unripe and closed).

(2) **Severe pre-eclampsia** with a tendency of prolonged induction—delivery interval.

(3) **Associated complicating factors,** such as elderly primigravidae, contracted pelvis, malpresentation, etc.

Management during labor: Blood pressure tends to rise during labor and convulsions may occur due to stress hormones (intrapartum eclampsia). The patient **should be in bed**. **Antihypertensive drugs** are given if the blood pressure becomes high. **Blood pressure and urinary output are to be noted** frequently so as to detect imminent eclampsia. Prophylactic $MgSO_4$ is started when systolic BP >160 diastolic >110, MAP >125 mm Hg. **Careful monitoring of the fetal well-being** is mandatory. **Labor duration is curtailed by** low rupture of the membranes in the first stage; and forceps or ventouse in second stage. **Intravenous ergometrine following the delivery of the anterior shoulder is withheld** as it may cause further rise of blood pressure. However, there is no contraindication of syntocinon IM or slow IV and to keep the patient under close observation for several hours.

7. **Ans. (A) Apical defect**
    - **Sacrospinous ligament fixation:** The main indication for sacrospinous ligament fixation is to correct total procidentia or post-hysterectomy vaginal vault prolapse with an associated weak cardinal uterosacral ligament complex and to correct posthysterectomy enterocele. The contraindication for the procedure is a short vagina.
    - The principle of this procedure is the fixation of the vaginal vault to the sacrospinous ligament with nonabsorbable sutures. The fixation site is typically the right sacrospinous ligament. However, bilateral fixation is performed in patients with recurrent vault prolapse and with the goal of restoring a vaginal axis and sexual life. The routes of entry to the sacrospinous ligament may be posterior and anterior. Usually, a unilateral, right-sided, posterior approach is preferred.
    - This procedure has advantages, including success rates comparable to abdominal procedures, the ability to repair

concomitant pelvic floor defects, the absence of laparotomy, shorter hospital stays, and the preservation of vaginal length and function.

- The most common problem after this procedure is the high rate of postoperative cystocele, which approaches 20% to 33%, resulting from the deviation of the vaginal axis. Recurrent cystoceles have been reported in 6% to 92% of patients.
- Other disadvantages include difficulty in exposing the ligament, the potential need for excessive tensioning during tying, injury risk to the pudendal or inferior gluteal vessels and sciatic or pudendal nerve, alterations in the vaginal axis, and vaginal narrowing.
- Thomson et al. have reported that by placing the sutures through the sacrospinous ligament 2.5 cm more medially from the ischial spine along the superior border of the ligament and not through the full thickness of the ligament, the risk of complications is minimal.

8. Ans. (C) After Valsalva pessary do not come out

Pessary treatment of prolapse: The ring pessary for prolapse is nearly a thing of the past when majority of elderly women and very young women desirous of childbearing received this treatment. With modern anesthesia and good preoperative care, advanced age is no longer a contraindication to permanent surgical procedure. The pessary treatment of prolapse has certain limitations:

- It is never curative and can only be palliative.
- It can cause vaginitis.
- Pessary needs to be changed every 3 months.
- The wearing of a pessary is not comfortable to some women and may cause dyspareunia.
- If the vaginal orifice is very patulous, the pessary is often not retained.
- A forgotten pessary can be the cause of ulcer, and in rare cases, carcinoma of the vagina and a vesicovaginal fistula.
- A pessary does not cure urinary stress incontinence.

Current *indications* for use of pessary are:

- A young woman planning a pregnancy.
- During early pregnancy.
- Puerperium.
- Temporary use while clearing infection and decubitus ulcer.
- A woman unfit for surgery.

- In case a woman refuses for surgery.
- The ring pessary made of soft plastic polyvinyl chloride material is available in different sizes. In a young woman planning to conceive in the near future, the operation is better postponed till after the childbirth, because a good surgical result could be ruined by vaginal delivery.
- Similarly, a pregnant woman with prolapse needs a ring pessary in the first trimester of pregnancy. As the uterus grows abdominally, the prolapse gets reduced, and the pessary can then be removed.
- Pessary treatment may be needed in a puerperal woman with severe degree of prolapse and distressing symptoms, while the conservative measures are being carried out in the first few months after delivery.

How to know if pessary fits well: Successful fitting usually means that the largest possible size device is fitted and sits comfortably within the vagina when you are standing upright. Pessaries are available in a various sizes and styles to suit women's individual differences and prolapse needs.

- When lying flat pessary may move down within vagina when patient cough, sneeze or hold breath and strain however it should not move back when relax. If device moves back when patient relax, that means need refitting with a larger size.
- A well fitting pessary will not cause pelvic discomfort when standing up and walking. When patient cough, bend forwards, squat or hold her breath and strain the device should not move down out of vagina. If the pessary moves to the entrance or out of vagina she may require refitting with a larger size.
- The pessary should stay in place when patient empty her bladder. It should not cause any change in bladder emptying such as difficulty initiating bladder emptying, slowing the flow of urine or feeling unable to completely empty the bladder.
- A well fitting pessary will not cause bladder control problems.
- The pessary should not cause constipation or difficulty completely emptying bowels.
- A well fitting pessary will not be felt within the vagina. When fitted, pessaries should not cause low abdominal or vaginal discomfort or pain in any upright or lying down position. Some women feel slight pelvic discomfort caused by the process of being fitted.

- A well fitting pessary should not be too tight against the walls of vagina. This can be checked by ensuring by running a fingertip between the outer edge of the pessary and the vaginal walls.
- Vaginal bleeding when wearing a prolapse can be a sign of erosion of the vaginal walls.

9. Ans. (D) Start ART immediately and continue lifelong

The summary of the Technical Guidelines and Options for the more efficacious PPTCT regimen

National Guidelines for Prevention of Parent-to-Child Transmission of HIV

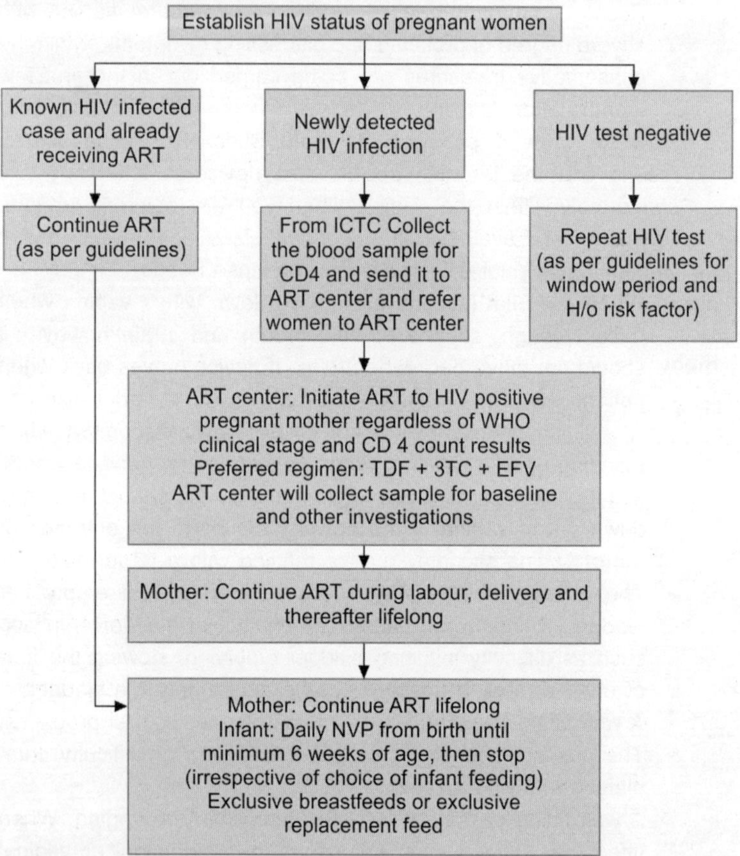

10. Ans. (B) Kroener procedure

The technique of fimbriectomy as described by Kroener employs the ligation of the distal ampulla of the tube with two permanent sutures and then division and removal of the infundibulum of the tube (See Figure below). Ligation and hemostasis are accomplished simultaneously. The simplicity with which this excisional procedure is performed on the distal portion of the tube accounted for its early popularity, especially when the sterilization was being performed through a colpotomy incision.

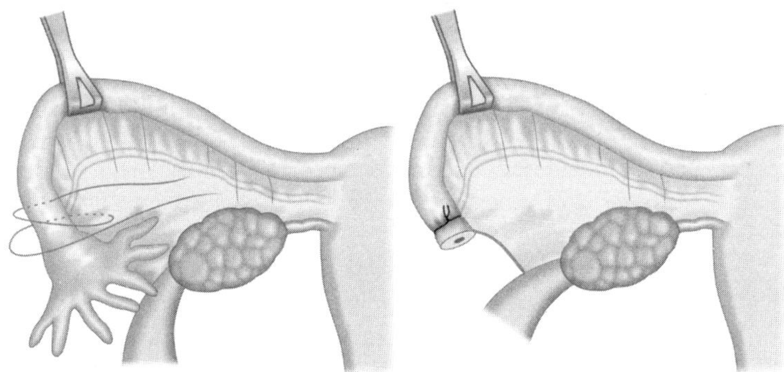

Kroener fimbriectomy. **Left.** A suture is anchored in the mesosalpinx and placed around the tube in the distal ampulla. A second suture may be placed adjacent to the first, and the infundibulum of the tube is excised. **Right.** The tube as it appears following excision of the distal segment.

11. Ans. (A) Ovulation is stopped completely

- Low-dose progestogen-only pill (POP), called 'minipill', is administered daily. Under the influence of progestogen, the cervical mucus becomes viscid and prevents penetration of sperms into the cervical canal. In addition, the pill inhibits ovulation in 40% and reduces fertility.
- The low-dose POP (norethisterone 350 mcg, norgestrel 75 mcg or LNG 30 mcg) have been introduced to avoid the side effects of estrogen in the combined pills. The tablet is taken daily without a break. The pill should be started within 5–7 days of the menstruation and taken at the same time with a leeway of 3 h on either side of the fixed time each day.If this regime is not observed any day, the woman continues with POP but observes extra precaution for 48 h.
- POP is started 21 days postpartum and soon after abortion. The woman needs to take precaution in the first 48 h in the first cycle.
- Minipill does not have some of the major side effects of the combined pill and *it is well suited for lactating women*; some

progestogens, in fact, increase milk secretion. However, it has a pregnancy rate of 2–3 per 100 woman years which is higher than that of the combined pill though comparable to an IUCD and is higher in obese women. Strict daily compliance is a drawback. Other drawbacks are irregular bleeding (20%), amenorrhoea, depression, headache, migraine and weight gain, ectopic pregnancy, functional ovarian cysts besides a higher failure rate.

- The use of newer generation of synthetic progestogen, namely desogestrel, has been encouraging. It has no androgenic effect, no adverse effect on carbohydrate and lipid metabolism, and is considered to be safe, especially for lactating women. *However, the incidence of thromboembolism is higher with these progestogens.*
- **Contraindications:** Contraindications to POP are previous ectopic pregnancy, ovarian cyst, breast and genital cancers, abnormal vaginal bleeding, active liver and arterial disease, porphyria, liver tumor, valproate, spironolactone and meprobamate. *Because of osteopenia, it is contraindicated in adolescents and young women.*
- **Advantages:** Advantages of POP are that they can be recommended to:
  - Lactating women
  - Women over 35 years
  - Those with focal migraine
  - Those intolerant to estrogen or estrogen contraindicated
  - Diabetic, hypertensive woman, sickle cell anemia. As regards to return of fertility, it is faster than in COC users because ovulation is not suppressed in all cases (suppressed in 40%)
- **Mode of Action of Minipills:**
  - Cerazette suppresses ovulation in 97–100%, whereas other progesterone only pills suppress ovulation in only 40%.
  - It forms a thick plug of mucus in the cervical canal and acts as a barrier to sperms.
  - It increases tubal peristalsis and fertilized egg reaches the uterine cavity too early for implantation.

12. Ans. (B) Fertilization of two or more ova in different intercourses in same menstrual cycle

- **Superfecundation** is the fertilization of two different ova released in the same cycle, by separate acts of coitus within a short period of time.

- **Superfetation** is the fertilization of two ova released in different menstrual cycles. The nidation and development of **one fetus over another fetus** is theoretically possible until the decidual space is obliterated by 12 weeks of pregnancy.

13. **Ans. (C) 3–5 weeks**

Fetal viability and gestational age is determined by detecting the following structures by **transvaginal ultrasonography**.

- *Gestational sac and yolk sac* by 5 menstrual weeks
- *Fetal pole and cardiac activity* — 6 weeks
- *Embryonic movements* by 7 weeks
- Fetal gestational age is best determined by measuring the CRL between 7 and 12 weeks (variation ± 5 days).
- **Doppler effect of ultrasound can pick up the fetal heart rate reliably by 10th week.** The instrument is small, handy and cheap. The gestational sac (true) must be differentiated from pseudogestational sac.

14. **Ans. (A) Previous history of manual removal of placenta**

The high risk factors in pregnancy: **Pregnancy**

Reproductive history	*Medical disorders in pregnancy*	*Previous surgery*
• Two or more previous miscarriage or previous induced abortion. • Previous stillbirth, neonatal death or birth of babies with congenital abnormality • Previous preterm labor or birth of a IUGR or macrosomic baby • Grand multiparity • Previous cesarean section or hysterotomy • Third stage abnormalities (PPH) • Previous infant with Rh-isoimmunization or ABO incompatibility	Diseases— • Pulmonary disease –TB • Renal disease • (Pyelonephritis) • Thyroid disorders • Psychiatric illness • Cardiac disease • Epilepsy • Viral hepatitis • Pre-eclampsia • Eclampsia • Anemia • Infections in pregnancy	• Myomectomy • Repair of complete perineal tear • Repair of vesicovaginal fistula • Repair of stress incontinence • **Family History** • **Socioeconomic status**—Patients belonging to low socioeconomic status have a higher incidence of anemia, preterm labor, growth retarded babies • **Family history** of diabetes, hypertension or multiple pregnancy and congenital malformation

15. Ans. (A) Pelvic inflammatory disease (PID)

- Dilatation and curettage is a minor gynecological procedure of dilatating the cervix and curetting (scraping) the endometrial tissue from the uterine cavity. It is mainly a diagnostic procedure, rarely done for therapeutic purpose (mainly obstetric). Dilatation of the cervix alone is required in the following conditions:
  - Prior to curettage (commonest).
  - For cervical stenosis.
  - To prevent cervical stenosis following Manchester operation for prolapse of the uterus.
  - To prevent postoperative cervical stenosis in cauterization of cervical erosion and conization.
  - To drain hematometra.
  - To drain pyometra.
  - Prior to insertion of radium into the uterine cavity in cancer of the cervix and endometrial cancer.
  - Prior to removal of embedded intrauterine contraceptive device (IUCD).
  - Prior to breaking uterine adhesions in Asherman syndrome.
  - Prior to endocervical curettage for endocervical cancer.
  - Prior to hysteroscopy.
  - To diagnose incompetent os. If no. 9 dilator goes in easily, the internal os of the cervix is considered as an incompetent os with the risk of habitual abortion and preterm labor.
- **Obstetric indications are:** Prior to evacuation in missed abortion, incomplete abortion, evacuation of hydatidiform mole. It is also necessary in medical termination of pregnancy. Curettage is mainly diagnostic. This is required in:
  - Abnormal uterine bleeding (AUB) to study the hormonal pattern causing abnormal bleeding.
  - Secondary amenorrhea to detect tubercular endometritis.
  - Postmenopausal bleeding to rule out endometrial cancer.
  - Endometrial cancer to study the endocervical tissue and the extent of spread. This helps in staging and deciding on treatment.
  - **Infertility:** Until recently, D&C was performed premenstrually to detect if ovulation has occurred. Secretory endometrium indicates that ovulation has occurred. Proliferative endometrium in the premenstrual phase indicates non-ovulation. Now, ultrasound has replaced D&C for monitoring

ovulation. It is however required if tubercular endometriosis is suspected. The endometrial tissue is preserved in saline for culture. The tissue is also subjected to polymerase chain reaction. Corpus luteal phase defect is diagnosed when the endometrial histology lags behind the menstrual date by 2 days.
  - A menopausal woman on hormonal replacement therapy; she should be watched for endometrial hyperplasia and cancer.
  - A woman on tamoxifen for breast cancer should undergo curettage 6-monthly to diagnose endometrial hyperplasia and cancer.
- Therapeutic D&C is indicated:
  - To remove endometrial polyp (polypectomy).
  - Obstetric indications mentioned for dilatation of cervix.
- Contraindications to D&C are:
  - Suspected pregnancy
  - Lower genital tract infection
- Sequelae of D&C:
  - Infection of upper genital tract.
  - Asherman syndrome

16. **Ans. (D) Estrogen is secreted by placenta**

The umbilical cord: The umbilical cord forms the connecting link between the fetus and the placenta through which the fetal blood flows to and from the placenta. It extends from the fetal umbilicus to the fetal surface of the placenta.

- **Development:** The umbilical cord is developed from the connective stalk or body stalk which is a band of mesoblastic tissue stretching between the embryonic disc and the chorion. Initially, it is attached to the caudal end of the embryonic disc, but as a result of cephalocaudal folding of the embryo and simultaneous enlargement of the amniotic cavity the amnio-ectodermal junction converges on the ventral aspect of the fetus. As the amniotic cavity enlarges out of proportion to the embryo and becomes distended with fluid, the embryo is carried more and more into the amniotic cavity with simultaneous elongation of the connective stalk, the future umbilical cord.
- **Structures:** The constituents of the umbilical cord when fully formed are as follows:
  - **Covering epithelium:** It is lined by a single layer of amniotic epithelium but shows stratification like that of fetal epidermis at term.

  - **Wharton's jelly:** It consists of elongated cells in a gelatinous fluid formed by mucoid degeneration of the extraembryonic mesodermal cells. It is rich in mucopolysaccharides and has got protective function to the umbilical vessels.
  - **Blood vessels:** Initially, there are four vessels—two arteries and two veins. The arteries are derived from the internal iliac arteries of the fetus and carry the venous blood from the fetus to the placenta. Of the two umbilical veins, the right one disappears by the 4th month, leaving behind one vein which carries oxygenated blood from the placenta to the fetus. Presence of a single umbilical artery is often associated with fetal congenital abnormalities.
  - **Remnant of the umbilical vesicle (yolk sac) and its vitelline duct:** Remnant of the yolk sac may be found as a small yellow body near the attachment of the cord to the placenta or on rare occasion, the proximal part of the duct persists as Meckel's diverticulum.
  - **Allantois:** A blind tubular structure may be occasionally present near the fetal end which is continuous inside the fetus with its **urachus** and bladder.
  - **Obliterated extraembryonic coelom:** In the early period, intraembryonic coelom is continuous with extraembryonic coelom along with herniation of coils of intestine (midgut). The condition may persist as **congenital** umbilical hernia or exomphalos.
- **Characteristics:** It is about 40 cm in length with a usual variation of 30–100 cm. Its diameter is of average 1.5 cm with variation of 1–2.5 cm. Its thickness is not uniform but presents nodes or swelling at places. These swellings (false knots) may be due to kinking of the umbilical vessels or local collection of Wharton's jelly.
- The umbilical arteries do not possess an internal elastic lamina but have well-developed muscular coat. These help in effective closure of the arteries due to reflex spasm soon after the birth of the baby. Both the arteries and the vein do not possess vasa vasorum.
- **Attachment:** In the early period, the cord is attached to the ventral surface of the embryo close to the caudal extremity, but as the coelom closes and the yolk sac atrophies the point of attachment is moved permanently to the center of the abdomen at 4th month. Unlike the fetal attachment, the placental attachment is inconsistent.

- It usually attaches to the fetal surface of the placenta somewhere between the center and the edge of the placenta called eccentric insertion. The attachment may be central, marginal or even on the chorion laeve at a varying distance away from the margin of the placenta, called velamentous insertion.
- Whartons jelly, a gelatinous substance rich in hyaluronic acid is present in the umbilical cord and not placenta.

17. Ans. (A) 3rd trimester

- Jaundice peculiar to pregnant state occurs in:
  - Intrahepatic cholestasis (obstetric hepatosis)—may be recurrent
  - Severe preeclampsia, eclampsia,
  - HELLP syndrome
  - Acute fatty liver (acute yellow atrophy of the liver)
  - Severe hyperemesis gravidarum
  - Endotoxic shock—disseminated intravascular coagulation (DIC)
- **Obstetric cholestasis (OC) is the second most common cause of jaundice in pregnancy**, **the first one being viral hepatitis**. Overall incidence is 1.2–1.5% of pregnant Indian women. The stasis of bile in the bile canaliculi with rise in conjugated bilirubin is probably due to excess circulating estrogen.
- The manifestations usually appear in the last trimester. The onset is insidious; generalized pruritus is the predominant symptom; there may be weakness, nausea or even vomiting. Jaundice is slight.
- There is rise in the levels of AST, ALT and serum alkaline phosphatase. Bilirubin level rarely exceeds 5 mg%.
- Liver biopsy shows no evidence of necrosis but shows the features of intrahepatic cholestasis.
- **There are increased risks of** preterm labor, low birth weight babies, meconium stained liquor, IUD and postpartum hemorrhage. Prothrombin time should be monitored. The features subside within two weeks postpartum.
- Cholestyramine is effective for itching. All women with OC should be given vitamin K to reduce postpartum hemorrhage and neonatal bleeding. The neonate should be given vitamin K as a routine. Combined oral contraceptives should be avoided in women with history of obstetric cholestasis.
- Prothrombin time should be monitored. Ursodeoxycholic acid (UDCA) is found helpful. It increases bile acid excretion. It improves pruritus.
- **Recurrence** rate is high (50–60%).

18. Ans. (A) Placenta previa

- **Secondary postpartum hemorrhage:** The bleeding usually occurs between 8th and 14th day of delivery.
- **The causes of late postpartum hemorrhage are:**
  - Retained bits of cotyledon or membranes (most common),
  - Infection and separation of slough over a deep cervicovaginal laceration,
  - Endometritis and subinvolution of the placental site—due to delayed healing process,
  - Secondary hemorrhage from cesarean section wound usually occur between 10–14 days. **It is probably due to**—(a) separation of slough exposing a bleeding vessel or (b) from granulation tissue,
  - Withdrawal bleeding following estrogen therapy for suppression of lactation,
  - Other rare causes are: chorionepithelioma—occurs usually beyond 4 weeks of delivery; carcinoma cervix; placental polyp; infected fibroid or fibroid polyp and puerperal inversion of uterus.
- **Diagnosis:** The bleeding is bright red and of varying amount. Rarely it may be brisk. Varying degree of anemia and evidences of sepsis are present. Internal examination reveals evidences of sepsis, subinvolution of the uterus and often a patulous cervical os. **Ultrasonography** is useful in detecting the bits of placenta inside the uterine cavity.
- **Management:**
  - Blood transfusion, if necessary,
  - To administer methergine 0.2 mg intramuscularly, if the bleeding is uterine in origin,
  - To administer antibiotics (clindamycin and metronidazole) as a routine.
  - If the bleeding is slight and no apparent cause is detected, a careful watch for a period of 24 hours or so is done in the hospital.
  - **It is preferable to explore the uterus urgently under general anesthesia**. One should not ignore the small amount of bleeding; as unexpected alarming hemorrhage may follow sooner or later. The products are removed by ovum forceps.
  - Gentle curettage is done by using flushing curette.

- Methergine 0.2 mg is given intramuscularly. **The materials removed are to be sent for histological examination.**
- Presence of bleeding from the sloughing wound of cervico-vaginal canal should be controlled by hemostatic sutures.
- **Secondary hemorrhage following cesarean section** may at times require laparotomy. The bleeding from uterine wound can be controlled by hemostatic sutures; may rarely require ligation of the internal iliac artery or may end in hysterectomy.

19. Ans. (C) 15–20 weeks

Second Trimester Screening: It is done between 15 weeks and 22 weeks.

- **MSAFP:** This test is done between 15 weeks and 20 weeks. MSAFP value of 2.5 multiples of the median (MOM) when adjusted with maternal weight and ethnicity is taken as cut-off point. Elevated MSAFP detects 85% of all neural tube defects. Cases with such high values are considered for high resolution ultrasound imaging and/or amniocentesis. Very low MSAFP levels are associated with increased rates of miscarriage, stillbirth and neonatal death.
- **Triple test:** It is a combined biochemical test which includes MSAFP, hCG and uE3 (unconjugated estriol). Maternal age in relation to confirmed gestation age is also taken into account. It is used for detection of Down's syndrome. In an affected pregnancy, levels of MSAFP and uE3 tend to be low while that of hCG is high. It is performed at 15–22 weeks. It gives a risk ratio and for confirmation CVS/amniocentesis has to be done. The result is considered to be screen positive if the risk ratio is 1:250 or greater.
- **Quadruple (Quad) screening includes four biochemical analytes:**
  - Maternal serum alpha fetoprotein (MSAFP)
  - Unconjugated estriol (uE3)
  - Dimeric inhibin-A and
  - hCG.
- Quadscreen can detect trisomy 21 in 85% of cases with a false-positive rate of 0.9%. Levels of serum analytes in cases with trisomy 21: hCG—increased; uE3—reduced; inhibin A—elevated; MSAFP—reduced.

20. Ans. (A) Dexamethasone

- **Glucocorticoid therapy:** Maternal administration of glucocorticoids is advocated where the pregnancy is less than 34 weeks.

- This helps in fetal lung maturation so that the incidence of RDS, IVH and NEC are minimized. This is beneficial when the delivery is delayed beyond 48 hours of the first dose. Benefit persists as long as 18 days.
- Either betamethasone (Betnesol) 12 mg IM 24 hours apart for two doses or dexamethasone 6 mg IM every 12 hours for 4 doses is given. Betamethasone is the steroid of choice.
- **Risks of antenatal corticosteroid use:** (a) Premature rupture of the membranes especially with evidence of infection as the infection may flare-up; (b) Insulin-dependent diabetes mellitus where patients need insulin dose readjustment; (c) Transient reduction of fetal breathing and body movements.

21. Ans. (A) Hot flushes

- **Hot flushes:** Almost 60–70% women go through menopausal period without problems. Rest need guidance and treatment.
- They are the waves of vasodilation affecting the face and the neck and these last for 2–5 min each. These are followed by severe sweating. Several of these flushes occur in a day, but are more severe during the night, and can disturb sleep.
- They are sometimes preceded by headache. Palpitation and anginal pains may be felt. Mental depression due to disturbed sleep or otherwise, irritability and lack of concentration are noticed. With passage of time, the frequency and severity of flushes diminish over a period of 1–2 years.
- They are caused by noradrenaline, which disturbs the thermoregulatory system. Estrogen deficiency reduces hypothalamic endorphins, which release more norepinephrine and serotonin. This leads to inappropriate heat loss mechanism.
- Other causes that can be associated with the symptom of hot flushes include: thyroid disease, epilepsy, pheochromocytoma, carcinoid syndromes, autoimmune disorders, mast cell disorders, insulinoma, pancreatic tumors and even leukemias.
- The vasomotor symptoms are more severe in surgical menopause than natural menopause.
- **Uses of HRT:**
  - Short term—hot flushes, vasomotor symptoms
  - Dyspareunia, libido
  - Urethral syndrome
  - Long term—osteoporosis
  - Cardiovascular
  - Alzheimer's disease

22. **Ans. (D) Round**

- **Position of the Uterus:** The uterus normally lies in a position of anteversion and anteflexion. The body of the uterus is bent forwards on the cervix approximately at the level of the internal os, and this forward inclination of the body of the uterus on the cervix constitutes anteflexion. The direction of the axis of the cervix depends upon the position of the uterus.
- It is difficult to explain why the uterus is normally anteverted and anteflexed. The round ligaments do not maintain this position on their own, although they are used to correct the retroversion during surgery. It appears that the position of the uterus in relation to the cervix is largely inherent in the uterine myometrium.
- In anteversion, the external os is directed downwards and backwards so that on vaginal examination the examining fingers find that the lowest part of the cervix is the anterior lip.
- When the uterus is retroverted the cervix is directed downwards and forwards, and the lowest part of the cervix is either the external os or the posterior lip. As a result of its normal position of anteflexion, the body of the uterus lies against the bladder. The pouch of peritoneum that separates the bladder from the uterus is the uterovesical pouch. The peritoneum is reflected from the front of the uterus on to the bladder at the level of the internal os.
- Posteriorly, a large peritoneal pouch lies between the uterus and the rectosigmoid colon. If the uterus is pulled forwards, two folds of peritoneum can be seen to pass backwards from the uterus to reach the parietal peritoneum lateral to the rectum. These folds, the uterosacral folds, lie at the level of the internal os and pass backwards and upwards. The uterosacral ligaments are condensation of the pelvic cellular tissues and lie at a lower level and within the uterosacral folds.
- The pouch of peritoneum below the level of the uterosacral folds, which is bounded in front by the peritoneum covering the upper part of the posterior vaginal wall and posteriorly by the peritoneum covering the sigmoid colon and the upper end of the rectum, is the pouch of Douglas.
- The posterior fornix of the vagina is in close relation to the peritoneal cavity, as only the posterior vaginal wall and a single layer of peritoneum separate the vagina from the peritoneal cavity. Collection of pus in the pouch of Douglas can therefore be evacuated without difficulty by incising the vagina in the region of the posterior fornix.

16 Skin

1. A 22-year old male developed pigmentation over upper chest for the last 2 years as shown in image. What is the diagnosis?

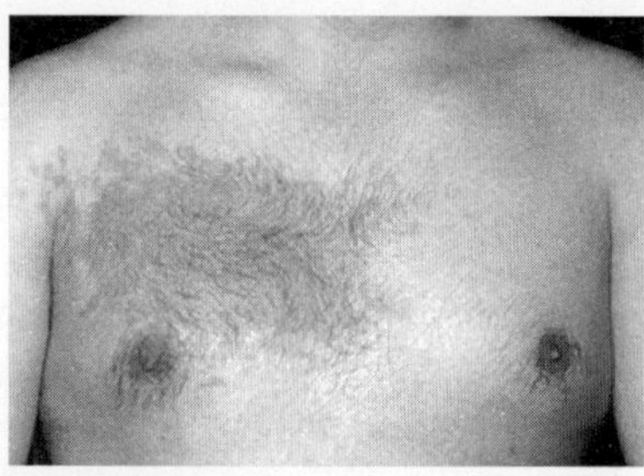

A. Becker nevus
B. Drug reaction
C. Post inflammmatory pigmentation
D. Congenital nevus

2. Identify the nerve thickened here in a leprosy patient?

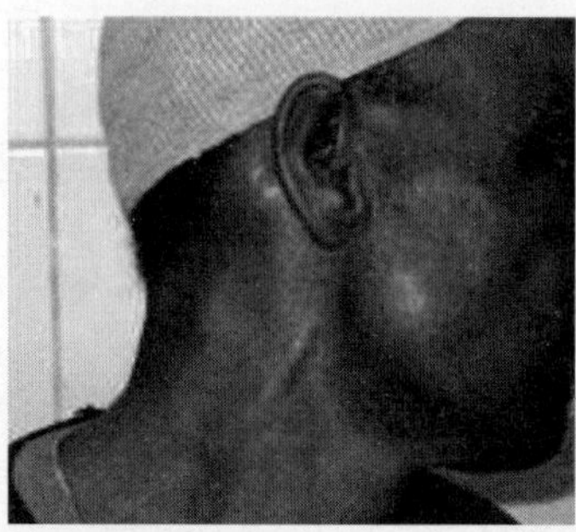

A. Greater auricular nerve
B. Facial nerve
C. Trigemeral nerve
D. Occipital nerve

3. Epithelium of hard palate is:

A. Keratinised, submucosal layer, minor salivary gland
B. Keratinised, absent submucosal layer, minor salivary gland
C. Non-keratinised, submucosal layer, minor salivary gland
D. Non-keratinised, submucosal layer, absent minor salivary gland

4. Shingles is caused by:

A. VZV
B. HSV
C. HPV
D. CMV

5. Virus of H. Zoster resides in:

A. Regional lymph node
B. Skin
C. Posterior root ganglion
D. Blood

6. A child has rash on elbow as shown with family history of asthma. What is the most probable diagnosis?

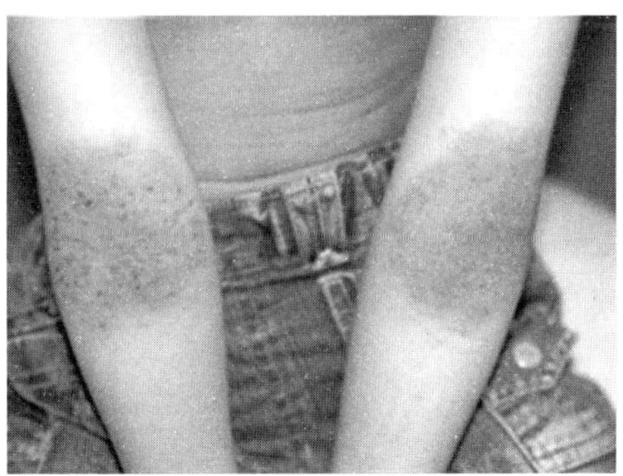

A. Atopic dermatitis
B. Contact dermatitis
C. Allergic dermatitis
D. Seborrheic dermatitis

7. Warthin Finkeldey cells are seen in:

A. Measles
B. Mumps
C. Rubella
D. Yellow fever

8. An anaerobe causing multiple abscess with discharging sinuses, demonstrating sulphur granules in pus are used to diagnose:

A. Actinomycetes
B. Nocardia
C. Salmonella
D. Tularemia

9. Cutis marmorata occurs due to exposure to:

A. Cold temperature
B. Dust
C. Hot temperature
D. Humidity

10. Which of the following condition is NOT caused by Parvovirus B19?

A. Roseola infantum
B. Aplastic anemia in sickle cell disease
C. Fetal hydrops
D. Erythema infectiosum

11. Genital warts are caused by which virus?

A. Herpes simplex
B. Human papilloma
C. Cytomegalovirus
D. Varicella zoster

Answers with Explanations

1. **Ans. (A) Becker nevus**
   - **Becker's nevus** (also known as "**Becker's melanosis**", "**Becker's pigmentary hamartoma**", "**pigmented hairy epidermal nevus**") is a skin disorder predominantly affecting males.
   - The nevus can be present at birth, but more often shows up around puberty. It generally first appears as an irregular pigmentation (melanosis or hyperpigmentation) on the torso or upper arm (though other areas of the body can be affected), and gradually enlarges irregularly, becoming thickened and often hairy (hypertrichosis). The nevus is due to an overgrowth of the epidermis, pigment cells (melanocytes), and hair follicles.
   - The pathophysiology of Becker's nevus remains unclear. While it is generally considered an acquired rather than congenital disorder.
   - There is so far no evidence of higher malignancy rates in Becker's nevi versus normal skin.
   - **Treatment:** As Becker's nevus is considered a benign lesion, treatment is generally not necessary except for cosmetic purposes. Shaving or trimming can be effective in removing unwanted hair, while electrology or laser hair removal may offer a longer-lasting solution. Different types of laser treatments may also be effective in elimination or reduction of hyperpigmentation, though the results of laser treatments for both hair and pigment reduction appear to be highly variable.
2. **Ans. (A) Greater auricular nerve**

   Lepra reactions comprise several common immunologically mediated inflammatory states that cause considerable morbidity. Some of these reactions precede diagnosis and the institution of effective antimicrobial therapy; indeed, these reactions may precipitate presentation for medical attention and diagnosis.

   A. **Type 1 Lepra Reactions (Down grading and Reversal Reactions):** It occurs in almost half of patients with borderline forms of leprosy but not in patients with pure lepromatous disease. Manifestations include classic signs of inflammation within previously involved macules, papules, and plaques and, on occasion, the appearance of new skin lesions, neuritis, and (less commonly) fever—generally low-grade. The nerve trunk most frequently involved in this process is the ulnar nerve at the elbow, which may be painful and exquisitely tender. If patients with affected nerves are not treated promptly with glucocorticoids, irreversible nerve damage may result in as little as 24 h. The most dramatic manifestation is footdrop, which occurs when the peroneal nerve is involved. When type 1 lepra reactions precede the initiation of appropriate antimicrobial therapy, they are termed *downgrading reactions*, and the case becomes histologically more lepromatous; when they occur after the initiation of therapy, they are termed *reversal reactions*, and the case becomes more tuberculoid. Reversal reactions often occur in the first months or years after the initiation of therapy but may also develop several years thereafter. Edema is the most characteristic microscopic feature of type 1 lepra lesions, whose diagnosis is primarily clinical. Reversal reactions are typified by a TH1 cytokine profile, with an influx of CD4+ T helper cells and increased levels of IFN-γ and IL-2. In addition, type 1 reactions are associated with large numbers of T cells bearing γ/δ receptors—a unique feature of leprosy.

B. **Type 2 Lepra Reactions (Erythema Nodosum Leprosum):** It occurs exclusively in patients near the lepromatous end of the leprosy spectrum (BL/LL), affecting nearly 50% of this group. Although ENL may precede leprosy diagnosis and the initiation of therapy (sometimes, in fact, prompting the diagnosis), in 90% of cases it follows the institution of chemotherapy, generally within 2 years. The most common features of ENL are crops of painful erythematous papules that resolve spontaneously in a few days to a week but may recur; malaise; and fever that can be profound. However, patients may also experience symptoms of neuritis, lymphadenitis,uveitis, orchitis, and glomerulonephritis and may develop anemia, leukocytosis, and abnormal liver function tests (particularly increased aminotransferase levels). Individual patients may have either a single bout of ENL or chronic recurrent manifestations. Bouts may be either mild or severe and generalized; in rare instances, ENL results in death. Skin biopsy of ENL papules reveals vasculitis or panniculitis, sometimes with many lymphocytes but characteristically with polymorphonuclear leukocytes as well.

3. Ans. (A) Keratinised, submucosal layer, minor salivary gland

Lips: Vermilion zone	Thin, orthokeratinized, stratified squamous epithelium	Numerous narrow papillae; capillary loops close to surface in papillary layer	Mucosa firmly attached to underlying muscle; some sebaceous glands in vermilion border, minor salivary glands and fat in intermediate zone
Lips: Intermediate zone	Thin, parakeratinized, stratified squamous epithelium	Long irregular papillae; elastic and collagen fibers in connective tissue	No distinct layer, mucosa firmly attached by collagen fibers to cementum and periosteum of alveolar process (mucoperiosteum)
Masticatory mucosa gingiva	Thick (250 um), orthokeratinized or parakeratinized, stratified squamous epithelium often showing stippled surface	Long, narrow papillae, dense collagenous connective tissue; long capillary loops with numerous anastomoses	Dense collagenous connective tissue attaching mucosa to periosteum (mucoperiosteum) fat and minor salivary glands are packed into connective tissue in regions where mucosa overlies lateral palatine neurovascular bundles
Hard palate	Thick, orthokeratinized (parakeratinized, in parts), stratified squamous epithelium thrown into transverse palatine ridges (rugae)	Long papillae; thick, dense collagenous tissue, especially under rugae; moderate vascular supply with short capillary loops	No distinct layer; mucosa is bound to connective tissue surrounding musculature of tongue
Specialized mucosa Dorsal surface of tongue	Thick, keratinized, and non-keratinized, stratified squamous epithelium forming three types of papillae, some bearing taste buds	Long papillae; minor salivary glands in posterior portion; rich innervations, particularly near taste buds; capillary plexus in papillary layer, large vessels lying deeper	

4. Ans. (A) VZV

- Varicella-zoster virus (VZV) causes two distinct clinical entities: Varicella (chickenpox) and herpes zoster (shingles). Chickenpox, a ubiquitous and extremely contagious infection, is usually a benign illness of childhood characterized by an exanthematous vesicular rash.
- With reactivation of latent VZV (which is most common after the sixth decade of life), herpes zoster presents as a dermatomal vesicular rash, usually associated with severe pain.
- Herpes zoster (shingles) is a sporadic disease that results from reactivation of latent VZV from dorsal root ganglia. Recurrent herpes zoster is exceedingly rare except in immunocompromised hosts, especially those with AIDS.
- Herpes zoster is characterized by a unilateral vesicular dermatomal eruption, often associated with severe pain. The dermatomes from T3 to L3 are most frequently involved. If the ophthalmic branch of the trigeminal nerve is involved, *zoster ophthalmicus* results.
- The onset of disease is heralded by pain within the dermatome,which may precede lesions by 48–72 h; an erythematous maculopapular rash evolves rapidly into vesicular lesions.
- The total duration of disease is generally 7–10 days; however, it may take as long as 2–4 weeks for the skin to return to normal.
- *Zoster ophthalmicus* is usually a debilitating condition that can result in blindness in the absence of antiviral therapy.
- Postherpetic neuralgia is uncommon in young individuals; however, at least 50% of zoster patients over age 50 report some degree of pain in the involved dermatome for months after the resolution of cutaneous disease.
- The characteristic rash and a history of recent exposure should lead to a prompt diagnosis.
- Both HSV and coxsackievirus infections can cause dermatomal vesicular lesions. Supportive diagnostic virology and fluorescent staining of skin scrapings with monoclonal antibodies are helpful in ensuring the proper diagnosis.
- In the prodromal stage of herpes zoster, the diagnosis can be exceedingly difficult and may be made only after lesions have appeared or by retrospective serologic assessment.
- **Laboratory findings:** Unequivocal confirmation of the diagnosis is possible only through the isolation of VZV in susceptible

tissue-culture cell lines, the demonstration of either seroconversion or a fourfold or greater rise in antibody titer between acute-phase and convalescent-phase serum specimens, or the detection of VZV DNA by PCR.

- A rapid impression can be obtained by a Tzanck smear, with scraping of the base of the lesions in an attempt to demonstrate multinucleated giant cells; however, the sensitivity of this method is low (~60%).
- The most frequently employed serologic tools for assessing host response are the immunofluorescent detection of antibodies to VZV membrane antigens, the fluorescent antibody to membrane antigen (FAMA) test, immune adherence hemagglutination, and enzyme-linked immunosorbent assay (ELISA). The FAMA test and the ELISA appear to be most sensitive.

5. Ans. (C) Posterior root ganglion

- **Varicella-zoster virus (VZV) causes two distinct clinical entities:** Varicella (chickenpox) and herpes zoster (shingles). Chickenpox, a ubiquitous and extremely contagious infection, is usually a benign illness of childhood characterized by an exanthematous vesicular rash.
- Herpes zoster (shingles) is a sporadic disease that results from reactivation of latent VZV from dorsal root ganglia.
- Recurrent herpes zoster is exceedingly rare except in immunocompromised hosts, especially those with AIDS.
- Herpes zoster is characterized by a unilateral vesicular dermatomal eruption, often associated with severe pain. The dermatomes from T3 to L3 are most frequently involved.

6. Ans. (A) Atopic dermatitis

- **Atopic dermatitis (AD)**, also known as **atopic eczema**, is a type of inflammation of the skin (dermatitis). It results in itchy, red, swollen, and cracked skin. Clear fluid may come from the affected areas, which often thicken over time.
- The condition typically starts in childhood with changing severity over the years. In children under one year of age much of the body may be affected. As children get older, the back of the knees and front of the elbows are the most common areas affected.
- In adults the hands and feet are the most commonly affected areas. Many people with atopic dermatitis develop hay fever or asthma.
- The cause is unknown but believed to involve genetics, immune system dysfunction, environmental exposures, and

difficulties with the permeability of the skin. If one identical twin is affected, there is an 85% chance the other also has the condition. While emotional stress may make the symptoms worse it is not a cause. The disorder is not contagious. The diagnosis is typically based on the signs and symptoms.

- Treatment involves avoiding things that make the condition worse, daily bathing with application of a moisturising cream afterwards, applying steroid creams when flares occur, and medications to help with itchiness. Phototherapy may be useful in some people. Antibiotics (either by mouth or topically) may be needed if a bacterial infection develops. Dietary changes are only needed if food allergies are suspected.
- AD commonly occurs on the eyelids where signs such as Dennie-Morgan infraorbital fold, infra-auricular fissure, periorbital pigmentation can be seen. Post-inflammatory hyperpigmentation on the neck gives the classic 'dirty neck' appearance. Lichenification, excoriation and erosion or crusting on the trunk may indicate secondary infection. Flexural distribution with ill-defined edges with or without hyperlinearily on the wrist, finger knuckles, ankle, feet and hand are also commonly seen.
- Many people with AD have a family history of atopy. Atopy is an immediate-onset allergic reaction (type 1 hypersensitivity reaction) that manifests as asthma, food allergies, AD or hay fever. The pathophysiology may involve a mixture of type I and type IV-like hypersensitivity reactions.

UK Diagnostic Criteria

- **People must have itchy skin, or evidence of rubbing or scratching, plus 3 or more of the following:**
  a. Skin creases are involved: flexural dermatitis of fronts of ankles, antecubital fossae, popliteal fossae, skin around eyes, or neck (or cheeks for children under 10)
  b. History of asthma or allergic rhinitis (or family history of these conditions if patient is a child ≤4 years old)
  c. Symptoms began before age 2 (can only be applied to patients ≥4 years old)
  d. History of dry skin (within the past year)
  e. Dermatitis is visible on flexural surfaces (patients ≥age 4) or on the cheeks, forehead, and extensor surfaces (patients < age 4)
- **Medication:** Topical corticosteroids, such as hydrocortisone have proven themselves effective in managing AD. If topical corticosteroids and moisturisers fail, short-term treatment with

topical calcineurin inhibitors like tacrolimus or pimecrolimus may be tried. Alternatively systemic immunosuppressants may be tried such as ciclosporin, methotrexate, interferon gamma-1b, mycophenolate mofetil and azathioprine.

7. **Ans. (A) Measles**
   - A **Warthin–Finkeldey cell** is a type of giant multinucleate cell found in hyperplastic lymph nodes early in the course of measles and also in HIV-infected individuals,as well as in Kimura disease, and more rarely in a number of neoplastic (e.g. lymphoma) and non-neoplastic lymph node disorders.
   - Their origin is uncertain, but they have previously been shown to stain with markers similar to those of follicular dendritic cells, including CD21. Under the light microscope, these cells consist of a large, grape-like cluster of nuclei.

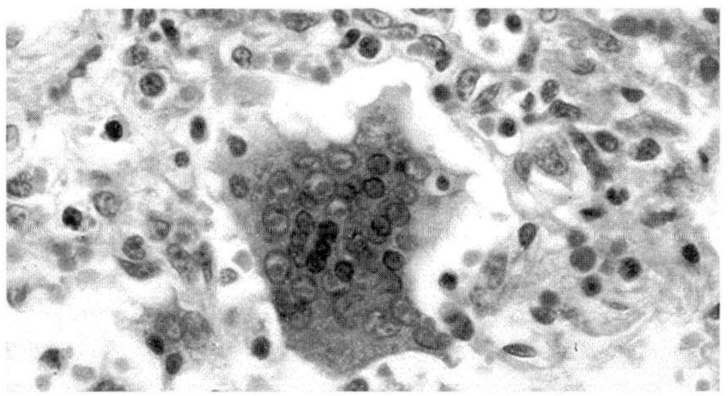

8. **Ans. (A) Actinomycetes**
   - Multiple discharging sinus foot. It is commonly due to mycetoma (Madura foot). It could also be due to tuberculosis, chronic pyogenic osteomyelitis or malignancy.
   - **Mycetoma (Madura foot)** is a disease of the tropics and subtropics and involves various species of fungus or actinomycetes. They gain access to the subcutaneous tissues, usually of the feet or legs, via a penetrating wound. The area becomes lumpy and distorted, later enlarging and developing multiple sinuses.
   - Pus exuding from these shows tiny diagnostic granules. Surgery may be a valuable alternative to the often poor results of medical treatment, which is with systemic antibiotics or antifungal drugs, depending on the organism isolated.
9. **Ans. (A) Cold temperature**
   - **Livedo reticularis:** This cyanosis of the skin is net-like (reticulated) or marbled and caused by stasis in the capillaries furthest

from their arterial supply: at the periphery of the inverted cone supplied by a dermal arteriole. It may be widespread or localized.

- *Cutis marmorata* is the name given to the mottling of the skin seen in many normal children. It is a physiologic vasospastic response to cold exposure and disappears on warming,whereas true livedo reticularis remains.

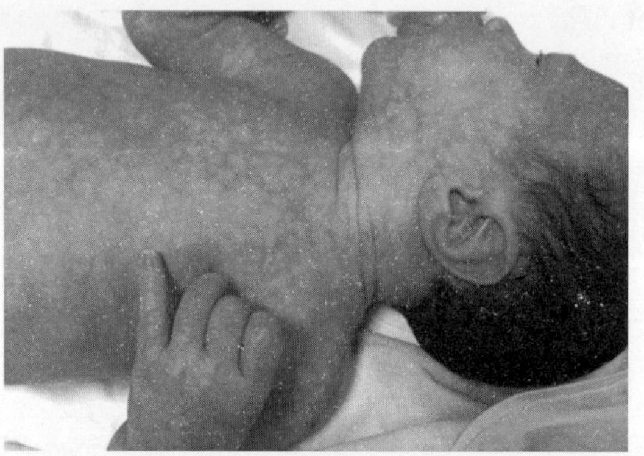

Fig. 16.1: Cutis marmorata

10. Ans. (A) Roseola infantum

Erythema infectiosum (fifth disease): This is caused by the human parvovirus B19 and occurs in outbreaks, often in the spring. A slapped cheek erythema is quickly followed by a reticulate erythema of the shoulders. The affected child feels well, and the rash clears over the course of a few days. Other features, sometimes not accompanied by a rash, include transient anaemia and arthritis.

11. Ans. (B) Human papilloma

- **Viral warts:** Warts are caused by the human papilloma virus (HPV), which has still not been cultured *in vitro*. Nevertheless, more than 70 'types' of the virus are now recognized by.
- HPV-1, 2 and 4, for example, are found in common warts, whereas HPV-3 is found in plane warts, and HPV-6, 11, 16 and 18 are most common in genital warts.
- Infections occur when wart virus in skin scales comes into contact with breaches in the skin or mucous membranes or when immunity is suppressed and dormant viruses escape from their resting place in the outer root sheaths of hairs.
- **Anogenital warts:** Two vaccines, a bivalent one against the high-risk HPV-16 and 18 and a quadrivalent vaccine which is

also effective against HPV-6 and 11 are now available. These are now part of the standard vaccination protocol for young women in many countries and have resulted in a marked fall in new cases of anogenital warts. Women with anogenital warts, or who are the partners of men with anogenital warts, should have their cervical cytology checked regularly as the wart virus can cause cervical cancer.

- The focus has shifted towards self-treatment using podophyllotoxin (0.5% solution or 0.15% cream) or imiquimod (5% cream). Both are irritants and should be used carefully according to the manufacturer's instructions. Imiquimod is an immune response modifier that induces keratinocytes to produce cytokines, leading to wart regression, and may help to build cell-mediated immunity for long-lasting protection. It is applied as a thin layer three times weekly and washed off with a mild soap 6–10 hours after application. Podophyllin paint (15%) is used much less often now. It should be applied carefully to the warts and allowed to dry before powdering with talcum. On the first occasion it should be washed off with soap and water after 2 hours but, if there has been little discomfort, this can be increased stepwise to 6 hours. Treatment is best carried out weekly by a doctor or nurse, but not by the patient. Podophyllin must not be used in pregnancy.

17 Anesthesia

1. 3-year-old undergoing squint surgery, initially heart rate was 140/min. After anesthesia and starting surgery heart rate is 40/min. Next appropriate step is:

A. Stop surgery
B. Decrease plane of anesthesia
C. Inj glycopyrrolate
D. Inj atropine

2. Circuit of choice for spontaneous ventilation is?

A. Mapleson A
B. Mapleson B
C. Mapleson C
D. Mapleson D

3. Most common nerve used for monitoring in anesthesia is?

A. Facial nerve
B. Median nerve
C. Radial nerve
D. Ulnar nerve

4. Murphys eye is a part of?

A. Endoscope
B. Endotracheal tubes
C. Ryle's tube
D. LMA

5. Modified Mallampati grading is used in assessment of?

A. Difficult intubation
B. Airway obstruction
C. Death due to aspiration
D. Intubation

6. Trilene is degraded by?

A. Enzymatic degradation
B. Nonenzymatic degradation
C. Chemical degradation
D. None

Answers with Explanations

1. Ans. (D) Inj atropine

- Squint surgery is done under general anesthesia. During GA excessive vagal activity, which causes severe bradycardia and hypotension can be life-threatening.
- The trigger can be painful stimulation of the bronchial, pharyngeal, laryngeal or esophageal mucosa. Prompt treatment is needed with urgent restoration of venous return by leg elevation, head down tilt and IV fluids, and the use of anticholinergic and sympathomimetic drugs. A pacemaker should be considered for patients with vasovagal syncope which is frequent and does not respond to medical treatment.
- The use of a temporary pacemaker for patients who develop bradycardia during general anesthesia is controversial.
- Profound bradycardia during eye surgery is potentially serious event. In clinical practice this oculocardiac reflex (OCR) is most often encountered during squint surgery.
- Atropine premedication in the patients of squint surgery under general anesthesia definitely obtunds OCR and prevents any untoward effects of dysrhythmias during eye surgery.

2. Ans. (A) Mapleson A

Mapleson A circuit is also known as Magills circuit.

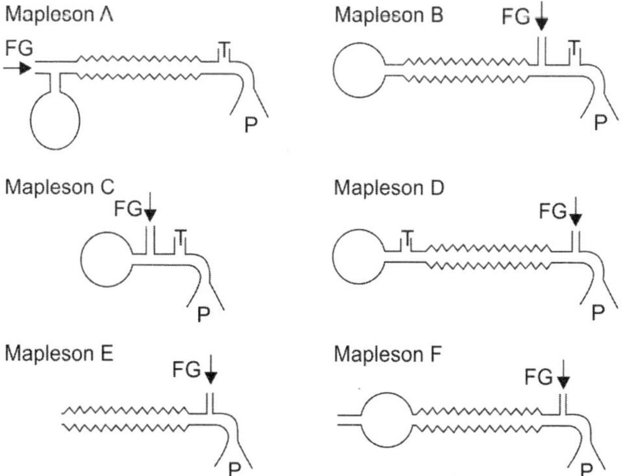

FG = Fresh gas, P = Patient

Advantages

- Best circuit for spontaneous respiration as no rebreathing occurs with adequate flows.
- Less fresh gas flow is required during spontaneous respiration.

Disadvantages

- Wastage of gases.
- Theater pollution by Magill circuit.
- Mechanical ventilator should not be used with this circuit because the entire system becomes dead space.

3. Ans. (D) Ulnar nerve

- Adductor pollicis muscle supplied by ulnar nerve is most commonly utilized muscle for neuromuscular monitoring.
- Facial nerve stimulation of orbicularis oculi is also very commonly used.
- **Neuromuscular monitoring**, also known as **train of four monitoring** is a technique used during recovery from the application of general anesthesia to objectively determine how well a patient's muscles are able to function.
- It involves the application of electrical stimulation to nerves and recording of muscle response using, for example, an acceleromyograph.
- The diaphragm, rectus abdominis, laryngeal adductors and orbicularis oculi muscles recover from neuromuscular blockage earlier than adductor pollicis.

4. Ans. (B) Endotracheal tubes

- Endotracheal tubes are used to establish and maintain airway patency, prevent aspiration into the lungs, i.e. 'secure' the airway, and allow mechanical ventilation.
- Most endotracheal tubes today are constructed of polyvinyl chloride, but specialty tubes constructed of silicone rubber, latex rubber, or stainless steel are also widely available.
- Most tubes have an inflatable cuff to seal the trachea and bronchial tree against air leakage and aspiration of gastric contents, blood, secretions, and other fluids.
- Uncuffed tubes are also available, though their use is limited mostly to pediatric patients (in small children, the cricoid cartilage, the narrowest portion of the pediatric airway, often provides an adequate seal for mechanical ventilation).
- Tubes larger than 6 mm ID usually have an inflatable cuff. Originally made from red rubber, most modern tubes are made from polyvinyl chloride. Those placed in a laser field may be flexometallic.

- Double-lumen endobronchial tubes for thoracic surgery allow single-lung ventilation while the other lung is collapsed to make surgery easier. Another type of endotracheal tube has a small second lumen opening above the inflatable cuff which can be used for suction of the nasopharngeal area and above the cuff to aid extubation (removal). This allows suctioning of secretions which sit above the cuff which helps reduce the risk of chest infections in long-term intubated patients.

  Its different parts are:

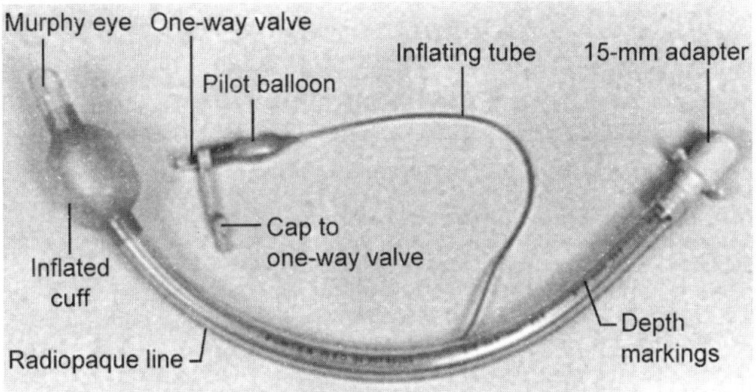

5. **Ans. (A) Difficult intubation**

   Mallampati scoring is used for assessing difficulty during intubation, its grades are:

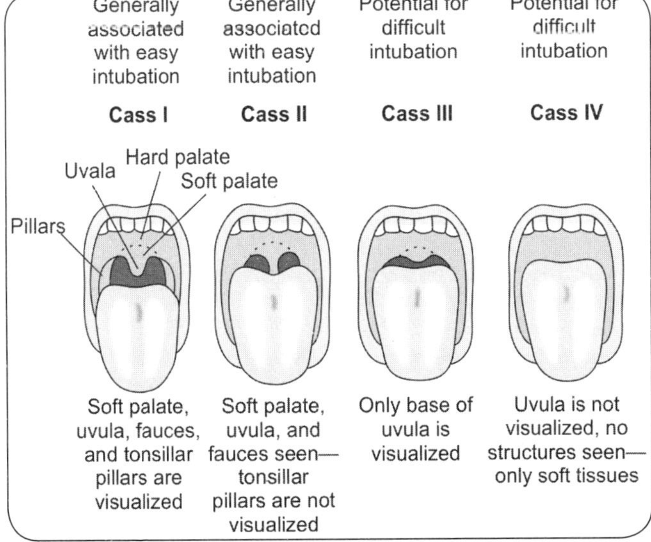

Modified Mallampati scoring

- Class I: Soft palate, uvula, fauces, pillars visible.
- Class II: Soft palate, uvula, fauces visible.
- Class III: Soft palate, base of uvula visible.
- Class IV: Only hard palate visible.

6. Ans. (C) Chemical degradation

- Trilene: It is a clear non-flammable liquid with a sweet smell.
- It was used as a volatile anesthetic and as an inhaled obstetrical analgesic.
- It is a potent analgesic.
- Soda lime produces toxic product dichloroacetylene which cause nerve palsies and produce phosgene gas along with it.
- Most common involved nerve is 5th.
- S/E is nausea and vomiting.

18 Radiology

1. Name the investigation shown in the given image.

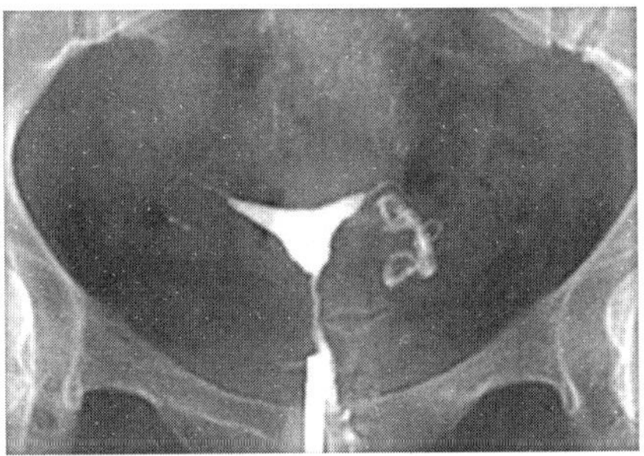

A. MR HSG
B. CT HSG
C. Conventional HSG
D. USG HSG

2. Child with bitemporal hemianopia. His IQ is normal. His visual acuity is diminished. The radiological image of this patient is shown below. What is the most likely diagnosis?

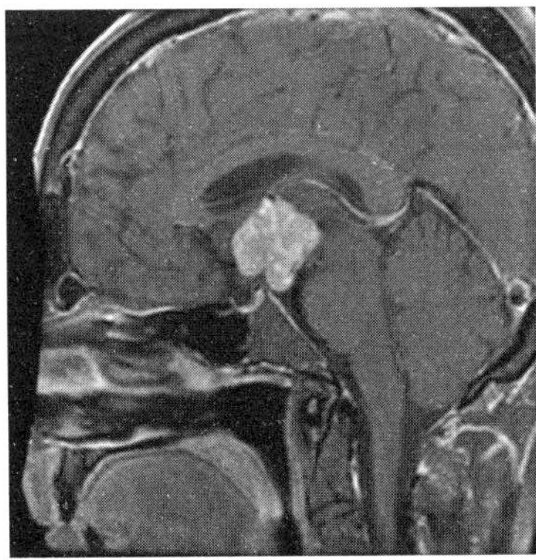

A. Craniopharyngioma
B. Optic glioma
C. Pineal tumor
D. Torus tubaris

3. A female having cervical lesion, which therapy is to be given after resection?

A. Electrons
B. Photons
C. Protons
D. X-rays

4. Identify the condition shown in the CT scan image below:

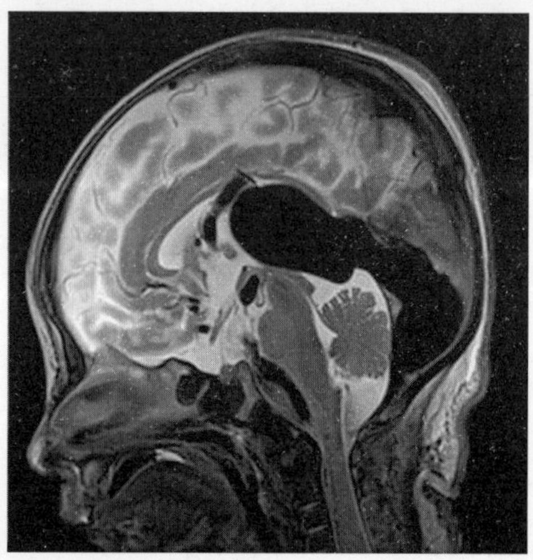

A. Dandy Walker syndrome
B. Vein of Galen malformation
C. Arnold-Chiari malformation
D. Cerebellar vermis malformation

5. What would be the contrast of choice in esophageal perforation?

A. Gadolinium
B. Iohexol
C. Barium
D. Iodine dye

6. After radical resection of chordoma which radiation therapy is best?

A. X-rays
B. Neutrons
C. Protons
D. Electrons

7. A 45-year-old female presented with chest pain and breathless in the ER and below is the representative CT section. What is the most likely cause of her symptoms?

A. Aortic dissection
B. Pulmonary embolism
C. Aortic aneurysm
D. Budd-Chiari syndrome

8. Braggs peak effect is seen in:

A. X-rays
B. Neutron
C. Protons
D. Electron

9. Which artery has been shown in the following CT angiographic image?

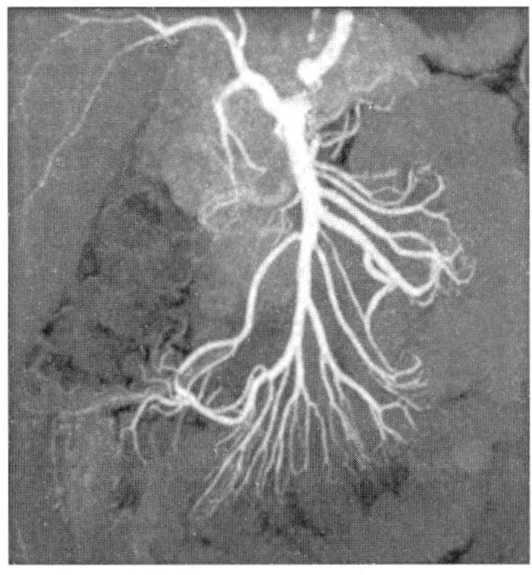

A. Superior mesenteric artery
B. Inferior mesenteric artery
C. Inferior rectal artery
D. Coeliac artery

10. CT scan of abdomen showing the structure marked is:

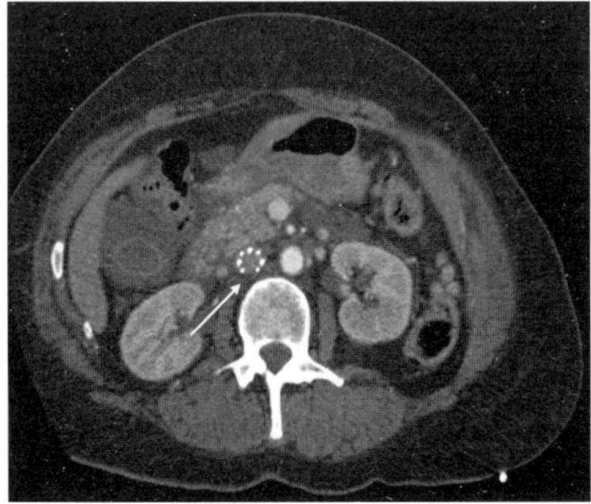

A. SVC
B. IVC
C. Aorta
D. Thoracic duct

Answers with Explanations

1. **Ans. (C) Conventional HSG**
   - **Hysterosalpingography (HSG):** Visualization of the uterine cavity and the fallopian tubes should be carried out by screening with the use of an image intensifier in an X-ray room using a Foley catheter, Rubin cannula or Leech-Wilkinson cannula for insufflation.
   - The investigation is performed between the end of the menstrual period and ovulation (usually the ninth or tenth day of the cycle).
   - After thoroughly cleaning the lower genital tract and with full aseptic precautions, a radiopaque dye is injected through the cannula into the uterine cavity under direct vision with a fluoroscopic screen; 15 mL of the medium is usually adequate to visualize the uterine cavity and the tubes.
   - If the tubes are patent, the medium will be seen to spill out of the abdominal ostia and smear the adjacent bowel. A hydrosalpinx will show as a large confined mass of dye without peritoneal spill.
   - If either tube is blocked, the site will be shown. At any stage of examination, radiographic pictures are taken for permanent record of the result.
   - A viscous water-soluble solution, 50% iodine with 6% polyvinyl alcohol in water, is the medium usually employed for HSG. It is rapidly absorbed, and the risk of tissue reaction and adhesion formation in the pelvis is minimal; even when intravasated into the uterine venous system, it is harmless. Although an oil-soluble medium gives a sharper and clearer picture and may have improved therapeutic effect, it is not preferred because of the occurrence of oil granuloma, peritoneal reaction, formation of pelvic adhesions and the need for a delayed film to be taken for detecting peritoneal spill. Besides, it causes pain. The pregnancy rate is slightly better than that with water-soluble dye.
   - Blockage of tube may be due to fibrotic block (stricture), spasms or inspissated amorphous material plugging the lumen.
   - Bilateral cornual block with extravasation of the dye is highly suggestive of tubercular salpingitis.
   - Apart from tubal anatomy, this examination excludes congenital abnormalities of the uterus, such as uterus bicornis, arcuate, septate uterus and fibroids.

- HSG has the advantage that it gives a permanent record and shows the site of tubal blockage. Among its complications are (i) pelvic infection, (ii) pain and collapse which can however be avoided by injecting atropine half an hour before the procedure and (iii) allergic reaction.
- HSG should not be performed (i) in the postovulatory period, (ii) in the presence of genital infection and suspected genital tuberculosis and (iii) if the patient is sensitive to iodine. HSG yields 25–30% salvage value and this enhancement of fertility is attributed to flushing and dislodgement of amorphous material that sometimes blocks its lumen. The amorphous material is an aggregate of histiocytes.

2. Ans. (A) Craniopharyngioma

- *Craniopharyngiomas:* They are rare, usually suprasellar, partially calcified, solid, or mixed solid-cystic benign tumors that arise from remnants of Rathke's pouch.
- They have a bimodal distribution, occurring predominantly in children but also between the ages of 55 and 65 years.
- They present with headaches, visual impairment, and impaired growth in children and hypopituitarism in adults.
- Craniopharyngiomas may be calcified and are usually hypodense, whereas gliomas are hyperdense on T2-weighted images.
- Treatment involves surgery, RT, or a combination of the two.

3. Ans. (A) Electrons

Clinical applications of radiotherapy in cancer of the cervix:

- Primary radiation therapy for cancer of the cervix combines teletherapy with brachytherapy. Radiation, like surgery, is a local therapy. It therefore influences only the tumor cells falling within the radiation volume.
- Intracavitary radiation by itself may therefore not be curative for patients in whom the tumor spread involves tissues beyond the effective radiation range and those with distant metastases.
- Additional external supplementary radiation to the pelvis is required to treat the pelvic lymph nodes. The tolerance of the normal tissues within the pelvis acts as the limiting factor in planning radiation therapy. Cervical cancer requires a radiation dose of 6000 cGy. The tolerance dose of irradiation for the urinary bladder is about 6000 cGy and for the rectum, it is about 5000 cGy. Doses in excess can damage these hollow viscera and cause radiation fistulae.

- The intracavitary radiation source is so calculated that it does not deliver a dose in excess of 8000 cGy to the point A located 2.0 cm above and lateral to the external cervical os. This point denotes the point of crossing of the ureter in the pelvis. The second point of consideration is point B located 5.0 cm laterally on the pelvic sidewalls where the obturator gland is located. The radiation dose at point B should not exceed 4500 cGy. This is to safeguard the bladder and rectum from over-irradiation.
- *Preoperative brachytherapy* is used in barrel-shaped endocervical growth of more than 2 cm. This is followed within a week or 4 weeks later by Wertheim's hysterectomy. Cisplatin prior to or during brachytherapy improves the response rate.
- Cisplatin acts as a radiosensitizer and is employed as a neoadjuvant or concomitant chemoradiation. The renal functions have to be checked. Cisplatin 40 mg/m^2 IV given within 1 hour prior to radiotherapy weekly improves the response rate of the latter. Other radiosensitizers are 5-FU, gemcitabine and taxol, carboplastin.
- Postoperative external radiotherapy is required when the surgery has been incomplete or lymph nodes prove positive for malignancy.
- Primary radiotherapy is mainly applied in advanced cancer of the cervix, but also preferred in Stages I and IIA by some gynecologists, alternative to Wertheim's hysterectomy. The cure rates achieved in early stages are comparable by either method.
- However, realizing that radiotherapy causes vaginal stenosis leading to dyspareunia, ovarian destruction with menopausal symptoms, and osteoporosis and cervical stenosis causing pyometra, the choice of treatment in young women is Wertheim's hysterectomy.
- In a few cases, radiotherapy fails to irradiate the pelvic nodes completely, and recurrence occurs. In such cases, surgery is preferable to repeat radiotherapy, provided the woman is surgically fit.
- In primary radiotherapy normally, brachytherapy is applied first followed by external teletherapy. If the growth is large, first teletherapy is applied to shrink the tumor followed by brachytherapy.
- In endocervical cancer, the best survival is seen when the concomitant cisplatin weekly and weekly pelvic radiotherapy

for 6 weeks is followed by surgery. Postoperative radiotherapy is required if pelvic lymph nodes prove positive for cancer.

4. **Ans. (B) Vein of Galen malformation**
   - **Vein of Galen aneurysmal malformations (VGAMs)**, termed as **median prosencephalic arteriovenous fistulas**, are uncommon intracranial anomalies that tend to present dramatically during early childhood with features of a left-to-right shunt and high-output cardiac failure.
   - **Pathology:** The anomaly is actually due to a cerebral arteriovenous fistula of the median prosencephalic vein (MPV) (a precursor of the vein of Galen) occurring at 6–11 weeks gestation and not a malformation. The MPV fails to regress and becomes aneurysmal. It drains via the straight sinus (present only in 50%) or a persistent falcine sinus, and the vein of Galen does not form.
   - **Radiographic features:**
     - **Antenatal ultrasound:** The dilated median prosencephalic vein (MPV) appears as an anechoic structure in the midline posteriorly and demonstrates prominent flow on Doppler examination.
     - **CT and MRI:** Both CT and MRI can be used to delineate the malformation cross-sectionally.
     - **CT angiography:** CTA in neonates with high output cardiac failure is technically-challenging due to the small volumes of contrast and very rapid passage of contrast through the circulation.
     - **MR angiography:** The dilated feeding and draining vessels appear as flow voids on T2. MRA may also be performed which would better delineate vascular anatomy.
     - **Angiography:** Angiography remains the gold standard in full characterisation of the lesion. It enables to individually catheterise feeding vessels. Venous drainage is via the median prosencephalic vein (MPV), the straight sinus (if present) and then out via the transverse/sigmoid sinuses.
   - **Treatment and prognosis:** Prior to endovascular intervention, the prognosis was dismal, with 100% mortality without treatment and 90% mortality following surgical attempts. Ideally, embolisation is deferred until 6 months of age for choroidal VGAM and later for mural types, to allow the cavernous sinus to mature. If cardiac failure is refractory to medical management, embolisation may be performed sooner. Both venous and arterial embolisation is possible, depending on

the number of feeders, and controversy persists in regards to the optimal approach. The prognosis is determined mainly by the presence or absence of cardiac failure. Thus choroidal types and those presenting in the neonatal period do poorly.

5. **Ans. (B) Iohexol**
   - Thoracic esophageal perforation is most commonly caused by instrumentation of a diseased esophagus, usually after attempted dilatation of a distal esophageal obstruction. Spontaneous rupture of the distal esophagus can occur after violent retching and emesis (Boerhaave syndrome).
   - Historically, patients with a Boerhaave's tear present in a more clinically dramatic fashion and have a worse prognosis due to greater contamination from spillage of gastric contents.
   - Workup starts with plain X-rays, which may demonstrate pneumomediastinum and pleural effusion. An upper GI swallow and CT scan are helpful in determining the extent of injury and infection. Assessment for the presence of concomitant esophageal disease is needed to help determine optimal surgical management.
   - Treatment options include expectant medical management or surgical intervention. Much has been mentioned on nonoperative management with antibiotics, nasogastric drainage, and distal tube feeds or parental nutrition. However, nonoperative management should be the exception, and not the rule, as specific criteria need to be met for medical management of esophageal perforation. They include a limited perforation with drainage of contrast back into the esophagus, with no clinical signs of infection and no pleural effusion.
   - Surgical principles for managing esophageal perforation include good debridement of infected tissues, two-layer repair of the mucosa, and muscularis layer with reinforcement using a pedicled intercostal flap.
   - **Different contrast agents are:**
     - **Ionic:** Water soluble iodide dyes like *Sodium diatrizoate, Meglumine iothalamate (Conray, Urograffin, Angiograffin)*. They are cheaper but often toxic and cause anaphylaxis.
     - **Non-ionic are** safer but expensive, like *Iohexol (Omnipaque), Iopamiro.*

- In abdominal CT, contrast agents can be given orally to delineate bowel properly.
- **Iohexol**, sold under the trade names **Omnipaque**, is a contrast agent used during X-rays.
- It is typically used intravenously for CT scans, pyelograms, and so on; it is very well tolerated whether given intrathecally, intravascularly, intracavitarily, or orally.
- Barium causes mediastinitis/fibrosis and gastrografin causes pneumonitis, that's why avoided.

6. Ans. (C) Protons

- **Chordoma:** They are rare, malignant bone tumors of the skull-base and axial skeleton arising from the remnants of notochord.
- It is seen in:
    - Sacrococcygeal region
    - Sphenoid sinus region
    - Around the foramen magnum.
- **Resection of recurrent or progressive disease:** For mobile spine and sacral tumors, the goal of salvage surgery with curative intent should be to achieve en-bloc resection with negative surgical margins (IV-B). Particular attention should be paid to avoid tumor rupture, as this is associated with significant risk of tumor seeding. Recurrences in the skull-base or neck, as well as in the intrathoracic, intra-abdominal or intra-pelvic areas, are usually not amenable to margin negative/R0 resections, and therefore surgery should be aimed at a gross total resection (IV-B). For skull-base tumors R1 resection should be the goal of surgical treatment in all cases, in order to reduce tumor volume and increase the effectiveness of subsequent RT (V-A).
- When no prior RT had been delivered, postoperative RT should be considered, especially when microscopic margins were positive/R1. A component of preoperative RT can also be considered.
- **RT can be delivered both with curative or palliative intent.**
- Since chordomas are radioresistant, a dose of at least 74 GyE should be delivered, using conventional fractionation (1.8–2 GyE) for photon and proton therapy; moderately hypofractionated schedules can be used with carbon ions with dose per

fractions ranging between 3 and 4.4 Gy RBE and total doses ranging from 60 and 70.4 Gy RBE.

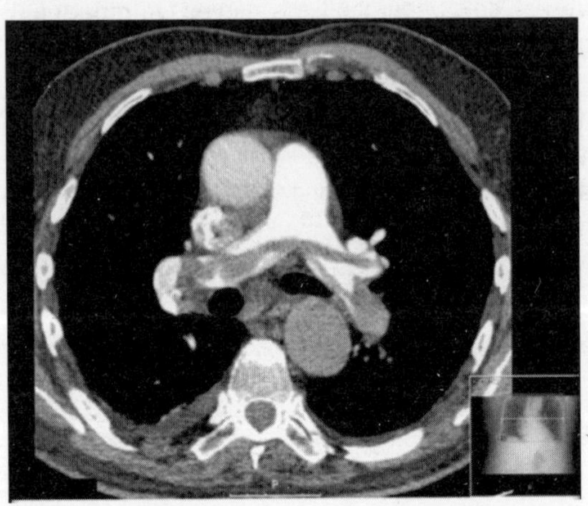

7. **Ans. (B) Pulmonary embolism**
   - CT of the chest with intravenous contrast is the principal imaging test for the diagnosis of PE. Multidetector row spiral CT acquires all chest images with ≤1 mm of resolution during a short breath hold. Sixth order branches can be visualized with resolution superior to that of conventional invasive contrast pulmonary angiography. The CT scan also provides an excellent four chamber view of the heart. RV enlargement on chest CT indicates an increased likelihood of death within the next 30 days compared with PE patients who have normal RV size. When imaging is continued below the chest to the knee, pelvic and proximal leg DVT also can be diagnosed by CT scanning. In patients without PE, the lung parenchymal images may establish alternative diagnoses not apparent on chest X-ray that explain the presenting symptoms and signs such as pneumonia, emphysema, pulmonary fibrosis, pulmonary mass, and aortic pathology. Sometimes asymptomatic early stage lung cancer is diagnosed incidentally.
   - Chest CT with contrast has virtually replaced invasive pulmonary angiography as a diagnostic test. Invasive catheter-based diagnostic testing is reserved for patients with technically unsatisfactory chest CTs and for those in whom an interventional procedure such as catheter-directed thrombolysis is planned.
   - A definitive diagnosis of PE depends on visualization of an intraluminal filling defect in more than one projection.

Secondary signs of PE include abrupt occlusion ("cutoff") of vessels, segmental oligemia or avascularity, a prolonged arterial phase with slow filling, and tortuous, tapering peripheral vessels.

8. **Ans. (C) Protons**
   - The **Bragg peak** is a peak on the *Bragg curve* which plots the energy loss of ionizing radiation during its travel through matter. For protons, α-rays, and other ion rays, the peak occurs immediately before the particles come to rest. This is called Bragg peak, after William Henry Bragg who discovered it in 1903.
   - When a fast charged particle moves through matter, it ionizes atoms of the material and deposits a dose along its path. A peak occurs because the interaction cross section increases as the charged particles energy decreases. Energy lost by charged particles is inversely proportional to the square of their velocity, which explains the peak occurring just before the particle comes to a complete stop.
   - The proton is a heavy and charged particle that gradually loses its speed as it interacts with human tissue. It is easily controlled and delivers its maximum dose at a precise depth, which is determined by the amount of energy it was given by the cyclotron (via acceleration), and can go as far as 32 cm. The proton is very fast when it enters the patient's body and deposits only a small dose on its way. The absorbed dose increases very gradually with greater depth and lower speed, suddenly rising to a peak when the proton is ultimately stopped. This is known as the Bragg peak.
   - The behavior of the proton can be precisely determined and the beam can be directed so the Bragg peak occurs exactly within the tumor site. Immediately after this burst of energy, the proton completely stops to irradiate. Proton therapy therefore allows to target tumors inside the body, precisely localize the radiation dosage and spare the patient's healthy cells, offering a much less invasive alternative to treat cancer.

9. **Ans. (A) Superior mesenteric artery**
   - **Superior mesenteric artery:** It is the artery of the midgut. It supplies all derivatives of the midgut, namely (1) the lower part of the duodenum below the opening of the bile duct, (2) jejunum, (3) ileum, (4) appendix, (5) cecum, (6) the ascending colon, (7) the right two-third of the transverse colon, and (8) the lower half of the head of the pancreas.

- **Origin and course:** It arises from the front of the abdominal aorta, behind the body of the pancreas, at the level of vertebra LI, one centimeter below the celiac trunk. It runs downwards and to the right, forming a curve with its convexity towards the left.
- At its origin it lies first behind the body of the pancreas and then in front of the uncinate process. Next it crosses the third part of the duodenum, enters the root of mesentery, and runs between its two layers. It terminates in the right iliac fossa by anastomosing with a branch of the ileocolic artery.
- **Relations: A.** *Above the root of the mesentery:* (a) *Anteriorly,* it is related to the body of the pancreas and to the splenic vein; (b) *posteriorly,* to the aorta, the left renal vein, the uncinate process and the third part of the duodenum. **B.** *Within the root of the mesentery*: (a) It crosses the inferior vena cava, the right ureter, and the right psoas. Throughout its course it is accompanied by the superior mesenteric vein which lies on its right side. The artery is surrounded by the superior mesenteric plexus of nerves.
- **Branches:** It gives off five sets of branches both from its right and left sides. a. Those arising from its right side are (1) inferior pancreaticoduodenal, (2) middle colic, (3) right colic, and (4) ileocolic. b. Those arising from its left side are 12–15 jejunal and ileal branches.

10. Ans. (B) IVC

Below is a labelled CT scan of abdomen showing all structures in cut section. In the question you can also see the filter in the IVC so that you can identify the IVC easily.

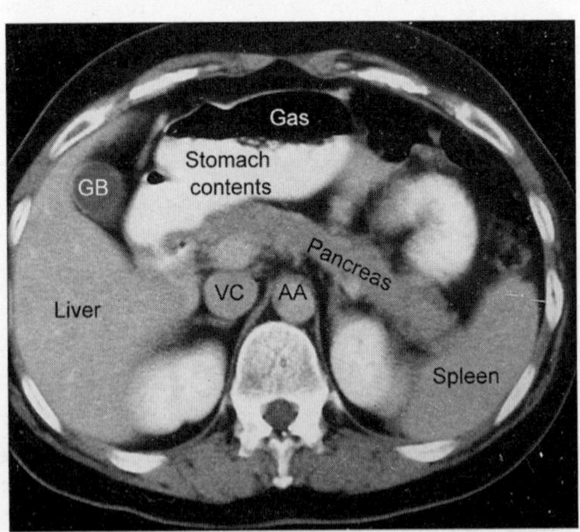

19 Psychiatry

1. Habit disorders are all except:

A. Thumb sucking
B. Nail biting
C. Temper tantrums
D. Tics

2. What is the new name for mental retardation according to the American association of Mental Retardation?

A. Mental handicap
B. Intellectual disability
C. Subnormal intelligence
D. Lunatic person

3. Stereotypic movements are:

A. Sustained posture against gravity
B. Passive inducible movements
C. Repetitive non-functional behavior
D. Repetitive functional behavior

4. Antipsychotic causing prolactinoma:

A. Ziprasidone
B. Clozapine
C. Olanzapine
D. Risperidone

5. Nowadays Down syndrome is considered under which category disorder?

A. Submental disorder
B. Oligophrenia
C. Madness
D. Mentally unstable

6. Semen squeeze technique is used for:

A. Premature ejaculation
B. Erectile dysfunction
C. Retrograde ejaculation
D. Oligospermia

7. Minimal dysfunction syndrome is seen in:

A. Dyslexia
B. ADHD
C. Mental subnormality
D. Down's syndrome

8. A patient with a history of RTA before 2 months presents with complaints of dreams of accidents. He is able to visualize the same scene whenever he visits the place and is afraid to go back to the accident site. Identify the type of disorder that he might be suffering from?

A. Adjustment disorder
B. PTSD
C. Anxiety disorder
D. OCD

9. Expression and consequent release of previously repressed emotion is called as:

A. Regression
B. Dissociation
C. Abreaction
D. All of the above

10. Freud's theory of dream includes all except?

A. Displacement
B. Condensation
C. Symbolisation
D. Correlation

11. A 55-year-old chronic alcoholic male presented with irrelevant talks, tremor and sweating. He had his last drink 3 days back. What will be the probable diagnosis?

A. Delirium tremens
B. Korsakoff psychosis
C. Post-acute withdrawal syndrome
D. Discontinuation syndrome

12. What differentiates delirium from dementia?

A. Confusion
B. Hallucination
C. Memory loss
D. Hypoactive psychomotor disorder

Answers with Explanations

1. **Ans. (C) Temper tantrums**
   - **Habit disorders:** These are stereotyped disorders which are intentionally and repetitively produced but serve no constructive or socially acceptable function.
   - The common habit disorders include thumb sucking, nail biting, pulling out of hair (*trichotillomania*), head banging, masturbation, teeth grinding, picking of nose, biting parts of the body, skin-scratching, body rocking, breath-holding, and swallowing of air (*aerophagia*). These habits range from normal to abnormal, depending on the severity of occurrence and the time of presentation during the developmental period (what is normal in infancy, may be abnormal in later childhood).
   - Many of habit disorders, particularly those which are self-stimulating in nature, are called as *gratification habits*. These have been considered by some as *masturbatory equivalents*. These habit disorders tend to be commoner in individuals with mental retardation or learning disability.
   - **Treatment:** The treatment is by behavior modification techniques and treatment of underlying psychopathology, if present.
2. **Ans. (B) Intellectual disability**
   - Intellectual disability (intellectual developmental disorder) is a disorder with onset during the developmental period that includes both intellectual and adaptive functioning deficits in conceptual, social, and practical domains.
   - Intellectual disability (intellectual developmental disorder) as a DSM-5 diagnostic term replaces 'mental retardation' used in previous editions of the manuals. In addition, the parenthetical name '(intellectual developmental disorder)' is included in the text to reflect deficits in cognitive capacity beginning in the developmental period. Together, these revisions bring DSM into alignment with terminology used by the World Health Organization's International Classification of Diseases, other professional disciplines and organizations, such as the American Association on Intellectual and Developmental Disabilities, and the US Department of Education.
   - DSM-5 emphasizes the need to use both clinical assessment and standardized testing of intelligence when diagnosing intellectual disability, with the severity of impairment based on adaptive functioning rather than IQ test scores alone. By

removing IQ test scores from the diagnostic criteria, but still including them in the text description of intellectual disability, DSM-5 ensures that they are not overemphasized as the defining factor of a person's overall ability, without adequately considering functioning levels.

- In DSM-5, intellectual disability is considered to be approximately two standard deviations or more below the population, which equals an IQ score of about 70 or below. The assessment of intelligence across three domains (conceptual, social and practical) will ensure that clinicians base their diagnosis on the impact of the deficit in general mental abilities on functioning needed for everyday life.

3. **Ans. (C) Repetitive nonfunctional behavior**
   - **Stereotypy:** Odd, repetitive and non-goal directed movement (can also be verbal).
   - **Stereotypic movement disorder (SMD)** is a motor disorder with onset in childhood involving repetitive, nonfunctional motor behavior (e.g. hand waving or head banging), that markedly interferes with normal activities or results in bodily injury.
   - The cause of this disorder is not known.
   - **Classification:** Stereotypic movement disorder is classified in DSM-5 as a motor disorder, in the category of neurodevelopmental disorders.
   - **Signs and symptoms:** Common repetitive movements of SMD include head banging, arm waving, hand shaking, rocking and rhythmic movements, self-biting, self-hitting and skin-picking; other stereotypies are thumbsucking, nail biting, trichotillomania, bruxism and abnormal running or skipping.
   - **Diagnosis:** There are no specific tests for diagnosing this disorder, although some tests may be ordered to rule out other conditions. SMD may occur with Lesch-Nyhan syndrome, intellectual disability, and fetal alcohol exposure or as a result of amphetamine intoxication. When diagnosing stereotypic movement disorder, DSM-5 calls for specification of:
     - With or without self-injurious behavior
     - Association with another known medical condition or environmental factor
     - Severity (mild, moderate or severe).
   - **Differential diagnosis:** Other conditions which feature repetitive behaviors in the differential diagnosis include autism spectrum disorders, obsessive–compulsive disorder, tic disorders (e.g. Tourette syndrome), and other conditions including dyskinesias. It is often misdiagnosed as tics or Tourette syndrome (TS).

- **Treatment:** There is no consistently effective medication for SMD, and there is little evidence for any effective treatment. In non-autistic or 'typically developing children', habit reversal training may be useful.
- Prognosis depends on the severity of the disorder. Recognizing symptoms early can help reduce the risk of self-injury, which can be lessened with meditations. Stereotypic movement disorder due to head trauma may be permanent.
- **Epidemiology:** Although not necessary for the diagnosis, individuals with intellectual disability are at higher risk for SMD. It is more common in boys, and can occur at any age.

4. Ans. (D) Risperidone

- Atypical antipsychotics
  - Clozapine
  - Aripiprazole
  - Risperidone
  - Ziprasidone
  - Olanzapine
  - Amisulpiride
  - Quetiapine
  - Zotepine
- **Risperidone:** Its antipsychotic activity has been ascribed to a combination of D2 + 5-HT2 receptor blockade. In addition it has high affinity for alpha 1 and apha 2 and H1 receptors: blockade of these may contribute to efficacy as well as side effects like postural hypotension. However, BP can rise if it is used with a SSRI.
- It is more potent D2 blocker than clozapine; extrapyramidal side effects are less only at low doses (< 6 mg/day). Prolactin levels rise disproportionately during risperidone therapy, but it is less epileptogenic than clozapine, though frequently causes agitation. Weight gain and incidence of new-onset diabetes is less than with clozapine. Caution has been issued about increased risk of stroke in the elderly.
- Hyperprolactinemia (due to D2 blockade) is common with typical neuroleptics and risperidone. This can lower Gn levels, but amenorrhoea, infertility, galactorrhea and gynecomastia occur infrequently after prolonged treatment. The atypical antipsychotics, except risperidone, do not appreciably raise prolactin levels.

5. **Ans. (B) Oligophrenia**
   - Oligophrenia is a group of nonprogressing psychic disorders of organic nature. General signs and symptoms are noticed in early childhood (either congenital or acquired) within the age of 3.
   - The diagnostic criteria for oligophrenia are:
     - Peculiar psychopathological structure of dementia with especially weak abstract thought processing and underdeveloped emotional sphere.
     - Nonprogressive character of intellect defect.
     - Slow psychic development of individual.
       - Therefore oligophrenia is not related to intellect disorders which occur as a result of progressive psychic diseases (schizophrenia and epilepsy) and as a result of severe organic defect occurring after 3 years of age (trauma, infection, intoxication etc.). Intelligence is determined polygenetically and environmentally.
       - Factors that cause oligophrenia may be divided into prenatal, perinatal, and postnatal.
   - **Prenatal abnormalities:** It may be due to genetic factors, congenital infections, teratogenic factors, radiation, etc. Chromosomal abnormalities and aberration comprises the largest number of known causes of oligophrenia. Examples are Edwards' syndrome (trisomy 18), Patau's syndrome (trisomy 13), Down syndrome (trisomy 21), Klinefelter's syndrome (XXY), Turner's syndrome (XO), etc. Trisomy 21 is the commonest. It occurs in 1/600 live births. The fragile X syndrome too cause mild familial oligophrenia. Genetic metabolic disorders which cause oligophrenia (MR) include X-linked recessive (Lesch-Nyhan, Hunter's disorders), autosomal recessive (phenylketonuria, galactosemia, maple-syrup disease, tuberous sclerosis, neurofibromatosis etc) and autosomal recessive lysosomal disorders (Tay-Sachs, Niemann-Pick, Gaucher's diseases etc).
   - Congenital infections are a major cause of MR. Rubella virus, cytomegalovirus, *Toxoplasma gondii*, treponema infections during pregnancy cause MR of child. Out of teratogenic factors, important are alcohol and drug addiction of parents and intake of medicines during pregnancy by mother.
   - Exogenic factors are excessive movements during pregnancy, psychological disturbances during pregnancy, intoxication, diabetes mellitus, toxicosis during pregnancy, rhesus conflicts, etc.

6. **Ans. (A) Premature ejaculation**
   - **Premature ejaculation:** It refers to repeated occurrences of ejaculation before or shortly after penetration, or with minimal sexual stimulation. The causes can be biological (relatively uncommon) or psychological (e.g. performance anxiety). It is a very common sexual complaint, which is often interpreted as sexual weakness; can cause considerable distress and dissatisfaction in the patient as well as in his partner. Sometimes the subject has unreasonable expectations about the optimal/desirable length of intercourse.
   - Most SSRIs and some TCAs, especially clomipramine have the common property of delaying and in some cases inhibiting ejaculation (this itself can cause sexual distress). The primary treatment of premature ejaculation is counselling and behavioral therapy, but this can be supplemented by drugs.
   - Dapoxetine is a SSRI which has been specifically introduced for this purpose. It acts rapidly; 60 mg taken 1 hour before intercourse has helped many subjects. Clomipramine 10–25 mg three times a day is a slow acting drug which needs to be taken regularly for maximum benefit. For on demand use, 25 mg may be taken 6 hours before sex.
   - **Squeeze technique (Semen's technique):** This has been used in treatment of premature ejaculation. The female partner is asked to manually stimulate the penis causing erection. When the male partner experiences 'ejaculatory inevitability', the female partner 'squeezes' the penis on the coronal ridge thus delaying ejaculation.There are similar simple techniques (such as orgasmic conditioning, desensitisation) for treatment of other psychosexual dysfunctions. The response rate is close to 80%, with maximum success in the treatment of premature ejaculation.

7. **Ans. (A) Dyslexia**
   - **Dyslexia**, also known as **reading disorder**, is characterized by trouble with reading despite normal intelligence. It may include difficulties in spelling words, reading quickly, writing words, 'sounding out' words in the head, pronouncing words when reading aloud and understanding what one reads. Often these difficulties are first noticed at school.
   - Dyslexia is believed to be caused by both genetic and environmental factors. Some cases run in families. It often occurs in people with attention deficit hyperactivity disorder (ADHD). It may begin in adulthood as the result of a traumatic brain injury,

stroke, or dementia. The underlying mechanisms of dyslexia are problems within the brain's language processing.

- Dyslexia is diagnosed through a series of tests of memory, spelling, vision, and reading skills. Dyslexia is separate from reading difficulties caused by hearing or vision problems or by insufficient teaching.
- Treatment involves adjusting teaching methods to meet the person's needs. Dyslexia is the most common learning disability and occurs in all areas of the world. It affects 3–7% of the population, however, up to 20% may have some degree of symptoms. While dyslexia is more often diagnosed in men, it has been suggested that it affects men and women equally.
- In early childhood, symptoms that correlate with a later diagnosis of dyslexia include delayed onset of speech and a lack of phonological awareness, as well as being easily distracted by background noise.

8. Ans. (B) PTSD

- **Post-traumatic Stress Disorder (PTSD):** According to ICD-10, this disorder arises as a delayed and/protracted response to an exceptionally stressful or catastrophic life event or situation, which is likely to cause pervasive distress in 'almost any person' (e.g. disasters, war, rape or torture, serious accident).
- The symptoms of PTSD may develop, after a period of latency, within six months after the stress or may be delayed beyond this period. PTSD is characterised by recurrent and intrusive recollections of the stressful event, either in flashbacks (images, thoughts, or perceptions) and/or in dreams. There is an associated sense of re-experiencing of the stressful event. There is marked avoidance of the events or situations that arouse recollections of the stressful event, along with marked symptoms of anxiety and increased arousal.
- The other important clinical features of PTSD include partial amnesia for some aspects of the stressful event, feeling of numbness, and anhedonia (inability to experience pleasure).
- The treatment consists of the following measures:
  - **Prevention:** Anticipation of disasters in the high risk areas, with the training of personnel in disaster management.
  - **Disaster management:** Here the speed of providing practical help is of paramount importance. This is also a preventive measure.
  - **Supportive psychotherapy.**
  - **Cognitive behavior therapy (CBT).**

- **Drug treatment:** Antidepressants and benzodiazepines (in low doses for short periods) are useful in treatment, if anxiety and/or depression are important components of the clinical picture.

9. Ans. (C) Abreaction

- Abreaction is an important procedure which brings to conscious awareness, for the first time, unconscious conflicts and associated emotions. The release of emotions is therapeutic. Although abreaction is an integral part of psycho analysis and hypnosis, it can be used independently also. Abreaction can be done with or without the use of medication.
- Earlier amphetamines, ether, nitrous oxide and lysergic acid diethylamide (LSD) have been used for abreaction. Particularly, intravenous amphetamines were very successful as they lead to a marked increase in productivity of speech, thus facilitating release of unconscious ideas and emotions. These agents are no longer commonly used in clinical practice, due to risk of dependence (in case of amphetamines and LSD) and/or side effects.
- Another method is the use of 5% solution of sodium amobarbital (amytal) or thiopentone sodium (pentothal), infused at a rate no faster than 1cc/min to prevent sleep as well as respiratory depression. This procedure must always be done very carefully with support from an anaesthetist who should be physically present.
- The abreactive procedure is begun with neutral topics at first, gradually approaching area(s) of conflicts. Usually about 150–350 mg (3–7 cc.) of amytal is sufficient for the purpose. In elderly and patients with organic brain disorder, even 75 mg of amytal may produce excessive drowsiness.
- The indications of amytal interview include:
  - Abreaction (mainly) e.g. in hysteria.
  - Interview with a mute patient.
  - Diagnostic test in catatonic syndrome.
  - Differentiating test in stupor (for differential diagnosis of depression, schizophrenia, hysteria and organic brain disorder).

There are certain contraindications for the use of amytal interview:

1. Airway disease including upper respiratory tract Infection.
2. Severe renal or hepatic disease.

3. History of porphyria.
4. Hypotension.
5. Dependence on barbiturates.
6. Psychosis (except for catatonia or stupor).

The other medications which have been used successfully for abreaction include diazepam and ketamine. The use of abreaction has declined considerably in the last three decades and the current practice and guidelines do not encourage its routine use.

10. Ans. (D) Correlation

Theory of Dreams

- Dream interpretation has been a major component of psychoanalysis. Beginning with his own dream experiences, freud analysed dreams as 'the royal road to the unconscious'. He believed dreams to be conscious expression of unconscious fantasies or impulses which are not accessible to the individual in wakefulness, thereby providing gratification by wish fulfilment. Since expression of unconscious forbidden fantasies can evoke considerable anxiety, these fantasies are considerably modified so as to preserve sleep on the one hand and provide gratification of the fantasies on the other. This modification is known as *dream work*.
- Here the unconscious forbidden fantasies or wishes which threaten to break sleep constitute the *latent dream content*, whereas the dream content modified by dream work constitutes the *manifest dream content*.
- According to Freud, the aim of dream interpretation is to get to the latent dream content from manifest dream content, via free association, in order to understand the 'real meaning' of the dream experience.
- According to this theory, the dream work consists of the following mechanisms:
  - Symbolism
  - Displacement
  - Condensation
  - Projection
  - Secondary elaboration (since dream content consists of *primary process thinking*, secondary elaboration is used to introduce logical thinking or *secondary process thinking* in the dream content).
- In addition to the unconscious impulses, wishes and fantasies, the dream content is also influenced by:

    - Nocturnal sensory stimuli (e.g. thirst, hunger, full bladder).
    - Day residue (residue of day experiences of previous one or several days).

11. Ans. (A) Delirium tremens

- Delirium tremens (DT) is the most severe alcohol withdrawal syndrome. It occurs usually within 2–4 days of complete or significant abstinence from heavy alcohol drinking in about 5% of patients, as compared to acute tremulousness which occurs in about 34% of patients.
- The course is short, with recovery occurring within 3–7 days. This is an acute organic brain syndrome (delirium) with characteristic features of:
    - Clouding of consciousness with disorientation in time and place.
    - Poor attention span and distractibility.
    - Visual (and also auditory) hallucinations and illusions, which are often vivid and very frightening. Tactile hallucinations of insects crawling over the body may occur.
    - Marked autonomic disturbance with tachycardia, fever, hypertension, sweating and pupillary dilatation.
    - Psychomotor agitation and ataxia.
    - Insomnia, with a reversal of sleep-wake pattern.
    - Dehydration with electrolyte imbalance.
- Death can occur in 5–10% of patients with delirium tremens and is often due to cardiovascular collapse, infection, hyperthermia or self-inflicted injury. At times, intercurrent medical illnesses such as pneumonia, fractures, liver disease or pulmonary tuberculosis may complicate the clinical picture.

12. Ans. (A) Confusion

Delirium is characterised by the following features:

- A relatively acute onset.
- Clouding of consciousness, characterised by a decreased awareness of surroundings and a decreased ability to respond to environmental stimuli.
- Disorientation (most commonly in time, then in place and usually later in person), associated with a decreased attention span and distractibility.
- The motor symptoms in delirium can include:
    - Asterixis (flapping tremor)
    - Multifocal myoclonus
    - Carphologia or floccillation (picking movements at cover-sheets and clothes)

- Occupational delirium (elaborate pantomimes as if continuing their usual occupation in the hospital bed)
- Tone and reflex abnormalities.
- Lability of affect is usually present.
- Motor and verbal perseveration, dysnomia, agraphia and impaired comprehension can also be seen.

A comparison of delirium and dementia

Features	*Delirium*	*Dementia*
1. Onset	Usually acute	Usually insidious
2. Course	Usually recover in 1 week may take up to 1 month	Usually protracted, although may be reversible in some cases
3. Clinical features		
a. Consciousness	Clouded	Usually normal
b. Orientation	Grossly disturbed	Usually normal; disturbed only in late stages
c. Memory	• Immediate retention and recall disturbed • Recent memory disturbed	• Immediate retention and recall normal • Recent memory disturbed • Remote memory disturbed only in late stages
d. Comprehension	Impaired	Imparied only in late stages
e. Sleep-wake cycle	Grossly disturbed	Usually normal
f. Attention and concentration	Grossly disturbed	Usually normal
g. Diurnal variation	Marked; sundowning may be present	Usually absent
h. Perception	Visual illusions and hallucinations very common	Hallucinations may occur
i. Other features	Asterixis; multifocal myoclonus	Catastrophic reaction perseveration